Emergency M

Editor

DAN MICHAEL TZIZIK

PHYSICIAN ASSISTANT CLINICS

www.physicianassistant.theclinics.com

Consulting Editors
KIM ZUBER
JANE S. DAVIS

January 2023 • Volume 8 • Number 1

ELSEVIER

1600 John F. Kennedy Boulevard • Suite 1800 • Philadelphia, Pennsylvania, 19103-2899

http://www.theclinics.com

PHYSICIAN ASSISTANT CLINICS Volume 8, Number 1
January 2023 ISSN 2405-7991, ISBN-13: 978-0-323-96067-0

Editor: Taylor Hayes
Developmental Editor: Axell Ivan Jade Purificacion

Physician Assistant Clinics (ISSN: 2405–7991) is published quarterly by Elsevier Inc., 360 Park Avenue South, New York, NY 10010-1710. Months of issue are January, April, July, and October. Periodicals postage paid at New York, NY and additional mailing offices. Subscription prices are $150.00 per year (US individuals), $305.00 (US institutions), $100.00 (US students), $150.00 (Canadian individuals), $320.00 (Canadian institutions), $100.00 (Canadian students), $150.00 (international individuals), $320.00 (international institutions), and $100.00 (international students). Foreign air speed delivery is included in all *Clinics* subscription prices. All prices are subject to change without notice. POSTMASTER: Send address changes to *Physician Assistant Clinics*, Elsevier Periodicals Customer Service, 11830 Westline Industrial Drive, St. Louis, MO 63146. Customer Service Health Sciences Division, Subscription Customer Service, 3251 Riverport Lane, Maryland Heights, MO 63043. **Customer Service: 1-800-654-2452 (U.S. and Canada); 314-447-8871 (outside U.S. and Canada). Fax: 314-447-8029. E-mail: journalscustomerservice-usa@elsevier.com (for print support); journalsonlinesupport-usa@elsevier.com (for online support).**

Reprints. For copies of 100 or more, of articles in this publication, please contact the Commercial Reprints Department, Elsevier Inc., 360 Park Avenue South, New York, NY 10010-1710. Tel. 212-633-3874; Fax: 212-633-3820; E-mail: reprints@elsevier.com.

Physician Assistant Clinics is covered in *EMBASE/Excerpta Medica* and *ESCI*.

PROGRAM OBJECTIVE
The goal of the *Physician Assistant Clinics* is to keep practicing physician assistants up to date with current clinical practice by providing timely articles reviewing the state of the art in patient care.

TARGET AUDIENCE
Physician Assistants and other healthcare professionals

LEARNING OBJECTIVES
Upon completion of this activity, participants will be able to:
1. Review the etiologies and clinical manifestations of injuries, complaints, and traumas in the emergency room setting, including those in special patient populations.
2. Discuss the significance of using a stepped approach and evidence-based practice guidelines, as well as assessment tools and screenings, diagnostic tools and studies, to promote accurate diagnosis of an emergent medical condition.
3. Recognize the difficulties in diagnosing, and managing medical disorders encountered in the emergency room.

ACCREDITATION
The Elsevier Office of Continuing Medical Education (EOCME) is accredited by the Accreditation Council for Continuing Medical Education (ACCME) to provide continuing medical education for physicians.

The EOCME designates this journal-based CME activity for a maximum of 15 *AMA PRA Category 1 Credit*(s)™. Physicians should claim only the credit commensurate with the extent of their participation in the activity.

All other health care professionals requesting continuing education credit for this enduring material will be issued a certificate of participation.

DISCLOSURE OF CONFLICTS OF INTEREST
The EOCME assesses conflict of interest with its instructors, faculty, planners, and other individuals who are in a position to control the content of CME activities. All relevant conflicts of interest that are identified are thoroughly vetted by EOCME for fair balance, scientific objectivity, and patient care recommendations. EOCME is committed to providing its learners with CME activities that promote improvements or quality in healthcare and not a specific proprietary business or a commercial interest.

The planning committee, staff, authors, and editors listed below have identified no financial relationships or relationships to products or devices they or their spouse/life partner have with commercial interest related to the content of this CME activity:
Jason Ausmus, MS, PA-C; Allisyn Brady, PA-C; Adam Broughton, PA-C, MSc; Adam Burman, MPAS, PA-C; Kasey Dillon, DScPAS, PA-C; Brooke Dorval, PA-S; Courtney Dumont, PA-S; Belinda Felicia, PA-S; Meghan Fortier, PA-S; Loryn Fridie, PA-C, MS; Alison Fulton, PA-S; Katherine Gardella, PA-S; Betsy Garnick, PA-S; James A. Johanning, MPAS, PA-C; Karla Juvonen, MPAS; PA-C; Pradeep Kuttysankaran; Mary Masterson, MPAS, PA-C, CAQ-EM, DFAAPA; Jennine McAuley, PA-C; Vidya Paray, PA-C; John Ramos, MMS, PA-C, CAQ-EM; Amanda Smith, DMSc, MMS, PA-C, CAQ-EM; Michael Smith, MS, PA-C; Lori J. Stack, MD, FACOG; Doreen Thomas-Payne, MSN, BSN, RN, PMHNP-BC; Dan Michael Tzizik, MPAS, MPH; Heather Wolek, MPAS, PA-C

UNAPPROVED/OFF-LABEL USE DISCLOSURE
The EOCME requires CME faculty to disclose to the participants:
1. When products or procedures being discussed are off-label, unlabelled, experimental, and/or investigational (not US Food and Drug Administration [FDA] approved); and
2. Any limitations on the information presented, such as data that are preliminary or that represent ongoing research, interim analyses, and/or unsupported opinions. Faculty may discuss information about pharmaceutical agents that is outside of FDA-approved labelling. This information is intended solely for CME and is not intended to promote off-label use of these medications. If you have any questions, contact the medical affairs department of the manufacturer for the most recent prescribing information.

TO ENROLL
The CME program is available to all *Physician Assistant Clinics* subscribers at no additional fee. To subscribe to the *Physician Assistant Clinics*, call customer service at 1-800-654-2452 or sign up online at www.physicianassistant.theclinics.com.

METHOD OF PARTICIPATION

In order to claim credit, participants must complete the following:

1. Complete enrolment as indicated above
2. Read the activity
3. Complete the CME Test and Evaluation. Participants must achieve a score of 70% on the test. All CME Tests and Evaluations must be completed online

CME INQUIRIES/SPECIAL NEEDS

For all CME inquiries or special needs, please contact elsevierCME@elsevier.com.

Contributors

CONSULTING EDITORS

KIM ZUBER, PAC, MS
American Academy of Nephrology PAs, St Petersburg, Florida

JANE S. DAVIS, DNP
Division of Nephrology, The University of Alabama at Birmingham, Birmingham, Alabama

EDITOR

DAN MICHAEL TZIZIK, MPAS, MPH, PA-C
Associate Director of Didactic Education, Assistant Professor of Medicine, Boston University School of Medicine Physician Assistant Program, Boston, Massachusetts

AUTHORS

JASON AUSMUS, MS, PA-C
Department of Emergency Medicine, NewYork-Presbyterian Weill Cornell Medicine, New York, New York

ALLISYN BRADY, PA-C, Chief Physician Assistant, Cambridge Health Alliance, Department of Obstetrics and Gynecology, Cambridge, Massachusetts

ADAM BROUGHTON, MScpa, PA-C
Assistant Clinical Professor, Northeastern University PA Program, Lahey Beverly Hospital Emergency Department Physician Assistant

ADAM BURMAN, MPAS, PA-C
Assistant Professor, Saint Catherine University, Saint Paul, Minnesota

KASEY DILLON, DScPAS, PA-C
Physician Assistant Studies, MCPHS University, Manchester, New Hampshire

BROOKE DORVAL, PA-S
MCPHS University, Manchester, New Hampshire

COURTNEY DUMONT, PA-S
MCPHS University, Manchester, New Hampshire

BELINDA FELICIA, PA-S
MCPHS University, Manchester, New Hampshire

MEGHAN FORTIER, PA-S
MCPHS University, Manchester, New Hampshire

LORYN FRIDIE, MPAS, PA-C
Emergency Department, New York, New York

ALISON FULTON, PA-S
MCPHS University, Manchester, New Hampshire

KATHERINE GARDELLA, PA-S
MCPHS University, Manchester, New Hampshire

BETSY GARNICK, PA-S
MCPHS University, Manchester, New Hampshire

JAMES A. JOHANNING, MPAS, PA-C
Assistant Professor of Didactic Training, St. Catherine University, Henrietta Schmoll
School of Health, Physician Assistant Program, St Paul, Minnesota

KARLA JUVONEN, MPAS, PA-C
Department of Psychiatry and Addiction Medicine, Allied HealthCare Physicians, Bronx,
New York

MARY MASTERSON, MPAS, PA-C, CAQ-EM, DFAAPA
Department of Emergency Medicine, Johns Hopkins Bayview Medical Center, Baltimore,
Maryland

JENNINE MCAULEY, PA-C
Physician Assistant, Department of Emergency Medicine, Weill Cornell Medicine, New
York, New York

VIDYA PARAY, MS, PA-C
Physician Associate, Neurosciences ICU at Yale New Haven Hospital, New Haven,
Connecticut

JOHN RAMOS, MMS, PA-C, CAQ-EM
Division of Emergency Medicine, Department of Surgery, Duke University Hospital,
Durham, North Carolina

AMANDA SMITH, DMSc, PA-C, CAQ-EM
Department of Emergency Medicine, Johns Hopkins Bayview Medical Center, Baltimore,
Maryland

MICHAEL SMITH, MS, PA-C
Associate Director of Clinical Education, Boston University School of Medicine Physician
Assistant Program, Boston, Massachusetts

LORI J. STACK, MD, FACOG
Center for Fetal Diagnosis and Treatment, Children's Hospital of Philadelphia,
Philadelphia, Pennsylvania

DAN MICHAEL TZIZIK, MPAS, MPH, PA-C
Associate Director of Didactic Education, Assistant Professor of Medicine, Boston
University School of Medicine Physician Assistant Program, Boston, Massachusetts

HEATHER WOLEK, MPAS, PA-C
Division of Emergency Medicine, Department of Surgery, Duke University Hospital,
Durham, North Carolina

Contents

> Among emergency department patients with chest pain, more than 50% patients are diagnosed with a noncardiac condition and 5.1% are diagnosed with acute coronary syndrome (ACS). ACS is suggested by a suspicious history (chest pain characteristics and risk factors) and either electrocardiogram or troponin abnormalities consistent with myocardial ischemia. In the absence of an indication for emergent reperfusion, risk stratification is often used in the emergency department to identify patients who would benefit from advanced cardiac testing or intervention.

> Pearls and Pitfalls of Trauma Management tackle select, relevant issues of importance today as it pertains to emergency medicine staff providers. Trauma itself is one of the most common and important presentations ER providers face on a daily basis. Standard workup guides and algorithms are touched upon while the focus of our chapter is a closer examination of specific elements of trauma care. This includes hemorrhage, use of point of care ultrasound in the trauma setting, unique considerations in pediatric trauma, key components of secondary/tertiary surveys, and "ouchless ER" pearls of wisdom.

> Abdominal pain is a common and challenging chief complaint. Signs and symptoms often overlap, and the differential includes both serious and self-limited conditions. This article reviews the differential diagnoses for adult patients with abdominal pain, distinguishing features of the history and physical examination, and diagnostic tests used to identify or exclude serious illness.

> Case studies of ischemic and hemorrhagic shocks with etiology, clinical manifestations, and management options.

pneumonia continues to be prevalent and clinical decision-making tools are useful aids to assist the appropriate disposition of patients.

Altered mental status (AMS) is not a singular diagnosis but rather a clinical sign that is representative of an extensive list of differential diagnoses ranging from benign to life threatening and causes that are reversible versus not reversible. It is essential to have a systematic approach to evaluate patients presenting with AMS that allows immediate life-threatening causes to be quickly identified and treated. This article defines AMS, delirium, and dementia highlighting key differences between these pathologies. Underlying causes of AMS are reviewed and categorized. With this background in mind, a systematic approach to evaluating and treating these patients is reviewed.

Pain is a common component of most patient presentations to the emergency department. There should be no surprise that analgesics are the most prescribed class of medications in emergency medicine. Current data support that pain represents up to 75% of emergency department visits annually. Manifestations of pain can be either acute or chronic in nature. Pain can have immediate and long-term effects on behavioral, physiologic, and social implications including impacts on the patient's employment and interpersonal relationships. In the emergency department, the concept of oligoanalgesia is difficult to obtain, as pain is often not initially addressed upon arrival and infrequently reassessed. Providers should have a number of methods to approach the management of pain in the emergency department. The overall goal should be directed toward identifying the underlying cause with an open and honest discussion on the goals of pain management and frequent reassessment of the patient's pain response to analgesia using established pain scales. Common initial analgesics include oral, parenteral, or topical medications in step-wise a balanced approach, but there are a number of other approaches to pain management that may be underutilized in the emergency department. Regional nerve blocks are a proven adjunct that can provide an advantage over traditional approaches in certain situations.

One in five adults experience mental illness annually, according to the National Institutes of Health. The rates are even higher among the drug or alcohol dependent, homeless, and those incarcerated or in detention centers. A concise chapter summarizing such emergencies follows, limited by length to only the most serious situations and the immediate management of those situations. This section does not provide recommendations for ongoing psychiatric management other than recommendations for referrals nor does it include mental illnesses outside of the realm of emergent.

Kasey Dillon

Sepsis and septic shock are medical emergencies, and the early recognition and management of both processes are critical for emergency medicine providers. Screening tools, although imperfect, are recognized as crucial to reducing mortality from sepsis, as these tools drive time-sensitive intervention. The Surviving Sepsis Guidelines are regularly updated and are considered the standard of care in the management of sepsis and septic shock. Given the varied clinical presentation of patients with sepsis and septic shock, emergency medicine clinicians must be diligent in using sepsis screening tools, understanding established recommendations, and confidently combining experience and expertise with set standards.

Michael Smith and James A. Johanning

Can't Miss Orthopedic Emergencies is a unique article for the emergency room provider highlighting optimal recognition and workup of specific orthopedic conditions we classify as "Can't Miss." This is must know information for the ED provider as each condition reviewed has the potential of high morbidity and both limb or life loss if not recognized and acted on without delay. This article will give the emergency room provider a unique and concise approach to these pathologic conditions emphasizing early recognition with stepwise and accurate approach to the appropriate workup in the emergency setting.

Adam Broughton

Point-of-care ultrasound (POCUS) is increasingly used in emergency medicine. The availability of cheaper, smaller machines makes it possible to transfer the use of POCUS in the hospital setting to prehospital care. Multiple protocols are used by emergency department clinicians. New protocols attempt to integrate POCUS into the care of out-of-hospital cardiovascular arrest to identify reversible causes during cardiopulmonary resuscitation and found to be feasible to teach and use.

PHYSICIAN ASSISTANT CLINICS

FORTHCOMING ISSUES

April 2023
Pharmacology
Rebecca Maxson, *Editor*

July 2023
Emerging and Re-Emerging Infectious Diseases
Gerald Kayingo, *Editor*

October 2023
Allergy, Asthma, and Immunology
Gabriel Ortiz, *Editor*

RECENT ISSUES

October 2022
Nutrition in Patient Care
Corri Wolf, *Editor*

July 2022
Obstetrics and Gynecology
Elyse Watkins, *Editor*

April 2022
The Kidney
Kim Zuber and Jane Davis, *Editors*

SERIES OF RELATED INTEREST

Primary Care: Clinics in Office Practice
https://www.primarycare.theclinics.com/

THE CLINICS ARE AVAILABLE ONLINE!
Access your subscription at:
www.theclinics.com

Foreword

Treat 'Em, Street 'Em, and Everything in Between

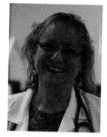 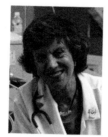

Kim Zuber, PAC, MS   Jane S. Davis, DNP
Consulting Editors

Bone fractures, chest pain, trauma—these events are unplanned and need immediate attention. The existence of emergency rooms (ER) is ingrained in our practice of medicine. It is less known that the practice of emergency medicine did not evolve until 1966 when physician groups in Virginia and Michigan developed the concept of emergency specialists.[1]

The public has long been fascinated by medical TV shows. Programs featuring emergency medicine have had long runs and enduring popularity. The drama of the rapid action and multiple crises has a lasting appeal. But *"No, Virginia, a patient does not come into the emergency room in organ failure and get sent to the OR immediately for a transplant,"* despite what we see on TV. In reality, while it can be fast paced and unpredictable, the ER is not all glamour and glory.

In 2017, 17.6% of all physician assistants (PAs) practiced in emergency medicine. This increased to 19% in 2021.[2] With almost one in five PAs working in emergency, whether in an urgent care center, acute care setting, or level 1 through level 5 ER, education of these practitioners is paramount. For this reason, we are excited to present this issue of *Physician Assistant Clinics*, led by an experienced emergency PA, Dan Tzizk, PA-C. Dan has trained many PAs in both PA school and clinical practice. He is here to guide us through the many specialties and encounters that make up a typical day in this 24-hour essential medical facility.

Practitioners need to be ready to address anything from a nosebleed to victims of an interstate five-car pileup. Since time is of the essence, practitioners must be prepared to recognize and act on a wide range of presenting symptoms and conditions. In addition, they must be able to differentiate the serious from the not so serious. Dan has put together an incredible list of emergency topics and experienced authors. We believe

Physician Assist Clin 8 (2023) xiii–xiv
https://doi.org/10.1016/j.cpha.2022.10.003
2405-7991/23/© 2022 Published by Elsevier Inc.

physicianassistant.theclinics.com

readers will gain new insight and appreciate of the decision-making skills of the ER practitioner; we know we did.

Kim Zuber, PAC, MS
American Academy of Nephrology PAs
131 31st Avenue North
Stain Petersburg, FL 33704, USA

Jane S. Davis, DNP
Division of Nephrology
University of Alabama at Birmingham
3605 Oakdale Road
Birmingham, AL 35223, USA

E-mail addresses:
zuberkim@yahoo.com (K. Zuber)
jsdavis@uabmc.edu (J.S. Davis)

REFERENCES

1. Suter RE. Emergency medicine in the United States: a systemic review. World J Emerg Med 2012;3(1):5–10.
2. National Commission on Certification of PAs. Specialty supplement report on secondary specialty. 2021. Available at: https://www.nccpa.net/wp-content/uploads/2022/09/2021-Specialty-supplement-v2.pdf. Accessed October 13, 2022.

Preface

Emergency Medicine: The Developing Nexus

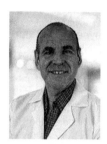

Dan Michael Tzizik, MPAS, MPH, PA-C
Editor

By its nature, the practice of Emergency Medicine involves all medical disciplines, and in addition, is a discipline unto itself. The Emergency Room is a point of confluence for all medical disciplines, often in a state of near extremis. The Emergency Medicine provider is in an unenviable position of having to know the warning signs to look for in conditions that are particular to each discipline while being knowledgeable about presentations and conditions that transcend a particular discipline and are applicable to all.

With that in mind, this issue on Emergency Medicine focuses on both specific conditions belonging to numerous disciplines and their approach from an Emergency Medicine perspective. This perspective considers the worst that a presentation possibly can be and stabilization with considerations for facilitating definitive care.

The topics I have included reflect an emphasis on some of the basics of Emergency Medicine practice while updating the treatment of common causes of morbidity and mortality. Chief complaints and medical conditions continue to evolve but, in a way, also remain the same. The difficult task in formulating the contents of this issue was not finding topics to include; it was narrowing down the topics to a minimum. There is a minimum of overlap between this issue and the previous one. Some topics are based on chief concerns to include the classic presentations of chest pain and abdominal pain, which have essentially remained the same and are worthy of review. In addition, the common concern of altered mental status is addressed systematically to aid in its emergent treatment. However, what often is a conundrum are those cases that do not present classically, that do not declare themselves conclusively. The disposition of atypical chest pain, for instance, has undergone several iterations and is reviewed here.

Other discipline-specific staples that are reviewed and updated include trauma management; burns; cerebral vascular accidents; eyes, ears, nose, and throat trauma;

Physician Assist Clin 8 (2023) xv–xvi
https://doi.org/10.1016/j.cpha.2022.10.002
2405-7991/23/© 2022 Published by Elsevier Inc.

high-stakes pediatrics; pain management; behavioral health; septic shock; and orthopedics.

Last, this issue also includes several cutting-edge topics. The burgeoning use of point-of-care ultrasound in the practice of Emergency Medicine cannot be overstated, and a broad review of its evidence-based applications is presented here. In addition, in between the last issue of this text and this one, the SARS-Cov-2 pandemic changed the way that Emergency Medicine is practiced for years to come. To include a thorough review of the systemic effects of COVID-19 is far beyond the scope of this text. But to deny its importance to the practice of Emergency Medicine is likewise inappropriate. Its effects on maternal health, in addition to hypertension during pregnancy and the etiologic overlap of the two, as well as its pulmonary effects are also addressed.

This text represents the effort of the editor and the authors to present content that is truly useful for the Emergency Medicine provider and not an examination of theoretical pathophysiology. It is my sincere wish that this text eventually will be a worn, well-used resource in many whitecoat pockets of both students and providers alike.

Dan Michael Tzizik, MPAS, MPH, PA-C
Boston University School of Medicine
Physician Assistant Program
72 East Concord Street
Suites L801 and L805
Boston, MA 02118, USA

E-mail address:
dmtzizik@bu.edu

Chest Pain
Evaluation and Management

John Ramos, MMS, PA-C, CAQ-EM[a],*, Heather Wolek, MPAS, PA-C[a]

KEYWORDS

- ACS • Acute coronary occlusion • HEART score • MACE • Chest pain • Troponin
- High sensitivity troponin • Clinical decision pathways

KEY POINTS

- 5.1% of emergency department patients with chest pain have acute coronary syndrome.
- Acute coronary artery occlusion is best managed with emergent reperfusion.
- Clinical decision pathways incorporating history, risk factors, electrocardiogram, and cardiac troponin are used to risk stratify patients without an indication for emergent reperfusion.
- Patients at low risk of acute coronary syndrome can be safely managed in the outpatient setting.
- Patients at intermediate risk may warrant cardiology consultation if they have previously abnormal cardiac tests, or if there is diagnostic uncertainty.

INTRODUCTION

Chest pain is a common chief complaint in the emergency department.[1] About 50% of patients with chest pain are ultimately diagnosed with a noncardiac condition, and the majority do not have a life-threatening illness.[2,3] In constrast, 5.1% of patients are diagnosed with acute coronary syndrome (ACS)—a spectrum of symptomatic occlusive coronary heart disease (CHD) and impaired myocardial perfusion.[3] Clinically, ACS is suggested by a suspicious history (chest pain characteristics and risk factors) and either electrocardiogram (ECG) or troponin abnormalities consistent with myocardial ischemia. Acute coronary occlusion (ACO) is frank or impending irreversible progression from myocardial ischemia to necrosis and is managed with emergent reperfusion (revascularization via percutaneous coronary intervention [PCI]). Although CHD affects more than 18 million adults and is a leading cause of death in the United States,[4] angioplasty is no panacea. Compared with optimized medical therapy alone, revascularization has not shown a clear benefit in reducing mortality or improving exercise

[a] Department of Emergency Medicine, Duke University Hospital, 2301 Erwin Road Suite 2600, Durham, NC 27710, USA
* Corresponding author.
E-mail address: john.ramos@duke.edu

Physician Assist Clin 8 (2023) 1–16
https://doi.org/10.1016/j.cpha.2022.08.006
2405-7991/23/© 2022 Elsevier Inc. All rights reserved.

Table 1 Acute coronary syndromes		
	Cardiac Biomarkers	**ECG Changes**
Unstable angina	Normal	TWI or ST depression
NSTE MI	Elevated	TWI or ST depression
STE MI	Normal or elevated	ST segment elevation, presumed new LBBB

Abbreviations: ECG, electrocardiogram; LBBB, left bundle branch block; MI, myocardial ischemia; NSTE, non-ST elevation; STE, ST segment elevation; TWI, T wave inversion.

tolerance among patients with stable CHD disease.[5] In the absence of evidence suggesting ACO, risk stratification is often used in the emergency department to identify patients who would benefit from advanced cardiac testing or intervention. Considering the therapeutic limitations of angioplasty, and the futility and harm from aggressive testing strategies, one challenge is the disposition of patients with chest pain who are at a low risk for ACO or major adverse cardiac events (MACE).[6,7]

DEFINITIONS

Myocardial injury occurs in occlusive and nonocclusive conditions whereby myocardial perfusion (supply of oxygen and nutrients) is insufficient relative to metabolic demand.[8,9] Occlusive conditions (coronary artery disease, thrombosis, vasospasm, dissection) obstruct the arterial blood supply of the heart, resulting in variably reversible hypoperfusion of the myocardium. Coronary artery disease (CAD), a leading contributor to CHD, is pathologically characterized by arterial vasoconstriction, mural thrombus formation, or, more commonly, lipid plaque formation, rupture, or erosion. Nonocclusive conditions include inadequate metabolic support (eg, hypoxemia, severe iron deficiency anemia), decreased coronary perfusion (eg, hypotension, hemorrhagic shock, sepsis), or increased myocardial oxygen demand (eg, fever, supraventricular or ventricular tachyarrhythmia, thyrotoxicosis).

The ACSs (**Table 1**) are symptomatic manifestations of CHD and are classically defined by symptoms (chest pain or anginal equivalent) and objective evidence of myocardial injury.[3] In an era before universal adoption of coronary angiography and PCI, ST segment elevation (STE) was retrospectively identified among patients who

Box 1 The fourth universal definition of myocardial infarction
An increase and/or decrease of cardiac troponin, with at least one value above the 99th percentile upper reference limit, and corroborative clinical evidence of infarction evidenced by at least 1 of the following: • Symptoms of myocardial ischemia • New ischemic electrocardiographic changes • Development of pathologic Q waves • Imaging evidence of new loss of viable myocardium or new regional wall motion abnormality in a pattern consistent with an ischemic cause • Identification of a coronary thrombus by angiography or autopsy *From* Thygesen K, Alpert JS, Jaffe AS, et al. Fourth Universal Definition of Myocardial Infarction (2018). Circulation. 2018;138(20):e618-e651; with permission.

Box 2
Risk factors for coronary heart disease

- Diabetes
- Hypertension
- Hyperlipidemia
- Human immunodeficiency virus
- Chronic kidney disease
- Coronary artery bypass graft
- Age (>45 years in men, >55 years in women)
- Early CAD in a first-degree relative
- Cerebral or peripheral arterial disease
- Sedentary lifestyle
- Obesity (Body Mass Index>30)
- Smoking history
- Cocaine and methamphetamine use

Data from Collet JP, Thiele H, Barbato E, et al. 2020 ESC Guidelines for the management of acute coronary syndromes in patients presenting without persistent ST-segment elevation. *Eur Heart J.* 2021;42(14):1289-1367; and Gulati M, Levy PD, Mukherjee D, et al. 2021 AHA/ACC/ASE/CHEST/SAEM/SCCT/SCMR Guideline for the Evaluation and Diagnosis of Chest Pain: A Report of the American College of Cardiology/American Heart Association Joint Committee on Clinical Practice Guidelines. Circulation. 2021;144(22):e368-e454.

---

benefitted from fibrinolytic reperfusion, and it is a central component of the classic ACS definitions.[10] The absence of STE does not exclude ACO or predict more favorable outcomes from nonemergent intervention.[11] The goal of the emergency evaluation is to distinguish noncardiac causes of chest pain from STE ACS and ACS with no STE (NSTE ACS). The American Heart Association has also established a broader definition (**Box 1**) for diagnosing myocardial infarction (MI).[8]

EVALUATION
History and Physical Examination

Acute onset chest pain or discomfort is the most common symptom reported by men and women who are ultimately diagnosed with ACS.[3] Referred pain in the shoulders, arms, jaw, neck, and upper abdomen should be considered anginal or chest pain equivalents. Acute chest pain is best defined as a noxious sensation that is either new in onset, or, for those with episodic symptoms, involves a change in the character, intensity, or duration of symptoms. Provoking events such as exertion and emotional stress are important to distinguish, especially among patients with episodic symptoms. The probability of myocardial ischemia is higher with specific features in location (central or retrosternal), quality (pressure, squeezing, gripping, heaviness, tightness), provoking factors (emotional stress and physical exertion), and relieving factors (rest, nitroglycerin). Anginal symptoms such as retrosternal pain, discomfort, or heaviness that occur at rest or with minimal exertion are strongly suggestive of ACS. ACS is less likely when symptoms increase or diminish with position, occur with inspiration (pleuritic), shift in location, or, are described as fleeting,

Box 3
Differential diagnoses of chest pain

Cardiac		Noncardiac

• Ischemic
  ◦ ACS
  ◦ Aortic Stenosis
  ◦ Chronic stable angina
  ◦ Coronary vasospasm
  ◦ Hypertrophic
    cardiomyopathy
  ◦ Unstable angina
	• Nonischemic
	  ◦ Aortic dissection
	  ◦ Mitral valve
	    prolapse
	  ◦ Myocarditis
	  ◦ Pericardial
	    tamponade
	  ◦ Pericarditis
		• Dermatologic
		  ◦ Herpes zoster/postherpetic
		    neuralgia
		• Chest wall
		  ◦ Costochondritis
		  ◦ Radicular pain
		  ◦ Rib pain
		  ◦ Nonspecific
		    musculoskeletal pain
		  ◦ Tietze syndrome
		• Gastrointestinal
		  ◦ Biliary colic
		  ◦ Boerhaave syndrome
		    (esophageal rupture)
		  ◦ Cholecystitis
		  ◦ Esophageal spasm
		  ◦ Gastroesophageal reflux disease
		  ◦ Peptic ulcer disease
		  ◦ Pancreatitis
		  ◦ Motility disorder
		• Pulmonary
		  ◦ Pleuritis
		  ◦ Pneumonia
		  ◦ Pulmonary embolism
		  ◦ Tension pneumothorax
		• Psychiatric
		  ◦ Anxiety
		  ◦ Depression
		  ◦ Panic disorder
		  ◦ Somatoform disorders
		• Other
		  ◦ Acute chest syndrome
		  ◦ Diabetic mononeuritis
		  ◦ Tabes dorsalis
		  ◦ Complex regional
		    pain syndrome (CRPS)

Data from Coté AP, Hodes JL, Voccia R. Low-Risk Chest Pain. Physician Assistant Clinics. 2017;2(3):537-556; and Yamasaki T, Fass R. Noncardiac chest pain: diagnosis and management. Curr Opin Gastroenterol. 2017;33(4):293-300; and Khan U, Robbins MS. Neurological Causes of Chest Pain. Curr Pain Headache Rep. 2021;25(5):32.

sharp, tearing, ripping, and burning. Associated symptoms such as shortness of breath, nausea, nonspecific abdominal pain, radiating discomfort, numbness, light-headedness, near or frank syncope, are more frequently described by women, patients aged older than 75 years, and those with diabetes. In addition to presenting symptoms, providers should consider risk factors for CHD (**Box 2**) from the past medical history, family, and social history.[3,9] The presence or absence of symptoms and risk factors are not sufficient to diagnose or exclude ACS.

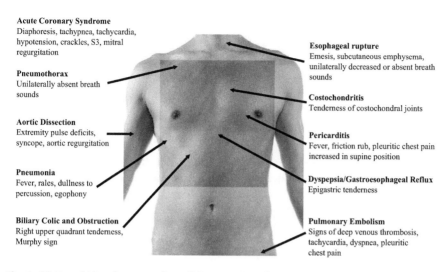

Acute Coronary Syndrome
Diaphoresis, tachypnea, tachycardia, hypotension, crackles, S3, mitral regurgitation

Pneumothorax
Unilaterally absent breath sounds

Aortic Dissection
Extremity pulse deficits, syncope, aortic regurgitation

Pneumonia
Fever, rales, dullness to percussion, egophony

Biliary Colic and Obstruction
Right upper quadrant tenderness, Murphy sign

Esophageal rupture
Emesis, subcutaneous emphysema, unilaterally decreased or absent breath sounds

Costochondritis
Tenderness of costochondral joints

Pericarditis
Fever, friction rub, pleuritic chest pain increased in supine position

Dyspepsia/Gastroesophageal Reflux
Epigastric tenderness

Pulmonary Embolism
Signs of deep venous thrombosis, tachycardia, dyspnea, pleuritic chest pain

Fig. 1. Distinguishing features of conditions causing chest pain. *From* Abrahams PH, Spratt JD, Loukas M, Van Schoor AN. Thorax. In: Abrahams' and McMinn's Clinical Atlas of Human Anatomy, 8th edition. Elsevier; 2019; with permission.

Box 4	
Ischemic patterns on electrocardiogram	
Q waves	• In leads V2–V3 >0.02 s or QS complex (negative deflection of QRS complex)
	• ≥0.03 s and ≥1 mm deep or QS complex in leads I, II, aVL, aVF or V4–V6 in any 2 leads of a contiguous lead grouping (I, aVL; V1–V6; II, III, aVF)
ST depression	• ≥0.5 mm in 2 contiguous leads, typically horizontal or downsloping
ST elevation	• ≥1 mm in all leads other than V2–V3
	• In leads V2-V3:
	○ ≥2 mm in men ≥40 y
	○ ≥2.5 mm in men <40 y
	○ ≥1.5 mm in women regardless of age
	• LVH may show deep S waves and ST segment elevation with a concave morphology, a convex morphology is more suggestive of concomitant ischemia
	• Terminal QRS distortion is the absence of S-wave preceding ST segment elevation (see **Fig. 2**)
T wave inversion	• >1 mm in 2 contiguous leads with prominent R wave or R/s ratio >1
	• Hyperacute T waves (**Fig. 3**)

Abbreviation: LVH, left ventricular hypertrophy.

Data from Thygesen K, Alpert JS, Jaffe AS, et al. Fourth Universal Definition of Myocardial Infarction (2018). Circulation. 2018;138(20):e618-e651; and Birnbaum Y, Bayés de Luna A, Fiol M, et al. Common pitfalls in the interpretation of electrocardiograms from patients with acute coronary syndromes with narrow QRS: a consensus report. J Electrocardiol. 2012;45(5):463-475; and Pendell Meyers H, Bracey A, Lee D, et al. Accuracy of OMI ECG findings versus STEMI criteria for diagnosis of acute coronary occlusion myocardial infarction. Int J Cardiol Heart Vasc. 2021;Apr 12;33:100767.

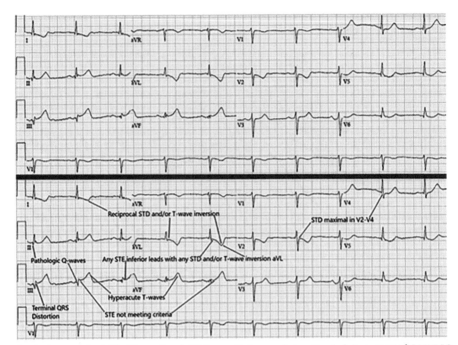

Fig. 2. Patterns in ACO. (*From*: Pendell Meyers H, Bracey A, Lee D, et al. Accuracy of OMI ECG findings versus STEMI criteria for diagnosis of acute coronary occlusion myocardial infarction. Int J Cardiol Heart Vasc. 2021;Apr 12;33:100767; with permission.)

ACS can be difficult to distinguish from the broad differential diagnoses associated with chest pain (**Box 3**).[12–14] The most common cause of recurrent or episodic chest pain is gastroesophageal reflux disease.[15] Physical examination abnormalities are often not specific to ACS, but can help distinguish alternative causes of chest pain (**Fig. 1**).[16–18]

DIAGNOSIS

Diagnostic testing in the workup of chest pain includes ECG, serology, and imaging. The initial evaluation for ACS includes ECG and troponin testing.

Electrocardiography

Electrocardiography provides a timely evaluation of the heart's electrical conduction and should be compared with previous ECGs, when available. As myocardial ischemia progresses, a host of proposed cellular effects (Adenosine triphosphate depletion, potassium leaking, late depolarization, faster repolarization) lead to characteristic changes on ECG (**Box 4, Fig. 2**).[19] Ischemic changes in anatomically contiguous leads and supplemental leads can localize culprit artery occlusion (**Fig. 4 , Tables 2** and **3**).[12,20–23] Left bundle branch blocks, left ventricular hypertrophy, and ventricular pacing can obscure typical findings of ischemia. The initial ECG is normal in more than 30% of patients ultimately diagnosed with NSTE ACS.[9] For patients with persistent symptoms and a nondiagnostic ECG, serial ECGs are recommended until more evidence is available to rule out myocardial ischemia.

Atypical patterns of STE-ACS (STEMI)

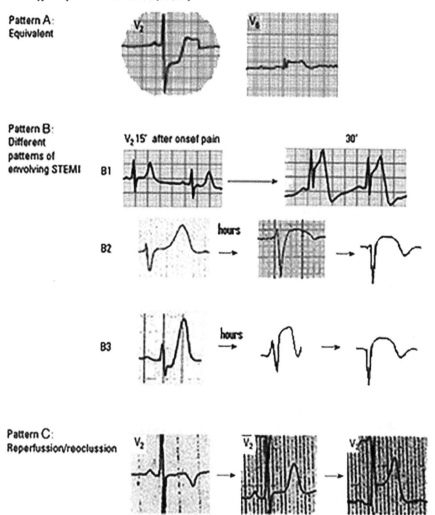

Pattern A:
Equivalent

Pattern B:
Different
patterns of
evolving STEMI

B1 — V_2 15″ after onset pain → 30′

B2 — hours →

B3 — hours →

Pattern C:
Reperfussion/reocclussion

V_2 → $\overline{V_2}$ → V_2

Fig. 3. Other patterns in ACO. Pattern A: ST depression (a mirror pattern of the ST elevation in leads facing the ischemic zone) in left circumflex and right coronary artery occlusion. Pattern B: Three patterns of positive peaked and symmetric T waves as a first sign of ischemia. B1: Transient peaked T waves followed by ST elevation a few minutes later. B2 and B3: Examples of persistent tall positive T waves (B3 with ST depression) lasting several hours, before complete occlusion and transmural involvement evolving to Q wave MI. Pattern C: Deep negative T waves (symptoms of ACO resolve), followed by pseudonormalization of the T wave (new occlusion or vasospasm), and then ST elevation evolves. (*From:* Birnbaum Y, Bayés de Luna A, Fiol M, et al. Common pitfalls in the interpretation of electrocardiograms from patients with acute coronary syndromes with narrow QRS: a consensus report. *J Electrocardiol.* 2012;45(5):463-475; with permission.)

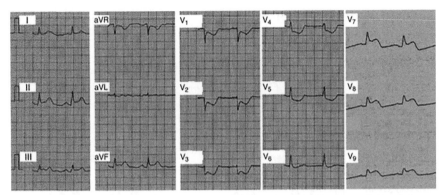

Fig. 4. ECG in left circumflex artery occlusion. ST depression in many precordial leads is seen (V1–V5) without a final positive T wave, and with ST elevation in II, III, avF, and V 7 to V9. (*From* Birnbaum Y, Bayés de Luna A, Fiol M, et al. Common pitfalls in the interpretation of electrocardiograms from patients with acute coronary syndromes with narrow QRS: a consensus report. *J Electrocardiol.* 2012;45(5):463-475; with permission.)

Cardiac Enzyme Testing

There are 3 types of cardiac troponin: troponin T, troponin I, and troponin C. Troponin T and I are specific to cardiac tissue, whereas troponin C can be found in both cardiac and skeletal tissues. Compared with creatinine kinase (CK), myoglobin, and CK myocardial band, troponins are detectable earlier, remain elevated for a longer duration, and are more sensitive and specific (**Fig. 5**). Higher baseline troponins are expected in patients who are male, aged greater than 60 years, and those with chronic kidney disease. Troponin values greater than 5 times the upper limit of normal are associated with poor outcomes. High-sensitivity troponin (hs-cTn) has greater sensitivity and negative predictive values for myocardial injury, with a shorter interval of detection from the onset of chest pain. Recommendations for initial and serial testing vary based on troponin assay selection.[3,9]

Bedside Cardiac Ultrasonography

Focused cardiac ultrasonography by an experienced provider offers insight into cardiac function as well as volume status. Focal wall motion abnormalities such as hypokinesis correspond to occlusive lesions (**Fig. 6**).[24] Ultrasound may also identify

Table 2
Culprit artery occlusion and ischemic patterns on electrocardiogram

Location of MI	ECG Leads Most Likely to Show Changes	Culprit Artery Occlusion
Inferior	II, III, avF	RCA
Posterior	ST depression in V1, V2	Circumflex, RCA
Anteroseptal	V1, V2	LAD
Anterolateral	V3, V4	LAD
Lateral	I, avL, V5, V6	Circumflex

Abbreviations: ECG, electrocardiogram; LAD, left anterior descending; MI, myocardial infarction; RCA, right coronary artery.

From Coté AP, Hodes JL, Voccia R. Low-Risk Chest Pain. Physician Assistant Clinics. 2017;2(3):537-556; with permission.

Table 3
Patterns of ischemia on supplemental leads

Location of MI	Standard 12 Lead ECG Changes	Supplemental Leads
Left circumflex artery (see Fig. 4)	V1–V3 (ST-segment depression ≥0.5 mm)	V7, V8, and V9 (ST-segment elevation ≥0.5 mm)
Inferior and right ventricular	aVR or V1 (ST-segment elevation ≥1 mm)	V3R and V4R (ST-segment elevation ≥0.5 mm, or ≥1 mm for men < 30 y)

Abbreviation: MI, myocardial ischemia.
Data from Wong CK, White HD. Patients with circumflex occlusions miss out on reperfusion: how to recognize and manage them. Curr Opin Cardiol. 2012;27(4):327-330; and Lopez-Sendon J, Coma-Canella I, Alcasena S, Seoane J, Gamallo C. Electrocardiographic findings in acute right ventricular infarction: sensitivity and specificity of electrocardiographic alterations in right precordial leads V4R, V3R, V1, V2, and V3. J Am Coll Cardiol. 1985;6(6):1273-1279.

alternate conditions or complications of cardiac conditions, including pericardial effusion (pericarditis), aortic dissection, or right ventricular dilation (pulmonary embolism).

Additional Tests

Serologic tests are commonly used to investigate noncardiac causes in the differential, or, causes of nonocclusive myocardial ischemia (eg, hyperkalemia, sepsis, anemia). X-ray and computed tomography are used to identify or exclude other conditions that cause chest pain, ischemic ECG patterns, or elevated troponin (eg, pulmonary embolism, aortic dissection, stroke).[3,9]

Advanced Cardiac Tests

More advanced cardiac testing should be guided by individual patient risk for ACS and the probability of results that would otherwise change management. For low-risk

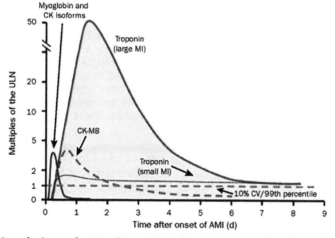

Fig. 5. Timing of release of various biomarkers after acute myocardial infarction. AMI, acute myocardial infarction; CV, coefficient of variation; ULN, upper limit of normal. (*From* Anderson JL, Adams CD, Antman EM, et al. ACC/AHA 2007 guidelines for the management of patients with unstable angina/non–ST-Elevation myocardial infarction. J Am Coll Cardiol 2007;50(7):e26; with permission.)

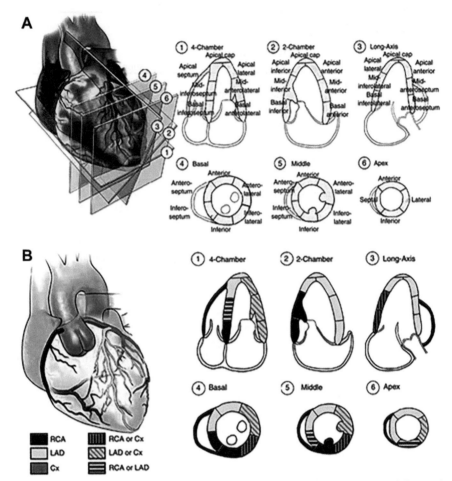

Fig. 6. Typical coronary artery distribution of blood flow in apical and parasternal short-axis views. (*A*) The Left ventricle segments. (*B*) The approximate and most common coronary arterial distributions related to these segments. Cx, circumflex; LAD, left anterior descending coronary artery; RCA, right coronary artery. (*From* Lang RM, Badano LP, Mor-Avi V, et al. Recommendations for cardiac chamber quantification by echocardiography in adults: an update from the American Society of Echocardiography and the European Association of Cardiovascular Imaging. *J Am Soc Echocardiogr.* 2015;28:1–39.e14; with permission.)

patients, there are suggested warranty periods of 2 years for a normal anatomic test (normal coronary angiogram, or coronary computed tomography angiogram [CCTA] with no stenosis or plaque), and 1 year for a normal stress test. Provided that previous cardiac testing was sufficiently performed (adequate imaging quality and exercise or pharmacologic stress) within the warranty period, there is limited value in repeat testing for a low-risk patient with a reassuring ECG and negative cardiac biomarkers.[3] Advanced cardiac testing is indicated for patients with higher than low risk or when there is a clinical concern for unstable CAD (**Figs. 7** and **8**).[3] CCTA is recommended for patients with known nonobstructive CAD (<50% stenosis) or an inconclusive or mildly abnormal stress test within the past year. Stress testing is recommended for

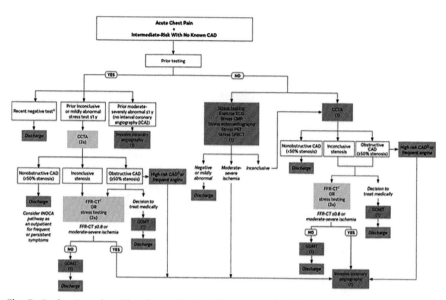

Fig. 7. Evaluation algorithm for patients with suspected ACS at intermediate risk with no known CAD. Test choice should be guided by local availability and expertise. [a]Recent negative test: normal CCTA 2 years or less (no plaque/no stenosis) OR negative stress test 1 year or less, given adequate stress. [b]High-risk CAD means left main stenosis 50% or greater; anatomically significant 3-vessel disease (≥70% stenosis). [c]For FFR-CT, turnaround times may affect prompt clinical care decisions. However, the use of FFR-CT does not require additional testing, as would be the case when adding stress testing. CAD, coronary artery disease; CCTA, coronary CT angiography; CMR, cardiovascular magnetic resonance imaging; CT, computed tomography; FFR-CT, fractional flow reserve with CT; GDMT, guideline-directed medical therapy; ICA, invasive coronary angiography; INOCA, ischemia and no obstructive coronary artery disease; PET, positron emission tomography; SPECT, single-photon emission CT. (*From* Gulati M, Levy PD, Mukherjee D, et al. 2021 AHA/ACC/ASE/CHEST/SAEM/SCCT/SCMR Guideline for the Evaluation and Diagnosis of Chest Pain: A Report of the American College of Cardiology/American Heart Association Joint Committee on Clinical Practice Guidelines. Circulation. 2021;144(22):e368-e454; with permission.)

patients with obstructive CAD (≥50%) or who are at intermediate risk without previous anatomic testing. Appropriate test selection should also consider contraindications such as exercise intolerance, hypertension or hypotension, concurrent medications, and acute illness (pulmonary embolism, aortic dissection, myocarditis, pericarditis).[3]

MANAGEMENT

Clinical decision pathways (CDPs; **Table 4**) incorporate clinical data to determine the risk of MACE or probability of ACS requiring emergent intervention.[9,25–29] In addition to risk stratification, CDPs reduce undertesting and overtesting in the ED.[3] The definition of MACE varies within studies, although most included index visit myocardial infarction or revascularization, or death. Other study specific variations include timing of troponin testing relative to symptom onset and CHD/CAD risk factors among the studied population. CDPs applicability may be limited by institutional variations in troponin assays and assay-specific cut-off levels. When there is diagnostic uncertainty or intermediate to high risk, cardiology consultation is essential for decisions

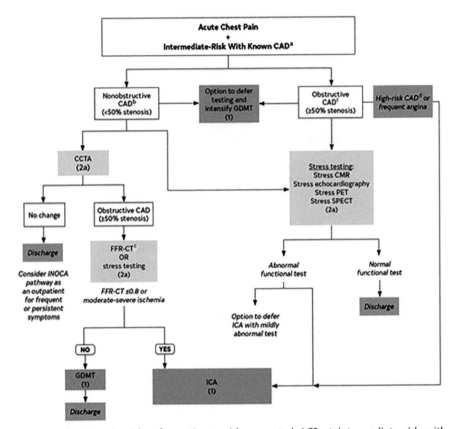

Fig. 8. Evaluation algorithm for patients with suspected ACS at intermediate risk with known CAD. Test choice should be guided by local availability and expertise. [a]Known CAD is prior MI, revascularization, known obstructive or nonobstructive CAD on invasive or CCTA. [b]If extensive plaque is present a high-quality CCTA is unlikely to be achieved, and stress testing is preferred. [c]Obstructive CAD includes prior coronary artery bypass graft/PCI. [d]High-risk CAD means left main stenosis 50% or greater; anatomically significant 3-vessel disease ($\geq$70% stenosis). ||FFR-CT turnaround times may affect prompt clinical care decisions. ACS, acute coronary syndrome; CAD, coronary artery disease; CCTA, coronary CT angiography; CMR, cardiovascular magnetic resonance; CT, computed tomography; FFR-CT, fractional flow reserve with CT; GDMT, guideline-directed medical therapy; ICA, invasive coronary angiography; INOCA, ischemia and no obstructive coronary artery disease; PET, positron emission tomography; SPECT, single-photon emission CT. (*From* Gulati M, Levy PD, Mukherjee D, et al. 2021 AHA/ACC/ASE/CHEST/SAEM/SCCT/SCMR Guideline for the Evaluation and Diagnosis of Chest Pain: A Report of the American College of Cardiology/American Heart Association Joint Committee on Clinical Practice Guidelines. Circulation. 2021;144(22):e368-e454; with permission.)

regarding advanced cardiac testing or intervention. Risk stratification for ACS or MACE does not exclude the presence of CAD.

Score-based risk stratification may lead to more unnecessary admissions or cardiac testing in select circumstances. That is, the risk of MACE is very low among patients with an undetectable hs-cTn, and patients with a reassuring ECG and biomarkers if

Table 4 Clinical decision pathways	
HEART	• History, ECG (1 point for LBB, new or unchanged repolarization disorders, 2 points for ST segment deviation), Age, risk factors, troponin (0, 3 h) • Low risk: Score ≤3, initial and serial cTn/hs-cTn < assay 99th percentile
EDACS	• History, Age, risk factors, sex, troponin (0, 2 h) • Low risk: Score ≤16; initial and serial cTn/hs-cTn < assay 99th percentile; No ischemic ECG changes
TIMI	• Age, ≥3 risk factors, Known CAD (stenosis ≥ 50%), ASA use in last 7 days, ≥2 episodes of severe angina in 24 h, ECG ST changes ≥0.5 mm, positive cardiac biomarker • Score of ≤1 = 5% risk of all cause mortality, new or recurrent MI, need for urgent revascularization at 14 d
ADAPT	• TIMI score, ECG, Troponin • Low risk: TIMI score 0; initial and serial cTn/hs-cTn < assay 99th percentile; No ischemic ECG changes (ST-segment depression ≥0.05 mV in ≥2 contiguous leads, including reciprocal changes; T-wave inversion ≥0.1 mV; Q waves ≥30 ms wide and ≥0.1 mV deep in ≥2 contiguous leads)
2020 ESC/hs-cTn	• History, ECG, hs-cTn (0, 1 or 2 h) • Low risk: Initial hs-cTn very low and CP onset >3 h before testing, or, initial hs-cTn low and 1-h or 2-h hs-cTn Δ is low[a]
2016 ESC/GRACE[b]	• Age, HR, SBP, serum Cr, cardiac arrest, ECG, cardiac biomarker, Killip class • Low risk: CP resolved; GRACE score <140; hs-cTn < ULN 0, 3 h with CP <6 h, or, 1 negative test with CP >6 h

Abbreviations: ACS, acute coronary syndrome; ADAPT, accelerated diagnostic protocol to assess chest pain using troponins; AMI, acute myocardial infarction; ASA, aspirin; CP, chest pain or equivalent; Cr, creatinine; cTn, cardiac troponin; ECG, electrocardiogram; ED, emergency department; EDACS, emergency department ACS; ESC, European Society of Cardiology; GRACE, global registry of acute coronary events; h, hour; HEART, history, ECG, age, risk factors, troponin; HR, heart rate; hs, high-sensitivity; MACE, major adverse cardiovascular events; neg, negative; SBP, systolic blood pressure; TIMI, Thrombolysis in myocardial infarction; ULN, upper limit of normal.
[a] The terms very low, low, and Δ refer to hs-cTn assay-specific thresholds in the ESC guideline.
[b] 30-d MACE sensitivity not studied.
Data from Gulati M, Levy PD, Mukherjee D, et al. 2021 AHA/ACC/ASE/CHEST/SAEM/SCCT/SCMR Guideline for the Evaluation and Diagnosis of Chest Pain: A Report of the American College of Cardiology/American Heart Association Joint Committee on Clinical Practice Guidelines. *Circulation.* 2021;144(22):e368-e454; and Mahler SA, Riley RF, Hiestand BC, et al. The HEART Pathway randomized trial: identifying emergency department patients with acute chest pain for early discharge. *Circ Cardiovasc Qual Outcomes.* 2015;8(2):195-203; and Than M, Flaws D, Sanders S, et al. Development and validation of the Emergency Department Assessment of Chest pain Score and 2 h accelerated diagnostic protocol. *Emerg Med Australas.* 2014;26(1):34-44; and Chase M, Robey JL, Zogby KE, Sease KL, Shofer FS, Hollander JE. Prospective validation of the Thrombolysis in Myocardial Infarction Risk Score in the emergency department chest pain population. *Ann Emerg Med.* 2006;48(3):252-259; and Than M, Cullen L, Aldous S, et al. 2-Hour accelerated diagnostic protocol to assess patients with chest pain symptoms using contemporary troponins as the only biomarker: the ADAPT trial. *J Am Coll Cardiol.* 2012;59(23):2091-2098; and Collet JP, Thiele H, Barbato E, et al. 2020 ESC Guidelines for the management of acute coronary syndromes in patients presenting without persistent ST-segment elevation. *Eur Heart J.* 2021;42(14):1289-1367; and Roffi M, Patrono C, Collet JP, et al. 2015 ESC Guidelines for the Management of Acute Coronary Syndromes in Patients Presenting Without Persistent ST-segment Elevation. *Rev Esp Cardiol (Engl Ed).* 2015;68(12):1125.

they have had a negative CCTA (<50% stenosis), ECG stress test, stress echocardiography, or stress myocardial perfusion scan in the past 12 months.[30,31] Patients who are at low risk for ACS or MACE can be safely discharged from the ED with appropriate follow-up.

SUMMARY

Between 2010 and 2016, there were more than 40 million ED visits for chest pain.[1] ACS has a high burden of morbidity and mortality, but is less frequently diagnosed than other emergent or noncardiac conditions.[2,3] Troponin and ECG are the best initial tests for ACS, and serial testing is sometimes indicated. In the absence of ACO or NSTE-ACS, risk stratification is used to determine a safe disposition for patients. CDPs risk stratify patients and guide judicious use of resources. Patients who are at low risk for ACS or MACE can be safely discharged from the emergency department with appropriate and timely follow-up (eg, primary care, cardiology). Patients at higher than low risk generally warrant cardiology consultation to select advanced cardiac tests and determine a safe disposition.

CLINICS CARE POINTS

- Among patients presenting to Emergency Departments with chest pain, 5.1% are diagnosed with ACS.
- Acute coronary syndrome is a spectrum of symptomatic CHD.
- Acute coronary artery occlusion is best managed with emergent reperfusion.
- CDPs incorporating history, risk factors, ECG, and cardiac troponin are used to risk stratify patients without an indication for emergent reperfusion.
- Patients at low risk can be safely managed in the outpatient setting.
- Patients at intermediate risk may warrant cardiology consultation if they have previously abnormal cardiac tests or if there is diagnostic uncertainty.

DISCLOSURE

The authors have no funding sources (beyond clinical employment), or, commercial or financial conflicts of interest.

REFERENCES

1. Aalam AA, Alsabban A, Pines JM. National trends in chest pain visits in US emergency departments (2006–2016). Emerg Med J 2020;37:696–9.
2. Hsia RY, Hale Z, Tabas JA. A national study of the prevalence of life-threatening diagnoses in patients with chest pain. JAMA Intern Med 2016;176:1029–32.
3. Gulati M, Levy PD, Mukherjee D, et al. 2021 AHA/ACC/ASE/CHEST/SAEM/SCCT/ SCMR Guideline for the Evaluation and Diagnosis of Chest Pain: A Report of the American College of Cardiology/American Heart Association Joint Committee on Clinical Practice Guidelines. Circulation 2021;144(22):e368–454.
4. Tsao CW, Aday AW, Almarzooq ZI, et al. Heart Disease and Stroke Statistics-2022 Update: A Report From the American Heart Association. Circulation 2022; 145(8):e153–639.
5. Teoh Z, Al-Lamee RK. COURAGE, ORBITA, and ISCHEMIA: Percutaneous Coronary Intervention for Stable Coronary Artery Disease. Interv Cardiol Clin 2020; 9(4):469–82.
6. Aldous S, Richards AM, Cullen L, et al. The incremental value of stress testing in patients with acute chest pain beyond serial cardiac troponin testing. Emerg Med J 2016;33(5):319–24.

7. Mahler SA, Lenoir KM, Wells BJ, et al. Safely identifying emergency department patients with acute chest pain for early discharge. Circulation 2018;138:2456–68.

8. Thygesen K, Alpert JS, Jaffe AS, et al. Fourth Universal Definition of Myocardial Infarction (2018). Circulation 2018;138(20):e618–51.

9. Collet JP, Thiele H, Barbato E, et al. 2020 ESC Guidelines for the management of acute coronary syndromes in patients presenting without persistent ST-segment elevation. Eur Heart J 2021;42(14):1289–367.

10. Indications for fibrinolytic therapy in suspected acute myocardial infarction: collaborative overview of early mortality and major morbidity results from all randomised trials of more than 1000 patients. Fibrinolytic Therapy Trialists' (FTT) Collaborative Group. Lancet 1994;343:311–22.

11. Aslanger EK, Yıldırımtürk Ö, Şimşek B, et al. Diagnostic accuracy of electrocardiogram for acute coronary occlusion resulting in myocardial infarction (DIFOCCULT study). IJC Heart & Vasculature 2020;30:100603.

12. Coté AP, Hodes JL, Voccia R. Low-Risk Chest Pain. Physician Assistant Clin 2017;2(3):537–56.

13. Yamasaki T, Fass R. Noncardiac chest pain: diagnosis and management. Curr Opin Gastroenterol 2017;33(4):293–300.

14. Khan U, Robbins MS. Neurological Causes of Chest Pain. Curr Pain Headache Rep 2021;25(5):32.

15. Dent J, El-Serag HB, Wallander MA, et al. Epidemiology of gastro-oesophageal reflux disease: a systematic review. Gut 2005;54:710–7.

16. McConaghy JR, Sharma M, Patel H. Acute Chest Pain in Adults: Outpatient Evaluation. Am Fam Physician 2020;102(12):721–7.

17. Stevens SM, Woller SC, Kreuziger LB, et al. Antithrombotic Therapy for VTE Disease: Second Update of the CHEST Guideline and Expert Panel Report. Chest 2021;160(6):e545–608.

18. Tsai TT, Trimarchi S, Nienaber CA. Acute aortic dissection: perspectives from the International Registry of Acute Aortic Dissection (IRAD). Eur J Vasc Endovasc Surg 2009;37(2):149–59.

19. Goldberger JJ, Albert CM, Myerburg RJ. Cardiac Arrest and Sudden Cardiac Death. In: Libby P, Bonow RO, Mann DL, et al, editors. Braunwald's heart disease: a textbook of cardiovascular medicine. 12th edition. Philadelphia: Elsevier; 2022. p. 1349–86.

20. Birnbaum Y, Bayés de Luna A, Fiol M, et al. Common pitfalls in the interpretation of electrocardiograms from patients with acute coronary syndromes with narrow QRS: a consensus report. J Electrocardiol 2012;45(5):463–75.

21. Pendell Meyers H, Bracey A, Lee D, et al. Accuracy of OMI ECG findings versus STEMI criteria for diagnosis of acute coronary occlusion myocardial infarction. Int J Cardiol Heart Vasc 2021;33:100767.

22. Wong CK, White HD. Patients with circumflex occlusions miss out on reperfusion: how to recognize and manage them. Curr Opin Cardiol 2012;27(4):327–30.

23. Lopez-Sendon J, Coma-Canella I, Alcasena S, et al. Electrocardiographic findings in acute right ventricular infarction: sensitivity and specificity of electrocardiographic alterations in right precordial leads V4R, V3R, V1, V2, and V3. J Am Coll Cardiol 1985;6(6):1273–9.

24. Lang RM, Badano LP, Mor-Avi V, et al. Recommendations for cardiac chamber quantification by echocardiography in adults: an update from the American Society of Echocardiography and the European Association of Cardiovascular Imaging. J Am Soc Echocardiogr 2015;28:1–39.e14.

25. Mahler SA, Riley RF, Hiestand BC, et al. The HEART Pathway randomized trial: identifying emergency department patients with acute chest pain for early discharge. Circ Cardiovasc Qual Outcomes 2015;8(2):195–203.

26. Than M, Flaws D, Sanders S, et al. Development and validation of the Emergency Department Assessment of Chest pain Score and 2 h accelerated diagnostic protocol. Emerg Med Australas 2014;26(1):34–44.

27. Chase M, Robey JL, Zogby KE, et al. Prospective validation of the Thrombolysis in Myocardial Infarction Risk Score in the emergency department chest pain population. Ann Emerg Med 2006;48(3):252–9.

28. Than M, Cullen L, Aldous S, et al. 2-Hour accelerated diagnostic protocol to assess patients with chest pain symptoms using contemporary troponins as the only biomarker: the ADAPT trial. J Am Coll Cardiol 2012;59(23):2091–8.

29. Roffi M, Patrono C, Collet JP, et al. 2015 ESC Guidelines for the Management of Acute Coronary Syndromes in Patients Presenting Without Persistent ST-segment Elevation. Rev Esp Cardiol (Engl Ed) 2015;68(12):1125.

30. Peacock W, Daniels L, Headdon G, et al. HEART, EDACS, and TIMI: Little Value After High-Sensitivity Troponin Testing. Ann Emerg Med 2021;78(4):S40–1.

31. Mehta P, McDonald S, Hirani R, et al. Major adverse cardiac events after emergency department evaluation of chest pain patients with advanced testing: Systematic review and meta-analysis. Acad Emerg Med 2022;29(6):748–64.

Pearls and Pitfalls of Trauma Management

James A. Johanning, MPAS, PA-C*, Adam Burman, MPAS, PA-C

KEYWORDS

- Trauma • Hemorrhage • Point of care ultrasound • POCUS • Pediatric trauma
- Traumatic brain injury • TBI • Ouchless ER

KEY POINTS

- Emergency trauma for the physician assistant or medical provider.
- Management of hemorrhage in the trauma setting.
- Use of Point of Care Ultrasound in the injured patient.
- Special Considerations in the emergent management of pediatric patients.
- Pearls of the Ouchless ER minimizing physical and emotional trauma in the ER setting.

INTRODUCTION

Trauma is one of the most common and important patient presentations in Emergency Medicine, and its management is a key component of an Emergency Medicine Physician Assistant's practice. In the United States, more than 41 million ED trauma visits occur annually and range widely in patient age, severity, and complexity. Several systems and heuristics have been developed to simplify this variety of presentations and guide workups to more successful outcomes. These include the primary survey (ABCDE - Airway, Breathing, Circulation, Disability, Exposure; MARCH - Massive Hemorrhage, Airway, Respirations, Circulation, Head Injury/Hypothermia), secondary survey (ie, a comprehensive head-to-toe assessment), and various clinical decision instruments like the NEXUS Criteria for C-spine evaluation and PECARN for evaluating the pediatric traumatic brain injury patient.

Beyond these well-known, core concepts of Emergency Medicine, we present a closer examination of specific elements involved with caring for the trauma patient. Recognition of various pearls and pitfalls in the management of these patients can improve their outcomes in the trauma setting.

Hemorrhage in Trauma

Hemorrhage is the quickest killer of trauma victims, and its rapid identification and intervention are crucial to optimizing patient outcomes. Every Emergency Medicine

Saint Catherine University, 2004 Randoplh Avenue, Saint Paul, MN 55105, USA
* Corresponding author.
E-mail address: Jjohanning994@stkate.edu

practitioner needs to know the signs of significant hemorrhage. The simplest of these are visual inspection of active bleeding on the primary survey, integration of vital signs and Illness Severity Score (ISS), and recognition of impending hypovolemic shock by physical examination (location and strength of peripheral pulses, capillary refill, skin color) and Point of Care Ultrasound (POCUS), for example, the FAST examination. It is important to recognize the limitations of these evaluations, however, and to avoid false reassurance by a normal heart rate in the beta-blocked patient, a negative FAST examination in a patient with retroperitoneal hemorrhage, or a pediatric trauma victim whose sympathetic tone may be able to compensate for blood loss approaching 30% total blood volume.[1]

To augment evaluation at the bedside, basic laboratory studies play a role in the workup of a trauma patient. Most commonly this will include the hemoglobin and/or hematocrit; however, these are concentration-based studies and not a true estimate of blood volume. A bleeding trauma patient presenting in the initial hours after injury may have a completely normal complete blood count (CBC), and only after crystalloid volume resuscitation and therefore blood dilution will a noticeable HGB drop occur. A more effective predictor for true hypovolemia, and therefore increased risk for morbidity and mortality, is the Arterial Base Excess (ABE),[2] commonly included as part of an arterial blood gas or basic metabolic panel. An ABE of greater than 6.5 mmol/L confers a > 3x risk of 1st-day mortality, and greater than 1.5x risk on day 7 after injury. Early recognition of this often overlooked laboratory abnormality may allow for earlier, more aggressive operative management in the bleeding patient, as opposed to blood product resuscitation only.[2]

Due to its potential to kill rapidly, massive hemorrhage must be addressed immediately, even when hemorrhage has not been positively confirmed. Any patient presenting with a significant mechanism of injury or with abnormal vital signs must have the following interventions provided immediately upon arrival to the ED:

1. Source control of identified hemorrhage with direct pressure, hemostatic dressings with direct pressure applied, and/or tourniquet application proximal to the extremity wound. Hemostatic dressings are placed into superficial and moderate depth wounds to encourage platelet activation and to serve as a physical lattice for clot formation. For deeper or more briskly bleeding wounds, a tourniquet must be immediately applied proximal to the wound. Strap and windlass type devices (Combat Application Tourniquet, Military Emergency Tourniquet, Special Operations Forces Tourniquet) seem to be the most effective and simple to use. Other types, such as strap and ratchet devices (Mechanical Advantage Tourniquet and the Ratcheting Medical Tourniquet) or those that use air pressure (Emergent Medical Tourniquet) are also effective but are limited in their relatively more complex mechanisms and reduced flexibility of use.

2. Large bore IV access. Adequate access to circulation is necessary for the administration of medications and fluids. The intraosseous device is effective for medication administration and functions essentially identically to a central venous catheter (CVC) in this regard. However, both the IO and CVC have relatively slower rates of flow compared with a proximally placed large bore peripheral IV catheter. A large bore 14 gauge IV placed in the AC fossa will flow at 240 mL/min, a standard 18 gauge IV at 100 mL/min, and a 16 gauge CVC distal port at 70 mL/min (all rates with gravity only).[3] In general, a larger bore and shorter length of tubing will allow for maximal flow rate.

3. Activation of blood bank resources and consideration of initiating massive transfusion protocols. Given the inherent delays of cross-matching and transporting blood

products, a multidisciplinary, hospital-wide approach is necessary to ensure rapid delivery of blood to the bedside. This can be circumvented by keeping a small supply of universal O-negative blood in the Emergency Department trauma bay, but this inherently resources intensive and will lead to spoilage of unused blood products.

Instituting these protocols within the first few minutes of ED arrival maximizes temporization of massive hemorrhage, and allows for more definitive management in the OR.

After initial stabilization has begun, attention can be turned to more specific bleeding management based on the patient's clinical condition. These can be divided into 4 groups:

1. Hemodynamic support with crystalloid fluids and consideration of pressor agents.
2. Hemodynamic support with blood products
3. Optimization of coagulation through the use of antifibrinolytic products and reversal of anticoagulation or other bleeding propensities
4. Reassessment of response to noninvasive methods

Crystalloid volume resuscitation is a mainstay of Emergency Medicine, though its use in the bleeding patient is limited and potentially harmful owing to its contribution to Trauma Induced Coagulopathy (TIC). Intravenous crystalloid contributes to the evolution of TIC via hypothermia from room temperature fluid administration, acidemia from hyperchloric metabolic acidosis when large volumes of normal saline are given, and dilution of coagulation factors. These lead to an increased risk of ongoing bleeding and ultimately death. Small volume crystalloid resuscitation (500–1000 mL) may be appropriate in the bleeding shock patient for transient circulation support, but volumes beyond that may cause harm. Vasopressors also play a mixed role in the hemorrhagic shock patient. On the one hand, they may be necessary to ensure adequate cerebral and vital organ perfusion. Conversely, it is important to remember the vascular physiology in the bleeding trauma patient. These patients are in a state of high endogenous catecholamine activity, with a high likelihood of significant peripheral vasoconstriction already at work. With this in mind, peripherally active vasopressors are not likely to improve the patient's actual perfusion, and therefore should be considered only when other noninvasive methods have failed.

Blood product transfusion is the more important method of volume resuscitation in the hemorrhaging patient. A combination of packed red blood cells (PRBC), fresh frozen plasma (FFP), and platelets (PLT) are the cornerstone of hemorrhagic shock management. Numerous studies have been performed in recent decades attempting to identify the ideal ratio of these products, with huge contributions coming from the United States Armed Services. Current recommendations are for administering a fixed ratio of 1:1:1 RBC:FFP:PLT in most bleeding trauma patients.[4] This strategy is most effective for improving outcomes, but due to logistical issues may contribute to FFP waste (owing to the inherent time taken to thaw, by which time it may no longer be necessary). Whole blood transfusion is another effective option and is commonly used by forward-deployed military personnel. However, due to significant costs, this is not feasible for most civilian settings. In addition to transfusion composition, transfusion rate is an important consideration. Most trauma victims will respond favorably to 1 to 2 units of blood, but those individuals with more worrisome clinical features (significant/active bleeding, presence of hemorrhagic shock, pre-existing coagulopathy) may require massive transfusion. This is defined as administering 6 or more units of blood in the first 4 hours of management. These individuals will require adequate vascular access, specific transfusion equipment, and close clinical monitoring. On this last point, it is important to remember that lab tests have almost no value in trending the response to massive transfusions; so much blood is given so quickly that the scenario has changed by the time the results return. There is, however, utility for bedside viscoelastic laboratory testing in these patients (see TEG/ROTEM, later in discussion).

While addressing the blood already lost due to hemorrhage, it is also important to consider underlying factors that may prevent adequate clot formation and address them. Most commonly, the pharmacologically anticoagulated patient, due to the preexisting condition, will need specific management. Warfarin has a direct antidote, vitamin K, which can be administered IV or PO in doses commensurate with their INR and clinical signs of hemorrhage. However, vitamin K is limited in its slow pharmacodynamic profile; onset of action occurs at 6 to 10 hours and it achieves peak effect at 24 to 48 hours. Moreover, vitamin K is specific to warfarin reversal and has no role in patients receiving direct oral anticoagulant medications (DOAC's). These also have specific antidotes for reversal; idarucizumab is approved for the reversal of dabigatran, and andexanet reverses apixaban and rivaroxaban (FXa inhibitors). These have a more rapid onset (within minutes) but are limited due to their specificity. Prothrombin complex concentrate (PCC) is a generalizable tool for anticoagulation reversal by administering clotting factors (II, IX, and X or II, VII, IX, and X) that otherwise have been inactivated. While currently only FDA-approved for warfarin-induced coagulopathy, it is widely and safely used for other anticoagulation causes as well, including DOAC's, congenital deficiencies, preoperative prophylaxis of bleeding, and trauma requiring massive transfusion. These are effective at achieving rapid correction of anticoagulation but come at a high monetary cost and their use must be carefully considered. FFP also contains small concentrations of clotting factor, including fibrinogen, but its use as monotherapy for anticoagulation reversal is inadequate. Finally, tranexamic acid (TXA) has been explored in the bleeding patient for its ability to prevent fibrinolysis, allowing the patient to keep the clot they have already formed. The CRASH trials[5,6] demonstrated relative safety and efficacy in hemorrhage control when TXA is administered within the first 1 hour of injury, and then again every 8 hours for the first 24 hours after injury. There may be an increased risk of venous thromboembolism (VTE) noted in the more recent HALT-IT trial, but owing to its overall safety, efficacy, and low cost, TXA is a common component of many hospitals' management of the massively bleeding patient.

If noninvasive methods fail to elicit appropriate hemodynamic response, operative management is required. Several markers exist to help identify patients who are failing or who will likely fail noninvasive management. First, a narrow pulse pressure (<30 mm Hg) is a predictor for more significant hypovolemia and can be tracked in real-time during the resuscitation.[7] Additionally, transient improvement in heart rate or blood pressure with volume resuscitation may indicate ongoing bleeding, which also may require surgical or interventional radiology treatment. Finally, the popularization of viscoelastic studies such as thromboelastography (TEG) and rotational thromboelastometry (ROTEM) allows the clinician to identify coagulopathy not noted by an abnormal PT/INR or aPTT, and also track a patient's coagulable state in real-time at the bedside.[8] These measures are particularly helpful in identifying patients who would benefit from a specific element of blood product transfusion, rather than using a 1:1:1 ratio in all patients. This more tailored approach may improve the odds of success with noninvasive management by minimizing iatrogenic contributions to a patient's coagulopathy of trauma.

POINT OF CARE ULTRASOUND IN THE INJURED PATIENT

Point of care ultrasound (POCUS) is a staple of Emergency Medicine practice. As its adoption by EM providers in the early 1990s through its development and expansion to today, POCUS skill has become the embodiment of a well-rounded EM provider. POCUS is useful in the trauma setting, particularly for identifying significant hemorrhage in hemodynamically unstable trauma patient. The FAST protocol (Focused Assessment of Sonography in Trauma) is commonly one of the first examinations learned by new EM providers, owing to its simplicity and value. This relatively cheap and easy procedure identifies intraperitoneal free fluid with a 62% to 96% sensitivity and 86.9% to 99.7% specificity.[9] Rapid identification of anechoic fluid in the Pouch of Douglas, Morison's Pouch, or the splenorenal fossa can meaningfully reduce time to transfer to the operating room for definitive management (64% reduction in time from ED to OR arrival[10]). Expanding the study to the eFAST protocol, which incorporates the subxiphoid cardiac window as well as thoracic windows, also allows for rapid identification of pericardial fluid (ie, tamponade in the crashing trauma patient) and/ or hemo/pneumothorax. Similarly, this allows for rapid treatment intervention at the bedside, temporizing the patient before more definitive operative management.

However, there are limitations to the FAST examination, and pitfalls exist in both positive and negative directions. When considering its positive predictive value, the FAST protocol is able to reliably identify hemoperitoneum only when volumes exceed 200 cc's,[11] potentially missing a developing bleeding problem that can later prove catastrophic. Additionally, obese body habitus will limit the quality of abdominal images obtained. Finally, the FAST examination has no ability to identify retroperitoneal bleeding, a critical space to consider in the potentially exsanguinating patient. Looking in the negative direction, the FAST examination is frequently (but inappropriately) used as a rule-out test. The absence of free fluid in the abdomen on POCUS does not preclude the existence of hemoperitoneum, and failure to recognize this limitation may contribute to missed thoracoabdominal hemorrhage. In the appropriate clinical setting, POCUS must be followed up with more advanced imaging such as CT. An unfortunate but necessary side effect of this logic then is that all negative FAST examinations in the significant trauma setting must be followed by CT to adequately overcome sensitivity limitations. This, therefore, leads to excess CT use, which carries with it the risk of excess radiation exposure, identification of clinically insignificant findings that will require further testing and other downstream effects, and added costs. This is of particular concern in the pediatric population, who otherwise would have benefited greatly from the lack of radiation exposure afforded by POCUS.

POCUS and particularly the FAST examination are of immense value in the hemodynamically unstable patient, and its use should be considered as an extension of the primary survey in that clinical setting.[12] However, stable or minor trauma patients receive little added benefit from it and are potentially exposed to the cascade effects of follow-up testing. Care must be taken to ensure the use of POCUS does not extend beyond its intended indication.

PEDIATRIC TRAUMA: SPECIAL CONSIDERATIONS

The pediatric patient provides a unique and special population in the trauma care setting with unique qualities and characteristics that differ from the adult patient. As the first half of the 20th century, advancements in medicine including improved public health, improved living standards, early detection, vaccination, use of antibiotics and interventional medicine have seen mortality rates due influenza, pneumonia, cancer, and congenital abnormalities decline and now give rise to injury as the number one killer of children and adolescents today.[13] This encompasses both unintentional and intentional injury from an array of sources including motor vehicle accidents, firearms, suffocation with homicide and suicide making up a portion of each. Given the preventable nature of pediatric trauma, childhood mortality is now a tragedy rather than the relative risk of living. That said, trauma itself is a disease process. Like other areas of medicine, trauma carries relative risk factors, socioeconomic implications, epidemiology, severity of disease, and predictors of outcomes in addition to the advancement in treatments improving both favorable outcomes and survival.

Pediatric trauma in the ER represents a wide array, from straightforward uncomplicated injuries to life-threatening illness. Here we will focus on our approach to the pediatric trauma patient and the two most lethal forms of youth trauma: Traumatic Brain Injury and Thoracic Trauma. We will specifically concentrate on unique aspects of the pediatric patient in relation to effective management.

GENERAL CONSIDERATIONS WHEN APPROACHING THE PEDIATRIC TRAUMA PATIENT:

Hemodynamics - Most pediatric trauma patients in the ED are awake and the condition is nonlife threatening. However, it is important to not be falsely reassured by a normal set of vital signs in significantly injured pediatric patient. Owing to their greater sympathetic reserve compared with adults, children are able to hemodynamically compensate for massive hemorrhage better and for longer than adults. However, once the child has exhausted their catecholamine supplies, they can rapidly and unexpectedly decompensate. This can be evidenced by sudden altered mental status or hypotension, requiring advanced resuscitation techniques. The necessary interventions should be ready in anticipation of this possible decline before they are needed.

Size variability - Injuries occur at all ages, and in the pediatric population, this means patients with a wide variety of sizes and weights. This is particularly salient for planning pharmacologic and procedural interventions, whereby the helpful dose for a teenager may be a fatal dose for an infant. Several tools exist to offload the need for rote memorization of doses and tube sizes. The Broselow tape uses a child's height to guide dosing, is conveniently organized and color-coded, and has been in wide use since the 1980s. More recent app-based platforms provide similar information, can incorporate the child's weight, and are easily accessed by anyone with a smartphone.

Communication barriers - The pediatric patient may not have sufficient language skills to describe their injury, or prior experience to accurately contextualize the severity of their symptoms. Seeking external sources of information (parents, caregivers, bystanders, EMS personnel) is an important technique to overcome these inherent communication barriers.

Emotional processing is another important consideration in communication. It is widely accepted that the human brain is not fully developed until about age 25.[14] Specifically, the prefrontal cortex is the latest in development and is responsible for rational thinking and modulation of intense emotions.[14] Because of this, the pediatric trauma patient processes this emotional and traumatic event differently than adults. The level of fear and paranoia often exceeds that of an adult and may be out of proportion to injury. The astute provider can take measures to mitigate and control these emotions while providing comfort to the patient and family while obtaining a higher quality history and examination. Practical examples are to address this concern first with reassurance that you are there to help. Assure the patient and family that your team successfully deals with pediatric injuries on a regular basis, providing the best possible outcomes (without false hope, of course). With children, kneeling or squatting so as to avoid towering over the patient may be helpful while having a parent or family member involved to give history or hold the child if available is invaluable. A slow approach to the physical examination and touch of the patient is paramount in gaining confidence in an awake toddler provided time is available.

Traumatic Brain Injury

Traumatic brain injury (TBI) results in greater mortality in youth than any other pathology today.[15] While motor vehicle accidents are responsible for the greatest proportion, bicycle accidents, contact sports, and violence (including injuries in the home or gunshot wounds) have significant contributions. While the approach to the pediatric patient with a potential TBI is similar to that of the adult, it is noteworthy that children respond exceedingly well to successful preservation of cerebral oxygen and perfusion.[16] The child and adolescent brain has great neuroplasticity with the ability to change and rewire in response to experience, behavior, and environment. While this persists throughout adult life, it is widely accepted this ability is greatest during childhood and adolescence.[14] Survival rates for moderate to severe TBI as well as favorable outcomes are better in children as compared with adults.[16]

Standard treatments for moderate to severe pediatric patients with TBI include controlled positive pressure ventilation settings, steroids, mannitol, and when indicated seizure prophylaxis with Phenytoin or Keppra. Goals of treatment include avoidance of hypotension and hypoxemia with a focus on the maintenance of Cerebral Perfusion Pressure (CPP) greater than 40 mm Hg or maintenance of intracranial pressure (ICP) less than 20 mm Hg, or both.[17] While CPP maintenance at $>/ = 40$ mm Hg has been demonstrated as a positive predictor of outcome, the Lund principle is also supported. The Lund principle focuses on ICP management and argues that ICP in a normotensive state is more important than a specific CPP threshold.[18] Here, the focus is on volume targeted therapy with antihypertensives to maintain normotension and normovolemia while maintaining ICP $</ = 20$ mm Hg. The Lund principle has shown improved outcomes and has gained greater acceptance over the past 25 years.[18,19]

Half or more pediatric patients with a head injury in the ED undergo CT scanning regardless of GCS score yet, only an estimated 1% require neurologic treatment.[20] The pediatric head trauma patient is unique in regards to the relative risk of radiation and its association with neural injury and increased cumulative effect and risk of malignancy later in life. Lifetime cancer mortality risk attributable to radiation exposure from head CT as a child of 0.07% has been reported and this is an order of one magnitude higher than that for adults.[21] The ALARA concept has been routinely adopted when ordering any radiographic studies in children. ALARA stands for "As Low As Reasonably Achievable and put into practice means that no matter the dose, if receiving it has no direct benefit or change in treatment then it should be avoided if possible. Also standard is the concept of time, distance, and shielding regarding radiation exposure if studies are necessary." In light of this, decision-making algorithms have been developed to aid clinicians regarding the decision to image pediatric head injuries. Three such algorithms have been recognized including PECARN (Pediatric Emergency Care Applied Research Network), CATCH (Canadian Assessment of Tomography in Childhood Head Injury), and CHALICE (Children's Head injury Algorithm for the prediction of Important Clinical Events). PECARN has come to the forefront after the comparison of these algorithms and is shown in (**Figs. 1** and **2**).[22] Judicious use of imaging in the pediatric patient can improve patient safety, eliminate unnecessary ionizing radiation while reducing health care costs, and improve overall efficiency in the delivery of health care.

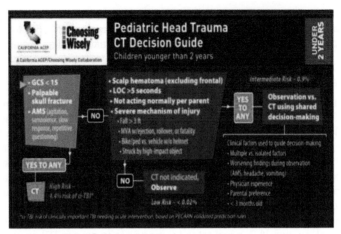

Fig. 1. PHTCT decision guide children less than 2 years of age.

Pediatric Thoracic Trauma

Pediatric thoracic trauma is the result of blunt or penetrating injury. While both can be ominous, penetrating trauma causes greater morbidity and mortality. Thankfully, this is less common than blunt force trauma. Overall thoracic trauma is relatively rare compared with head injury, spinal, and extremity trauma, yet it remains the second leading cause of death in the pediatric trauma patient largely due to the frequency of motor vehicle accidents.[16,23] Intrathoracic injuries secondary to thoracic trauma in children include pulmonary contusion, pneumothorax, hemothorax, lung laceration, and less commonly mediastinal injuries such as tracheobronchial tree, esophageal, or cardiovascular injury. Most pediatric thoracic trauma can be managed conservatively with observation or tube thoracostomy. Rarely is mechanical ventilation or surgery required.

The presence of fractures is often the most obvious feature of a providers' physical examination and initial chest x-ray. However, children pose a particular challenge in this regard as the bony thorax remains highly cartilaginous. This provides for pliability

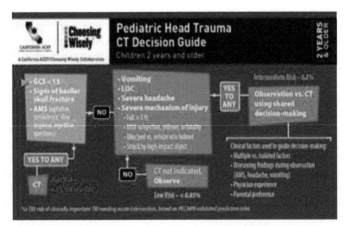

Fig. 2. PHTCT decision guide children greater than 2 years of age.

during the traumatic insult whereby bones can undergo plastic deformity and subsequent recoil into their normal anatomic configuration. Children are prone to significant intrathoracic injury without fracture. Physical examination techniques of inspection, palpation, percussion, and auscultation are inherently unreliable[16] due to this as well as patient compliance in the setting of trauma, fear, and emotional response. These unique features of children and adolescents make it critical for care providers to physically examine them meticulously. One should interpret any subtle radiographic findings as positive, and then scour initial imaging studies for more ominous pathology such as absent apical lung markings, tracheal deviation, blurring of the costophrenic angles, widening of the mediastinum and abnormal aortic contour in the absence of fractures. Further, this necessitates detailed ordering of imaging studies mentioning clinical features including the mechanism of injury. Providing clinical insight into your order details lends a hand to our partner radiologists in their over-reading of the study. In the writers' experience, this has been met with appreciation and readings that often specifically address the presence or absence of specific pathology or further imaging recommendations.

Pediatric Secondary and Tertiary Examination Pearls:

Also unique to pediatric trauma patients and important to the emergency medicine provider is children's ability to heal rapidly. Early recognition of injuries is important so as not to delay treatments. After initial stabilization and primary survey, a comprehensive secondary survey is indicated. Among the challenges to this are the child's emotional state, fear, and reaction to trauma discussed above. Physical examination during the secondary survey is again, inherently unreliable in this setting and should be conducted in as much detail as possible. Careful tertiary examination of the entire upper and lower extremities including inspection, palpation, range of motion, strength, and sensation is imperative so as not to miss a significant injury. This should include major joints, long bones, complex joints of the ankle and wrist as well as fingers and toes. Any focal area of swelling, skin breakdown, tenderness, lack of motion, pain upon motion, refusal to use, weakness, or numbness should be investigated thoroughly. Importantly, strength and sensation should be examined according to motor sensory innervations per peripheral nerve root, or in cases of spinal involvement, per spinal nerve root. Choose areas for light touch that follow peripheral nerve root and or spinal nerve root dermatomal patterns. Special considerations for the motor examination include testing muscles with focused neural inputs with movements that isolate that particular muscle. (**Tables 1** and **2**). For example, biceps strength is best tested via resisted forearm supination and is innervated per C6 > C5 spinal neural inputs and musculocutaneous peripheral neural input. A deficit is an immediate alert of a spinal or peripheral nerve injury and warrants further examination. Some pure motor inputs are particularly useful and less used. One is resisted abductor pollicis brevis strength with purely median nerve innervation. Another is resisted Flexor Digitorum Profundus (FDP) and Lumbrical function with C8-specific spinal nerve root inputs. (**Figs. 3** and **4**).

Pediatric Bone Considerations:

Noteworthy is the fact that pediatric bone is different from adult bone in several ways which allow for early clinical stability after fracture. These factors include the ability to compress rather than comminute under axial load, stronger periosteum allowing for greater subperiosteal hematoma formation and early callus formation, as well as the presence of hormones, growth plates and in general an ongoing environment of osteogenesis provides the setting for fracture healing even before injury.[24] Depending on

Table 1
Peripheral Nerve/Isolated muscle innervation/Action: Muscle innervations detailed are reliable groups to test against resistance. While there are mixed innervations, the peripheral nerve identified here is the nerve with the largest motor input. These tests or "actions" are appropriate testing and identification for the tertiary trauma survey

Peripheral Nerve	Motor Innervation	Action
Axillary	Deltoid Muscle	Resisted arm abduction
Musculocutaneous	Biceps Muscle	Resisted forearm supination
Radial	Extensor Pollicis Longus Muscle	Resisted Thumb extension
Median	Abductor Pollicis Brevis Muscle	Resisted Thumb volar extension (see inset).
Ulnar	Intrinsic muscle	Resisted finger abduction

age, musculoskeletal dislocations and fractures will rapidly begin healing as compared with an adult and if not identified until 7 to 14 days later, may have significant stiffness, scarring, calcification as well as possible chronic dislocation or malunion. This often culminates in the need for surgical intervention otherwise not required or that may have been dealt with at an index surgery for other pathology. Therefore, this can delay retrieval of function and final outcomes by weeks or months in an already trying situation. In rare cases, this could unnecessarily generate permanent disability.

THE OUCHLESS EMERGENCY DEPARTMENT

For a child, the Emergency Department can be a particularly stressful or scary place, and mismanagement of their care can add to their already traumatized state. Great strides have already been made to minimize child and family discomfort during the ED stay, including implementing Child Life specialists, the use of service animals, and the concept of "The Ouchless ED." These "ouchless" techniques encompass a range of equipment, tricks, and medications, presented here in no particular order:

The J tip device is an attachment to a syringe that allows for dermal delivery of any liquid medication (lidocaine, insulin, etc.) without the use of a needle. Instead, it uses a pressurized CO2 cartridge to propel the liquid to a depth of 8 mm, bestowing an anesthetized area about the size of a pencil eraser. This is particularly useful for IV starts and potentially lumbar puncture in the infant population. Limitations of the J tip are that it causes a loud and potentially startling popping noise as it is activated,

Table 2
Spinal Nerve/Muscle Innervation: Muscle innervations detailed are reliable groups to test against resistance. While there are mixed innervations, the spinal nerve identified here is the nerve with the largest motor input. These tests or "actions" are appropriate testing and identification for the secondary trauma survey

Spinal Nerve	Motor Innervation	Action
C5	Deltoid	Resisted arm abduction
C6	Biceps, ECR, ECU Muscles	Resisted forearm supination/Resisted wrist extension
C7	Triceps, FCR, FCU	Resisted elbow extension/Resisted wrist flexion
C8	Lumbricals, FDS, FDP	Resisted finger flexion in claw formation (see inset)

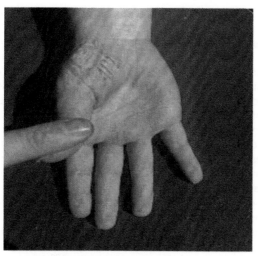

Fig. 3. Median nerve motor exam: Resisted APL function

availability in department stock/supply and slightly increased cost compared with traditional hypodermic needles ($0.98–4.10 vs ~$0.50 on average).

Topical anesthetic creams such as LMX or EMLA reach an anesthesia depth of 3 mm after 30 to 60 minutes (respectively). This can be of particular use in nonemergent procedures such as lumbar puncture, whereby injected lidocaine may otherwise obscure anatomic landmarks. Limits of topical anesthesia include its inability to be applied to open/broken skin, loss of effect if removed in under 30 minutes, and inherent delays to your intended procedure.

Buzzy Bee devices use the gate-theory of pain transmission to distract afferent pain nerve fibers in children receiving shots, such as vaccination but also for IV placement. The device is placed in the freezer for 10 minutes, then is applied to the skin ~5 cm proximal to the intended injection site and then turned on to activate its vibration feature. This combination, when initiated 1 minute before and continuing through the duration of the procedure, effectively reduces pain levels in children ages 3 to 18.[25]

The use of oral adjuncts to pain medications has long been shown to reduce procedure-related pain. Concentrated 24% oral sucrose solutions (Sweet-ease) 1 to

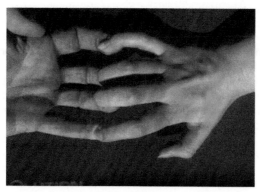

Fig. 4. C8 motor exam: simultaneous resisted FDP and Lumbrical function.

2 mL applied to the buccal mucosa, breast milk, or even active breast-feeding have been shown to meaningfully reduce pain in the 0 to 6-month-old infant undergoing IV placement, lumbar puncture, or vaccination.

In recent years, virtual reality headsets have been used to distract children during painful procedures with mixed results. Chan and colleagues[26] in 2019 showed a meaningful reduction in pain scores by virtually transporting the child to another location, but other studies have shown no significant reduction. This strategy also has the obvious barriers of cost and user experience.

Intranasal administration of sedating or dissociating medications is a safe and reliable method of reducing or even eliminating pain in the ED, particularly for more significant procedures like fracture reduction or abscess incision and drainage. Intranasal fentanyl 1.5 to 2 mcg/kg (max dose 100 mcg) provides good pain relief within 10 minutes and is sustained for 30 minutes. This has been shown to be as effective as IV morphine with an equivalent dose.[27] Midazolam 0.2 to 0.4 mg/kg (max dose 10 mg) also achieves good anxiolysis and light sedation within 15 minutes, and full recovery occurs at 50 minutes. Ketamine is helpful for both analgesia and sedation/dissociation depending on the dose. At a dose of 1 to 1.5 mg/kg it achieves good analgesia after 15 minutes and has comparable efficacy to IN fentanyl.[28] Sedation/dissociation with IN ketamine is more difficult to achieve owing to dose requirements and concentration limitations.[29] Typically, doses as high as 9 mg/kg are sedating, but most ketamine formulations exist in a 100 mg/mL concentration. For example, an average 12 kg toddler would require 108 mg of ketamine or just over 1 mL. As IN atomization volumes are optimally effective at 0.3 mL and maximized at 1 mL, any child larger than an average toddler will not receive adequate dissociative absorption of IN ketamine.

Given all of the tips and tools available to the EM provider, the Ouchless ED is a realistic and important standard to maintain in patient and family-centered care for the pediatric trauma patient.

VITAL SIGNS IN TRAUMA: PEARLS AND PITFALLS.

Recognition of abnormal vital signs is an important component of the initial trauma evaluation and should be tracked during the course of resuscitation as a marker for response to intervention. However, it is also important to recognize the limitations of vital signs and their ability to falsely reassure a trauma clinician.

Respiratory Rate: Respiratory Rate (RR) is an early predictor of preventable patient deterioration yet remains the most inaccurately measured and recorded vital sign.[30] Busy ED staff often do not take the time to take and report RR accurately. It is the first vital sign to increase in such conditions as sepsis, shock, severe inflammatory responses, or any condition leading to respiratory compromise. It is arguable that emergency room providers should routinely and accurately recheck and document respiratory rates to enhance recognition during the early phases of ominous pathology in patients.

Heart rate: will commonly rise in response to acute physiologic stress or hypovolemic state. However, a beta-blocked patient will have blunted sympathetic response to external stressors and will therefore maintain a normal heart rate for longer in the trauma setting and may never develop tachycardia.

Blood pressure: specifically hypotension is a late finding in the hypovolemic or hemorrhaging patient and should be treated aggressively. The presence of normal blood pressure does not preclude the presence of significant hypovolemia. Pulse pressure, the difference between systolic and diastolic pressure, can be a helpful indicator for ongoing hemorrhage when narrowed and will often precede the onset of hypotension.

Temperature: is important to control in the trauma setting, specifically to prevent hypothermia. However, a febrile trauma patient is also important to recognize as it may point to an underlying infectious process that may have precipitated the traumatic event.

Oxygen saturation[31]: is a common but suboptimal measure of breathing status, limited by both physiologic and logistical restraints. Oxygen saturation correlates with a wide range of Pao_2 values, will drop late in a disease process owing to inherent oxygen binding of the hemoglobin molecule and reserve volume within the lungs, and will be affected by inadequate tissue perfusion or transducer adherence to skin. End-tidal capnography (ETCO2) is a better evaluator of respiratory status as it is applied directly in line with airway adjuncts, will respond almost immediately to resuscitation interventions (or failure thereof), and is able to reflect the more helpful measure of tissue/organ perfusion. Even this is limited, however, in that it requires the patient to be spontaneously breathing; EtCO2 becomes unreliable owing to air washout when applying positive pressure ventilation with a bag-valve-mask (BVM) apparatus.

DISCLOSURE

We have no disclosures.

ACKNOWLEDGMENTS

David Dvorak M.D., MPH. Stephen Smith M.D. Emergency Medicine Physician Hennipen Healthcare, Professor of Emergency Medicine University of Minnesota.

REFERENCES

1. Gonzalez, et al. Hemorrhagic Shock. J Pediatr Intensive Care 2015;4(1):4–9. PMID: 6513149.

2. Hamed R, Mekki I, Aouni H, et al. Base Excess usefulness for prediction of immediate mortality in severe trauma patients admitted to the Emergency department. Tunis Med 2019;97(12):1357–61. PMID: 32173805.

3. Reddick A, Ronald J, Morrison W. Intravenous fluid resuscitation: was Poiseuille right? J Emerg Med 2011;28(3):201–2. PMID: 20581377.

4. Nascimento B, Callum J, Tien H, et al. Effect of a fixed-ratio (1:1:1) transfusion protocol versus laboratory-results-guided transfusion in patients with severe trauma: a randomized feasibility trial. CMAJ 2013;185(12):E583–9. https://doi.org/10.1503/cmaj.121986.

5. Roberts I, Shakur H, Coats T, et al. The CRASH-2 trial: a randomized controlled trial and economic evaluation of the effects of tranexamic acid on death, vascular occlusive events and transfusion requirement in bleeding trauma patients. Southampton (UK): NIHR Journals Library; 2013. https://doi.org/10.3310/hta17100. Health Technology Assessment, No. 17.10.) Available at: https://www.ncbi.nlm.nih.gov/books/NBK260390/.

6. Cap AP. CRASH-3: a win for patients with traumatic brain injury. Lancet 2019; 394(10210):1687–8.

7. Schellenberg M, Owattanapanich N, Getrajdman J, et al. Prehospital Narrow Pulse Pressure Predicts Need for Resuscitative Thoracotomy and Emergent Intervention After Trauma. J Surg Res 2021;268:284–90. Erratum in: J Surg Res. 2021;270:1. PMID: 34392182.

8. Abdelfattah K, Cripps MW. Thromboelastography and Rotational Thromboelastometry use in trauma. Int J Surg 2016 Sep;33(Pt B):196–201. https://doi.org/10.1016/j.ijsu.2015.09.036. Epub 2015 Sep 16. PMID: 26384835.

9. Savatmongkorngul S, Wongwaisayawan S, Kaewlai R. Focused assessment with sonography for trauma: current perspectives. Open Access Emerg Med 2017;9: 57–62. PMID: 28794661.

10. Melniker L, et al. Randomized controlled clinical trial of point-of-care, limited ultrasonography for trauma in the emergency department: the first sonography outcomes assessment program trial. Ann Emerg Med 2006 Sep;48(3):227–35. PMID 16934640.

11. Von Kuenssberg Jehle D, Stiller G, Wagner D. Sensitivity in detecting free intraperitoneal fluid with the pelvic views of the FAST exam. Ann Emerg Med 2003; 21(6):476–8. PMID: 14574655.

12. Stengel, et al. Emergency ultrasound-based algorithms for diagnosing blunt abdominal trauma. Cochrane Database Syst Rev 2015;(9):2015. :CD004446. PMID: 26368505.

13. Cunningham RM, Walton MA, Carter PM. The Major Causes of Death in Children and Adolescents in the United States. N Engl J Med 2018;379(25):2468–75.

14. Arain M, Haque M, Johal L, et al. Maturation of the adolescent brain. Neuropsychiatr Dis Treat 2013;9:449–61. https://doi.org/10.2147/NDT.S39776.

15. Araki T, Yokota H, Morita A. Pediatric Traumatic Brain Injury: Characteristic Features, Diagnosis, and Management. Neurol Med Chir (Tokyo) 2017;57(2):82–93. Epub 2017 Jan 20. PMID: 28111406; PMCID: PMC5341344.

16. Brian J. Considerations in Pediatric Trauma. Medscape J Med 2021. Retrieved 3/12/2022 Available at: https://emedicine.medscape.com/article/435031 Daley.

17. Rangel-Castilla L, Gopinath S, Robertson CS. Management of intracranial hypertension [published correction appears in Neurol Clin 2008 Aug;26(3). https://doi.org/10.1016/j.ncl.2008.02.003. xvii. Rangel-Castillo, Leonardo [corrected to Rangel-Castilla, Leonardo]]. Neurol Clin. 2008;26(2):521-x.

18. Nordström CH. Physiological and biochemical principles underlying volume-targeted therapy–the "Lund concept. Neurocrit Care 2005;2(1):83–95. https://doi.org/10.1385/NCC:2:1:083. PMID: 16174975.

19. Grände PO. Critical Evaluation of the Lund Concept for Treatment of Severe Traumatic Head Injury, 25 Years after Its Introduction. Front Neurol 2017;8:315. https://doi.org/10.3389/fneur.2017.00315.

20. Kuppermann N, Holmes JF, Dayan PS, et al. Pediatric Emergency Care Applied Research Network (PECARN), Identification of children at very low risk of clinically-important brain injuries after head trauma: A prospective cohort study. Lancet 2009;374:1160–70.

21. Brenner D, Elliston C, Hall E, et al. Estimated risks of radiation-induced fatal cancer from pediatric CT. AJR Am J Roentgenol 2001;176(2):289–96.

22. Babl FE, Borland ML, Phillips N, et al. Paediatric Research in Emergency Departments International Collaborative (PREDICT). Accuracy of PECARN, CATCH, and CHALICE head injury decision rules in children: a prospective cohort study. Lancet 2017;389(10087):2393–402. https://doi.org/10.1016/S0140-6736(17)30555-X.

23. Cooper A, Barlow B, DiScala C, et al. Mortality and truncal injury: the pediatric perspective. J Pediatr Surg 1994 Jan;29(1):33–8.

24. Lindaman LM. Bone Healing in Children. Clin Podiatr Med Surg 2001;18(1): 97–108.

25. Ballard A, et al. Efficacy of the Buzzy Device for Pain Management During Needle-related Procedures: A systematic Review and Meta-Analysis. Clin J Pain 2019;35(6):532–43.

26. Chan E, et al. all. Virtual Reality for Pediatric Needle Procedural Pain: Two Randomized Clinical Trials. J Pediatr 2019;209:160–7, e4. PMID: 31047650.

27. Mudd S. Intranasal fentanyl for pain management in children: a systematic review of the literature. J Pediatr Health Care 2011;25(5):316–22.

28. Graudins A, et al. The PICHFORK (Pain in Children Fentanyl or Ketamine) trial: a randomized controlled trial comparing intranasal ketamine and fentanyl for relief of moderate to severe pain in children with limb injuries. Ann Emerg Med 2015; 65(3):248–54. PMID: 25447557.

29. Canton K, et al. Intranasal Ketamine for Procedural Sedation and Analgesia in Children: A Systematic Review. J Pediatr 2018;141(1):350.

30. Loughlin PC, Sebat F, Kellett JG. Respiratory Rate: The Forgotten Vital Sign-Make It Count. Jt Comm J Qual Patient Saf 2018;44(8):494–9. https://doi.org/10.1016/j.jcjq.2018.04.014. Epub 2018 Jun 20. PMID: 30071969.

31. Mardirossian G, Schneider RE. Limitations of pulse oximetry. Anesth Prog 1992; 39(6):194–6. PMID: 2148612.

Abdominal Pain
The Differential Diagnosis, Classic Histories, and Diagnosis

John Ramos, MMS, PA-C, CAQ-EM*

KEYWORDS

- Abdominal emergencies • Abdominal pain • Emergency medicine
- Pelvic emergencies • Diagnostic imaging • Pathognomonic • Classic presentations
- Ureterolithiasis

KEY POINTS

- History and physical examination can distinguish serious causes of abdominal pain.
- Rarely, laboratory tests are diagnostic of conditions causing abdominal pain.
- Contrast-enhanced computed tomography is an ideal imaging modality for most emergent abdominopelvic complaints.
- Ultrasound is the test of choice for diagnosing cholecystitis, gonadal torsion, and ectopic pregnancy.

CASES

At the beginning of your shift in the emergency department (ED), you are taking care of the following patients:

Mohammed A. is a 58-year-old man with a history of diabetes mellitus type II and hypertension who presents with 3 days of left lower quadrant abdominal pain. Two days before arrival, he was seen at an outside clinic and prescribed amoxicillin-clavulanate. His pain has improved, but today he noticed a fever. His last bowel movement was 2 days ago. His temperature is 38.1 C, and the rest of his vitals are normal. On examination there is minimal tenderness to palpation in the left lower quadrant. His white blood cell count, lactate, and electrolytes are all within normal limits.

Gloria B. is a 79-year-old woman with a history of hypertension who presents with sudden-onset right-sided flank pain for 1 day. The pain lasts for a couple minutes, comes in waves, and is associated with intense nausea and emesis. During your interview she is retching violently. Her vitals show temperature 37.1 C, heart rate 104, and blood pressure 110/68 mm Hg. Her urinalysis shows 20 white blood cells and no red blood cells, nitrite, or bacteria.

Department of Emergency Medicine, Duke University Hospital, 2301 Erwin Road Suite 2600, Durham, NC 27710, USA
* Corresponding author.
E-mail address: john.ramos@duke.edu

Physician Assist Clin 8 (2023) 33–48
https://doi.org/10.1016/j.cpha.2022.08.008
2405-7991/23/© 2022 Elsevier Inc. All rights reserved.

Lisa Z. is a 42-year-old woman with a history of gastroesophageal reflux disease and cholelithiasis who presents with right upper quadrant pain. The pain started 3 days ago and was dull and aching. She tried taking over-the-counter antacids, which did not provide any relief. The pain worsened in the last 12 hours and is now described as intense pressure. Her vitals are normal, and her examination is remarkable for a positive Murphy sign.

Reggie J. is a 21-year-old woman with no past medical history who presents with severe abdominal bloating, pain, and vomiting for 1 day. She reports frequent loose, and often bloody, stools that started 3 weeks prior to arrival. In the last week she has also had at least one episode per night of rectal discharge that has blood and mucus. On examination she is febrile and tachycardic, with diffuse abdominal tenderness. Her rectal examination shows no bright bed blood or melanic stool. Her white blood cell count and lactate are elevated.

HEADING: INTRODUCTION

Beware, the abdomen is full of mischief. The abdominopelvic compartment is anatomically complex, the differential includes both serious and self-limited conditions, and signs and symptoms often overlap. Among adult patients presenting to EDs with abdominal pain, about 17% have a serious diagnosis or require hospitalization.[1] Establishing a safe disposition is often resource intensive requiring diagnostic testing, pharmacotherapeutics and reassessments, specialist consultation, and patient expectation management. Many patients can be safely discharged with modern access to timely laboratory testing and diagnostic imaging, even though a specific diagnosis is not achieved in as many as one-third of patients.[2] This article reviews the differential diagnoses for adult patients with atraumatic abdominal pain, distinguishing features of the history and physical examination, and diagnostic tests used to identify or exclude serious illness.

HEADING: ASSESSMENT

The history and physical examination alone inform an intentional approach to diagnostic testing and can lead to a correct diagnosis.[3] Providers should also take into account special considerations (**Table 1**) that increase a patient's risk of illness or contribute to relatively atypical presentations.[4–17] Timing, character, and location are important aspects of the history. The physical examination includes an assessment of vital signs, inspection, auscultation, palpation, and special maneuvers when indicated.

Defined by time of symptom onset, abdominal pain can be acute (within several days), subacute (less than 6 months), or chronic ($\geq$ 6 months). Acute abdominal pain that is sudden in onset, or achieves maximal intensity within 1 to 2 hours, is one characteristic of surgical emergencies.[14] Acute abdominal pain that develops over several hours suggests a medical condition, such as dyspepsia, infectious enterocolitis, and infections of the urinary or reproductive organs. Episodic symptoms can be seen with dyspepsia or biliary colic but may present with an acute exacerbation. Symptom onset is one piece of the history (**Table 2**) and providers should consider presentation variability to avoid representative bias and premature closer. For example, appendicitis frequently presents after 24 hours, gonadal torsion may occur in seconds, and volvulus may be episodic due to spontaneous detorsion.

The location of pain or objective tenderness further narrows the differential (**Table 3**).[18]

The character of abdominal pain is categorized into visceral, parietal, and referred pain.

Table 1
Special considerations

Risk factors for thromboembolic disease	Atrial fibrillation Exogenous estrogen or testosterone Past medical history of DVT (mesenteric venous thrombosis) Smoking tobacco (abdominal aortic aneurysm rupture)
Risk factors for spontaneous hemorrhage	Alcohol Steroidal and nonsteroidal antiinflammatory drugs Therapeutic anticoagulation
Risk factors for infection	Diabetes Chronic kidney disease Autoimmune conditions (eg, rheumatoid arthritis, systemic lupus erythematosus, multiple sclerosis) Chemotherapy (eg, immune checkpoint inhibitors) Chronic steroid use Immunomodulating drugs (eg, select monoclonal antibodies)
Critically ill (obtunded, intubated, hemodynamically unstable)	History and physical examination often unreliable
Elderly	Fever and peritoneal signs may be absent. More frequently hospitalized or observed
Pregnancy	A gravid uterus may displace abdominal structures, eg, migration of the appendix to the right hypochondrium or right flank. Appendicitis and cholecystitis are the most common nonobstetric surgical emergencies. Round ligament pain complicates about 30% of pregnancies, typically during the end of the first trimester and second trimester. Endomyometritis may develop up to 6 wk after delivery, and risk factors include cesarean delivery, and prolonged labor or rupture of amniotic membranes.
Previous abdominopelvic surgery	Surgically altered anatomy may obscure classic localization patterns. Adhesions are the most common cause of small bowel obstruction. Adhesions, hernias, and anastomotic breakdown are not uncommon after bariatric surgery. Dropped gallstones are relatively uncommon but more likely during laparoscopic cholecystectomies. Stump appendicitis is relatively uncommon (~1:50,000) but more likely following nonoperative management of appendiceal rupture.

Abbreviation: DVT, deep vein thrombosis.

Data from Harward T.R., Green D., Bergan J.J., et. al.: Mesenteric venous thrombosis. J Vasc Surg 1989; 9: pp. 328-333; and Altobelli E, Rapacchietta L, Profeta VF, Fagnano R. Risk Factors for Abdominal Aortic Aneurysm in Population-Based Studies: A Systematic Review and Meta-Analysis. Int J Environ Res Public Health. 2018;15(12):2805; and Aloysius MM, Perisetti A, Goyal H, et al. Direct-acting oral anticoagulants versus warfarin in relation to risk of gastrointestinal bleeding: a systematic review and meta-analysis of randomized controlled trials. Ann Gastroenterol. 2021;34(5):651-659; Barkun AN, Almadi M, Kuipers EJ, et al. Management of Nonvariceal Upper Gastrointestinal Bleeding: Guideline Recommendations From the International Consensus Group. Ann Intern Med. 2019;171(11):805-822; Wolfe C, McCoin N. Abdominal Pain in the Immunocompromised Patient. Emerg Med Clin North Am. 2021;39(4):807-820; Leuthauser A, McVane B. Abdominal Pain in the Geriatric Patient. Emerg Med Clin North Am. 2016;34(2):363-375; Ishaq A, Khan MJH, Pishori T, Soomro R, Khan S. Location of appendix in pregnancy: does it change?. Clin Exp Gastroenterol. 2018;11:281-287; Zachariah SK, Fenn M, Jacob K, Arthungal SA, Zachariah SA. Management of acute abdomen in pregnancy: current perspectives. Int J Womens Health. 2019;11:119-134; Beigi RH. Infections of the Female Pelvis. In: Bennett JE, Dolin R, Blaser MJ. Mandell, Douglas, and Bennett's Principles and Practice of Infectious Diseases, 2nd edition. Elsevier; 2020. p. 1477-1485; and Jackson P, Cruz MV. Intestinal obstruction: evaluation and management. Am Fam Physician. 2018;98(6):362–367; and Smith, Kurt. Abdominal pain. In: Walls RM, Hockberger RS, Gausche-Hill M. Rosen's Emergency Medicine: Concepts and Clinical Practice, 9th edition. Philadelphia: Elsevier; 2018. P.213-223; and Perrotti G, O'Moore P, Kirton O. Hey, you forgot something! The Management of Symptomatic Retained Gallstones. Surgery in Practice and Science. 2022;8; and Hadrich Z, Mroua B, Zribi S, Bouassida M, Touinssi H. Stump appendicitis, a rare but serious complication of appendectomy: A case report. Clin Case Rep. 2021 Sep 22;9(9):e04871; and Di Saverio S, Podda M, De Simone B, et al. Diagnosis and treatment of acute appendicitis: 2020 update of the WSES Jerusalem guidelines. World J Emerg Surg. 2020;15(1):27.

Visceral pain is a result of activated unmyelinated C type nerve fibers that innervate organ walls and capsules. Noxious stimuli include distention of hollow organs (eg, fluid or gas) or capsular stretching (eg, edema, blood, abscesses). Visceral pain is often dull, aching, or crampy and may be steady or intermittent/colicky. Intraperitoneal organs are bilaterally innervated, and the distribution of visceral afferents correlates to embryonic somatic segments. Thus, pain localizes to a specific spinal cord level or dermatome

Table 2
Timing of symptoms in emergent conditions

Time to Maximal Intensity of Symptoms	Conditions
Seconds to minutes	Esophageal rupture (Boerhave syndrome) Esophageal variceal bleeding Abdominal aortic aneurysm rupture Ectopic pregnancy rupture Mesenteric arterial embolism Myocardial infarction
1–2 h	Cholecystitis Pancreatitis Appendicitis Small bowel obstruction Ureteral colic Volvulus Strangulated hernia Ovarian or testicular torsion
Days	Diverticulitis Mesenteric arterial thrombosis

Table 3
Differential diagnosis based on location of abdominal pain

Location	Differential Diagnosis
RUQ	*Biliary*: cholecystitis, cholelithiasis, cholangitis *Hepatic*: hepatitis, hepatic abscess *Others*: pneumonia, pulmonary embolism, pancreatitis, peptic ulcer disease, retrocecal appendicitis
LUQ	*Splenic*: splenic infarct, splenic laceration *Cardiac*: myocardial infarction, pericarditis *Others*: pneumonia, pulmonary embolism, pancreatitis, peptic ulcer disease, diaphragmatic hernia
Epigastric	*Gastric*: peptic ulcer disease, gastritis *Pancreatic*: pancreatitis *Biliary*: cholecystitis, cholelithiasis, cholangitis
RLQ	*Colonic*: appendicitis, cecal diverticulitis, cecal volvulus *Genitourinary*: nephrolithiasis, ovarian torsion, PID, ectopic pregnancy, testicular torsion, inguinal hernia *Others*: mesenteric adenitis
LLQ	*Colonic*: sigmoid diverticulitis *Genitourinary*: nephrolithiasis, ovarian torsion, PID, ectopic pregnancy, testicular torsion, inguinal hernia *Others*: abdominal aortic aneurysm

Abbreviations: LLQ, left lower quadrant; LUQ, left upper quadrant; PID, pelvic inflammatory disease; RLQ, right lower quadrant; RUQ, right upper quadrant.
From: Natesan S, Lee J, Volkamer H, Thoureen T. Evidence-Based Medicine Approach to Abdominal Pain. *Emerg Med Clin North Am.* 2016;34(2):165-190; with permission.

and is experienced in the midline. For example, the sensation of a distended appendix is reported as midline epigastric or periumbilical pain (the T8 to T10 dermatomes).[19]

In contrast, somatic or parietal pain is caused by irritation of myelinated nerve fibers that innervate the parietal peritoneum. Thus, pain is better localized to the area of disease. For example, the wall of an obstructed appendix becomes inflamed and localizes at the right lower quadrant. Visceral pain initially manifests as tenderness and guarding and progresses to rigidity and rebound tenderness.

Referred pain may be visceral or somatic and occurs at a distance from the diseased organ, owing to shared segmental innervation of anatomically contiguous organs during embryonic development (**Fig. 1**). For example, pain at the right inferior scapula may be referred from the gallbladder and inguinal or testicular pain may be referred from an inflamed or distended ureter. Extraintestinal disease may be perceived as abdominal pain owing to shared efferent projections from the abdominal wall, for example, upper abdominal pain associated with parietal pleural irritation in pulmonary embolism or lower lobe pneumonia, or epigastric pain associated with myocardial infarction.[20,21]

FROM
Physical Examination

Vitals are the first objective assessment. A fever is defined as a temperature greater than or equal to 38°C, and a temperature greater than 38.3°C is associated with sepsis. A temperature less than 36°C may be present in severe infections.[22] Among the elderly, a fever may be defined as a single oral temperature greater than 37.8°C, repeated oral temperatures greater than 37.2°C, or repeated rectal temperatures greater than 37.5°C. Tachycardia and hypotension may be seen in severe infections,

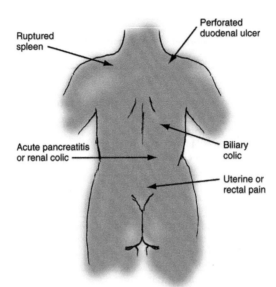

Ruptured spleen

Perforated duodenal ulcer

Acute pancreatitis or renal colic

Biliary colic

Uterine or rectal pain

Fig. 1. Locations of referred pain. (*From* Smith, Kurt. Abdominal pain. In: Walls RM, Hockberger RS, Gausche-Hill M. Rosen's Emergency Medicine: Concepts and Clinical Practice, 9th edition. Philadelphia: Elsevier; 2018. p. 213-223; with permission.)

hemorrhage, and dehydration. Tachycardia may be blunted in patients treated with β-blockers, opiates, or benzodiazepines. However, analgesia does not obscure examination findings or diagnostic accuracy.[23] An elevated respiratory rate may be in response to pain or compensation for metabolic acidosis.

The abdomen should be inspected for signs of trauma, distention, and surgical wounds or scars. Unilateral skin lesions in a dermatomal distribution are diagnostic for varicella zoster. Bowel sounds are transmitted throughout the abdomen and are best auscultated with the diaphragm of a stethoscope in one location. Bowel sounds may be increased in diarrheal illnesses or early intestinal obstruction. High-pitched tinkling corresponds to luminal air tension in early obstruction. Decreased sounds occur when bowel is hypotonic (eg, ileus, advanced bowel obstruction) or perforates.

Palpation is used to localize and quantify depth and severity of pain. Voluntary guarding is seen when a patient contracts their abdominal wall muscles to avoid intra-abdominal palpation. Voluntary guarding can be attenuated with analgesia, relaxation techniques, and patient positioning (raising the knees and head, patient's arms placed at sides or crossed over the chest). Involuntary guarding is a reflexive spasm of the abdominal wall occuring with peritoneal inflammation. Rebound tenderness is a more severe tenderness after the abrupt removal of the examiner's hand during palpation, resulting from movement of inflamed peritoneum. Special maneuvers are sometimes indicated for specific conditions (**Table 4**). Considering the generally low sensitivity of obturator, psoas, and Rovsing signs, their absence does not rule out appendicitis.

Genitourinary Examination

A pelvic examination is indicated for women with lower abdominal pain or genitourinary symptoms or when there is no reasonable alternative diagnosis.[24] Some research has shown poor reliability between individual examiners and poor correlation of examination and laparotomy findings.[25,26] However, abnormalities encountered during the

Table 4
Special maneuvers

Sign	Diseases	Description
McBurney	Acute appendicitis	Pain elicited when palpating McBurney's point (1.5–2 inches from the anterior superior iliac spine on an imaginary line drawn to the umbilicus).
Rovsing	Acute appendicitis	Deep palpation of the left lower quadrant provokes pain at McBurney's point.
Psoas	Acute appendicitis, pyelonephritis, psoas abscess	Although the patient lies on the opposite side, extension of the thigh on the affected side elicits pain. Patient may also flex their hip on the affected side to relieve pain.
Obturator	Acute appendicitis	Standing on the right side of the patient, the patient's right thigh is slightly flexed and internally rotated at the hip. Thigh flexion relaxes the psoas muscle. A positive test elicits hypogastric pain.
Murphy	Acute cholecystitis	Inspiratory arrest or inability to fully inspire with deep palpation of the right costal margin.

pelvic examination may prompt additional diagnostic testing or empirical treatment of conditions such as cervicitis (cervical friability or discharge) or pelvic inflammatory disease (cervical motion, uterine, or adnexal tenderness).

Male genitourinary examination is essential for evaluating testicular torsion, epididymitis/orchitis, inguinal hernia, and soft tissue infections. Among prepubertal men, abdominal pain is more frequently observed as an isolated symptom of testicular torsion.[27]

Rectal Examination

The rectal examination can yield useful information in select cases, but routine use in undifferentiated abdominal pain does not increase diagnostic accuracy (eg, appendicitis). Digital rectal examination is relatively contraindicated in the neutropenic or critically ill patient, out of concern for bacterial seeding. An empty rectal vault in the setting of constipation is concerning for large bowel obstruction or malignancy. Anoscopy is useful for visualizing hemorrhoids, mucosal lesions, and fistulous tract openings. A tender or boggy prostate on digital palpation indicates prostatitis.[28] Fecal inspection for bright red blood or melena should be performed in the appropriate clinical context; however, fecal occult blood testing is primarily used for outpatient colorectal cancer screening and rarely changes ED management.[29]

HEADING: ADDITIONAL TESTS

Laboratory tests are useful in select clinical indications (**Table 5**) but otherwise rarely establish a diagnosis. The white blood cell count is elevated in about 50% of patients with severe intraabdominal pathology, but a normal white blood cell count does not exclude serious pathology.[30] Hemoglobin and hematocrit are mostly useful for

Table 5
Clinical indications for laboratory testing

Tests	Clinical Indication
hCG, urinary or serum quantitative	Pregnancy
Lipase	Pancreatitis
Liver function tests	Biliary obstruction, hepatitis
Urinalysis Pathogen-specific testing	Urethritis, cervicitis, pelvic inflammatory disease
Lactate, blood gas analysis	Systemic inflammatory response syndrome, sepsis
Glucose, anion gap, ketones, osmoles	Hyperglycemia, diabetic ketoacidosis
Fecal calprotectin, leukocytes	Inflammatory bowel disease

decisions regarding transfusion and endoscopic interventions in the context of gastrointestinal bleeding. Further, anemia may not be present in early cases of gastrointestinal bleeding when clinical presentation may be more informative,[14] for example,: tachycardia, hypotension, new or worsened hypoxia, altered mental status, frank hematemesis, and bright red blood per rectum. Serum electrolytes are rarely abnormal, even in the context of severe emesis or diarrhea.[31]

Diarrheal illnesses are often self-limited, and enteropathogenic stool testing is reserved for patients in whom antimicrobial treatments may confer clinical benefit. Targeted stool tests are considered for patients with fever, bloody stools, greater than 6 unformed stools in 24 hours, traveler's diarrhea for 2 weeks or more, endemic exposure, and immunosuppression.[32] *Clostridium difficile* infection should be suspected in patients with unexplained and new-onset more than or equal to 3 unformed stools in 24 hours and a history of prolonged hospitalization or antibiotic treatment in the preceding 3 months.[33] Other risk factors for *C difficile* infection include age greater than 65 years, nursing home residence, proton pump inhibitor therapy, and immunosuppression.

HEADING: IMAGING

Contrast-enhanced computed tomographic (CT) imaging is often used for the diagnosis of infectious, inflammatory, and ischemic conditions. Contrast-induced nephropathy remains controversial, and there is no consensus recommendation for the safe use of intravenous contrast in patients with glomerular filtration rate (GFR) 15 to 30 who are not dialysis dependent. For patients with GFR 30 to 45, one should consider prophylactic volume expansion with isotonic fluids.[34]

Ultrasound (US) is considered the first-line imaging modality for biliary obstruction and infection (eg, symptomatic cholelithiasis, cholecystitis, choledocholithiasis). US is the test of choice for testicular and ovarian torsion and ectopic pregnancy.

Emergent endoscopy is diagnostic and therapeutic in the management of acute upper gastrointestinal bleeding and should typically be performed within 24 hours of presentation.[7] Urgent upper endoscopy is useful for patients with dyspepsia refractory to medical treatment or with worrisome features such as dysphagia, weight loss, or age greater than 50 years. Lower endoscopy is useful in the diagnosis of colorectal cancer and inflammatory bowel disease, and the evaluation of gastrointestinal bleeding and nonspecific CT findings of colitis. Colonoscopy is recommended for patients after clinical resolution of complicated diverticulitis if they have not had a recent colonoscopy.[35] Diverticulitis is considered complicated when there is an associated abscess, phlegmon, fistula, obstruction, bleeding, or perforation.

Classic presentations of abdominal emergencies

Differential Diagnosis	Classic History	Key Physical Exam Findings	Diagnosis
AAA, ruptured or leaking	Abdominal or back pain, limb ischemia	Pulsatile abdominal mass	CT, US
Appendicitis	Periumbilical or epigastric pain, may localize to RLQ, anorexia, nausea, obstipation	Fever (late finding), RLQ tenderness (LR+ = 8.0), Psoas sign (LR+ = 2.38)	US, CT
Bowel obstruction	Diffuse, colicky (early) or steady and localized (late) pain, nausea, anorexia, no passage of flatus and/or stool Etiology: Small bowel; adhesions, hernia, malignancy. Large bowel; malignancy, medications	Distention (LR+ = 5.6–16.8) Bowel sounds increased, high-pitched tinkling, or, decreased (late finding)	CT
Cholangitis	RUQ pain	Charcot's triad (50–70% of patients): Abdominal tenderness, fever, jaundice Reynold's pentad (≤30% of patients): Charcot's triad, hypotension, AMS	Bilirubin ≥2 mg/dL LFTs >1.5 x ULN Elevated WBC, CRP, ESR US, CT, MRCP, ERCP
Cholecystitis	RUQ pain, associated with fatty meals Risk factors: female-to-male ratio 3:1, multiparity, obesity, alcohol intake, oral contraceptives	Murphy sign (Sensitivities range 58-97%) RUQ tenderness (LR 1.6)	US, CT, HIDA LFTs abnormal in ~30% of patients
Diverticulitis	LLQ or suprapubic pain (partial relief with passing flatus or stool), constipation or loose stools	Localizing tenderness in LLQ, fever (late finding)	CT
Enterocolitis	Fevers, vomiting, diarrhea IBD: blood or mucous in stool, night time awakenings, extraintestinal manifestations (arthritis, uveitis, dermatitis)	Poorly localizing tenderness Toxic megacolon: peritoneal abdomen	Toxic megacolon/IBD: CRP, ESR, stool studies, CT, endoscopy

(continued on next page)

Table 6
(continued)

Differential Diagnosis	Classic History	Key Physical Exam Findings	Diagnosis
Ectopic pregnancy, ruptured	Lower abdominal pain, vaginal bleeding, amenorrhea Risk factors: nonwhite race, older age, history of STI or PID, infertility treatment, intrauterine contraceptive device placed within the past year, tubal sterilization, and previous ectopic pregnancy.	CMT, localized adnexal tenderness, hypotension (positional), tachycardia, bradycardia, AMS	Doppler US, laparoscopy
GI Bleed	UGIB: Coffee-ground or bloody emesis LGIB: Poorly localized discomfort, bright red blood per rectum. Risk factors: Peptic ulcer disease, gastritis, liver disease, therapeutic anticoagulation, alcoholism	Tachycardia and hypotension with severe blood loss.	Endoscopy
Hepatitis, acute	Dull or intense RUQ pain, worse with deep inspiration, anorexia, nausea	Jaundice, enlarged and tender liver	LFTs, virus specific Ag/Ab
Mesenteric ischemia	Sudden (AMAE) or insidious onset (AMAT, NOMI), postprandial pain (AMAT, NOMI) Risk factors: atherosclerosis (AMAT), low perfusion states such as sepsis or heart failure (NOMI) 50% are AMAE, 20-30% are NOMI	Objectively benign abdominal exam (out of proportion to subjective description), distention, peritoneal abdomen	CT or MR with angiography Endoscopy
Pancreatitis	Epigastric abdominal pain radiating to back, vomiting Most common etiologies: cholelithiasis, alcohol, hypertriglyceridemia	Low grade fever, hypotension, Flank or periumbilical ecchymosis in hemorrhagic or necrotizing pancreatitis.	2 of the following: Symptoms, lipase or amylase > 3 x UNL, radiographic evidence (US, CT, MR)
Pelvic inflammatory disease	Lower abdominal or pelvic pain, vaginal discharge or bleeding Etiology: Neisseria gonorrhea or Chlamydophila trachomatis (50% of cases)	CMT, uterine or adnexal tenderness, fever	Vaginal wet prep, pathogen specific tests, ESR, CRP CT (tubo-ovarian abscess), laparoscopy
Perforated viscus	Sudden onset generalized abdominal pain	Rebound, guarding, rigidity	CT

	Risk factors: receptive anal intercourse, HIV		specific testing
	diarrhea.		Endoscopy
Peptic ulcer disease	Burning or gnawing upper abdominal pain, postprandial pain or relief. Etiology: Helicobacter pylori, aspirin, NSAIDS	Epigastric tenderness	Endoscopy
Ovarian torsion	Colicky to constant unilateral abdominal pain	Adnexal tenderness or mass	Doppler US
Ureterolithiasis	Unilateral colicky flank or back pain, may radiate to groin or testicle	CVA tenderness	CT, US

Abbreviations: AAA, abdominal aortic aneurysm; AMAE, acute mesenteric arterial embolism; AMAT, acute mesenteric arterial thrombus; AMS, altered mental status; CMT, cervical motion tenderness; CRP, C-reactive protein; CT, computed tomography; ERCP, Endoscopic retrograde cholangiopancreatography; HIDA, hepatobiliary iminodiacetic acid scan; HIV, human immunodeficiency virus; IBD, inflammatory bowel disease; LFTs, liver function tests; LLQ, left lower quadrant; LR, likelihood ratio; MR, magnetic resonance; MRCP, magnetic resonance cholangiopancreatography; NOMI, non-occlusive mesenteric ischemia; NSAIDS, non-steroidal anti-inflammatory drugs; OMI; occlusive mesenteric ischemia; RLQ, right lower quadrant; RUQ, right upper quadrant; UC, ulcerative colitis; ULN, upper limit of normal; US, ultrasound; Sx, symptoms.

Data from Fink HA, Lederle FA, Roth CS, et al. The accuracy of physical examination to detect abdominal aortic aneurysm. *Arch Intern Med.* 2000;160(6):833-836; and 17. Di Saverio S, Podda M, De Simone B, et al. Diagnosis and treatment of acute appendicitis: 2020 update of the WSES Jerusalem guidelines. World J Emerg Surg. 2020;15(1):27; and Natesan S, Lee J, Volkamer H, Thoureen T. Evidence-Based Medicine Approach to Abdominal Pain. *Emerg Med Clin North Am.* 2016;34(2):165-190; and Jackson P, Cruz MV. Intestinal obstruction: evaluation and management. Am Fam Physician. 2018;98(6):362-367; Miura F, Okamoto K, Takada T, et al. Tokyo Guidelines 2018: initial management of acute biliary infection and flowchart for acute cholangitis. *J Hepatobiliary Pancreat Sci.* 2018;25(1):31-40; and Buxbaum JL, Buitrago C, Lee A, et al. ASGE guideline on the management of cholangitis. *Gastrointest Endosc.* 2021;94(2):207-221; and Smith, Kurt. Abdominal pain. In: Walls RM, Hockberger RS, Gausche-Hill M. Rosen's Emergency Medicine: Concepts and Clinical Practice, 9th edition. Philadelphia: Elsevier. P 213-223; and Sekimoto R, Iwata K.: Sensitivity of murphy's sign on the diagnosis of acute cholecystitis: is it really so insensitive. J Hepatobiliary Pancreat Sci 2019; 26: p.E10; and Padda M, Singh S, Tang S, et al. Liver test patterns with acute calculous cholecystitis and/or choledocholithiasis. Aliment Pharmacol Ther. 2009;29:1011-1018; and Pisano M, Allievi N, Gurusamy K, et al. 2020 World Society of Emergency Surgery updated guidelines for the diagnosis and treatment of acute calculus cholecystitis. *World J Emerg Surg.* 2020;15(1):61; and Sartelli M, Weber DG, Kluger Y, et al. 2020 update of the WSES guidelines for the management of acute colonic diverticulitis in the emergency setting. *World J Emerg Surg.* 2020;15(1):32; and Barkun AN, Almadi M, Kuipers EJ, et al. Management of Nonvariceal Upper Gastrointestinal Bleeding: Guideline Recommendations From the International Consensus Group. Ann Intern Med. 2019;171(11):805-822; and De Simone B, Davies J, Chouillard E, et al. WSES-AAST guidelines: management of inflammatory bowel disease in the emergency setting. *World J Emerg Surg.* 2021;16(1):23; and Crockett SD, Wani S, Gardner TB, Falck-Ytter Y, Barkun AN; American Gastroenterological Association Institute Clinical Guidelines Committee. American Gastroenterological Association Institute Guideline on Initial Management of Acute Pancreatitis. *Gastroenterology.* 2018;154(4):1096-1101; and Chappell CA, Wiesenfeld HC. Pathogenesis, diagnosis, and management of severe pelvic inflammatory disease and tuboovarian abscess. *Clin Obstet Gynecol.* 2012;55(4):893-903; and Moore CL, Carpenter CR, Heilbrun ME, et al. Imaging in Suspected Renal Colic: Systematic Review of the Literature and Multispecialty Consensus. J Am Coll Radiol. 2019;16(9):1132-1143; and Smith-Bindman R, Aubin C, Bailitz J, et al. Ultrasonography versus computed tomography for suspected nephrolithiasis. N Engl J Med. 2014;371(12):1100-10.

HEADING: CONSIDERATIONS
Appendicitis

Although CT is typically the test of choice, in the hands of an experienced sonographer US can diagnose acute uncomplicated appendicitis in patients with lean body habitus. US and MRI are also considered first-line imagihg options in pregnancy. Although a weak recommendation, CT may be avoided before laparotomy for adult patients younger than 40 years with strong signs and symptoms suggesting acute uncomplicated appendicitis, in conjunction with high-risk clinical scores (Appendicitis Inflammatory Response Score 9–12, Alvarado Score 9–10, and Adult Appendicitis Score ≥ 16).[17]

Diverticulitis

CT is the modality of choice for diagnosing acute diverticulitis. Clinical parameters (eg, previous history of diverticulitis or fever) and C-reactive protein (CRP) can exclude complicated (eg, abscess, perforation) or severe uncomplicated left-sided colonic diverticulitis.[36] Although a clinical diagnosis may reduce the need for CT imaging or ED visits, the extrapolation of this approach to the ED setting should done cautiously.

Ureterolithiasis

Ureteral colic is largely a self-limited condition, and urologic intervention is reserved for those with concomitant urinary tract infection, failure of medical expulsive therapy, or kidney injury disproportionate to anuria, dehydration, or obstruction. Stones greater than 5 to 10 mm are more likely to require urologic intervention. The gold standard for diagnosis is CT without contrast, offering more precise estimation of stone size, ureteral obstruction, and infection. Low-radiation-dose protocols can detect small stones (<2 mm) in non-obese patients. Contrast-enhanced CT can accurately detect clinically significant stones (ie, stones ≥ 3 mm) and augment operative planning for patients requiring surgical intervention.[37] Further, contrast-enhanced CT is useful in the diagnosis of alternative conditions with similar presentations. US detects signs of ureteral obstruction, rather than estimating stone size or location, and is unlikely to miss pathology requiring emergent intervention.[38] US, MRI, and intravenous pyelography (less frequently used) are alternative imaging modalities.

Case Resolution

Mohammed A.: a CT abdomen and pelvis with intravenous (IV) contrast shows sigmoid diverticulitis with a 3 cm × 2 cm fluid collection concerning for a contained perforation. He is admitted for intravenous antibiotics and analgesics, and interventional radiology is consulted for placement of a percutaneous drain.

Gloria B.: a CT abdomen and pelvis with IV contrast shows left-sided perinephric stranding and a 1.5 mm obstructing ureteral stone. Her serum creatinine is elevated, and analgesics and antiemetics do not effectively control her symptoms. Urology is consulted for percutaneous nephrostomy.

Lisa Z. has an US that shows multiple gall stones, pericholecystic fluid, and dilation of the common bile duct (1.2 cm). She is admitted for intravenous antibiotics and analgesics, and gastroenterology is consulted for endoscopic retrograde cholangiopancreatography.

Reggie J. has a CT abdomen pelvis with IV contrast that shows diffuse colonic dilation, concerning for toxic megacolon. Her CRP, fecal leukocytes, and fecal calprotectin are elevated. She is admitted for nasogastric decompression and IV antibiotics, fluids, analgesics, and antiemetics. Twelve hours later, she develops abdominal rigidity, worsening fevers, and hypotension. She is consented for a laparoscopic proctocolectomy.

HEADING: SUMMARY

Abdominal pain is the most common chief complaint encountered in the ED. Recognizing classic presentations (see **Table 6**) is essential for clinical reasoning, as well as selecting appropriate diagnostic tests[7,13,14,17,18,24,36–48].

CLINICS CARE POINTS

- History and physical examination can often distinguish serious causes of abdominal pain.
- Extremes of age and immunosuppression may blunt physiologic manifestations of serious illness.
- Sudden onset of pain is associated with surgical emergencies.
- Laboratory tests are sometimes diagnostic and more often identify sequela of acute and chronic diseases.
- Contrast-enhanced CT is an ideal imaging modality for most emergentabdominopelvic complaints.
- US is the test of choice for diagnosing cholecystitis, gonadal torsion, and ectopic pregnancy.

DISCLOSURE

The author has no funding sources (beyond clinical employment) or commercial or financial conflicts of interest.

REFERENCES

1. Bhuiya FA, Pitts SR, McCaig LF. Emergency department visits for chest pain and abdominal pain: United States, 1999-2008. NCHS Data Brief 2010;(43):1–8.
2. Cervellin G, Mora R, Ticinesi A, et al. Epidemiology and outcomes of acute abdominal pain in a large urban Emergency Department: retrospective analysis of 5,340 cases. Ann Transl Med 2016;4(19):362.
3. Peterson MC, Holbrook JH, Von Hales D, et al. Contributions of the history, physical examination, and laboratory investigation in making medical diagnoses. West J Med 1992;156(2):163–5.
4. Harward TR, Green D, Bergan JJ, et al. Mesenteric venous thrombosis. J Vasc Surg 1989;9:328–33.
5. Altobelli E, Rapacchietta L, Profeta VF, et al. Risk Factors for Abdominal Aortic Aneurysm in Population-Based Studies: A Systematic Review and Meta-Analysis. Int J Environ Res Public Health 2018;15(12):2805.
6. Aloysius MM, Perisetti A, Goyal H, et al. Direct-acting oral anticoagulants versus warfarin in relation to risk of gastrointestinal bleeding: a systematic review and meta-analysis of randomized controlled trials. Ann Gastroenterol 2021;34(5):651–9.
7. Barkun AN, Almadi M, Kuipers EJ, et al. Management of Nonvariceal Upper Gastrointestinal Bleeding: Guideline Recommendations From the International Consensus Group. Ann Intern Med 2019;171(11):805–22.

8. Wolfe C, McCoin N. Abdominal Pain in the Immunocompromised Patient. Emerg Med Clin North Am 2021;39(4):807–20.

9. Leuthauser A, McVane B. Abdominal Pain in the Geriatric Patient. Emerg Med Clin North Am 2016;34(2):363–75.

10. Ishaq A, Khan MJH, Pishori T, et al. Location of appendix in pregnancy: does it change? Clin Exp Gastroenterol 2018;11:281–7.

11. Zachariah SK, Fenn M, Jacob K, et al. Management of acute abdomen in pregnancy: current perspectives. Int J Womens Health 2019;11:119–34.

12. Bennett JE, Dolin R, Blaser MJ. Mandell, Douglas, and Bennett's Principles and Practice of infectious diseases. 2nd edition. Philadelphia: Elsevier; 2020. p. 1477–85.

13. Jackson P, Cruz MV. Intestinal obstruction: evaluation and management. Am Fam Physician 2018;98(6):362–7.

14. Smith Kurt. Abdominal pain. In: Walls RM, Hockberger RS, Gausche-Hill M, editors. Rosen's emergency medicine: Concepts and clinical Practice. 9th edition. Philadelphia: Elsevier; 2018. p. 213–23.

15. Perrotti G, O'Moore P, Kirton O. Hey, you forgot something! The Management of Symptomatic Retained Gallstones. Surg Pract Sci 2022;8.

16. Hadrich Z, Mroua B, Zribi S, et al. Stump appendicitis, a rare but serious complication of appendectomy: A case report. Clin Case Rep 2021 Sep 22;9(9):e04871.

17. Di Saverio S, Podda M, De Simone B, et al. Diagnosis and treatment of acute appendicitis: 2020 update of the WSES Jerusalem guidelines. World J Emerg Surg 2020;15(1):27.

18. Natesan S, Lee J, Volkamer H, et al. Evidence-Based Medicine Approach to Abdominal Pain. Emerg Med Clin North Am 2016;34(2):165–90.

19. Petroianu A, Villar Barroso TV. Pathophysiology of Acute Appendicitis. JSM Gastroenterol Hepatol 2016;4(3):1062.

20. Gantner J, Keffeler JE, Derr C. Pulmonary embolism: An abdominal pain masquerader. J Emerg Trauma Shock 2013;6(4):280–2.

21. Grief SN, Loza JK. Guidelines for the Evaluation and Treatment of Pneumonia. Prim Care 2018;45(3):485–503.

22. Rowe TA, McKoy JM. Sepsis in Older Adults. Infect Dis Clin North Am 2017;31(4):731–42.

23. Gavriilidis P, de'Angelis N, Tobias A. To Use or Not to Use Opioid Analgesia for Acute Abdominal Pain Before Definitive Surgical Diagnosis? A Systematic Review and Network Meta-Analysis. J Clin Med Res 2019;11(2):121–6.

24. Workowski KA, Bachmann LH, Chan PA, et al. Sexually Transmitted Infections Treatment Guidelines, 2021. MMWR Recomm Rep 2021;70(4):1–187.

25. Close RJ, Sachs CJ, Dyne PL. Reliability of bimanual pelvic examinations performed in emergency departments. West J Med 2001;175(4):240–5.

26. Padilla LA, Radosevich DM, Milad MP. Accuracy of the pelvic examination in detecting adnexal masses. Obstet Gynecol 2000;96(4):593–8.

27. Goetz J, Roewe R, Doolittle J, et al. A comparison of clinical outcomes of acute testicular torsion between prepubertal and postpubertal males. J Pediatr Urol 2019;15(6):610–6.

28. Sayuk GS. The Digital Rectal Examination. Gastroenterol Clin North Am 2022;51(1):25–37.

29. Drescher MJ, Stapleton S, Britstone Z, et al. A Call for a Reconsideration of the Use of Fecal Occult Blood Testing in Emergency Medicine. J Emerg Med 2020. https://doi.org/10.1016/j.jemermed.2019.09.026. S0736-4679(19)30809-1.

30. Kushimoto S, Akaishi S, Sato T, et al. Lactate, a useful marker for disease mortality and severity but an unreliable marker of tissue hypoxia/hypoperfusion in critically ill patients. Acute Med Surg 2016;3:293–7.

31. Laméris W, van Randen A, van Es HW, et al. Imaging strategies for detection of urgent conditions in patients with acute abdominal pain: diagnostic accuracy study. BMJ 2009;338:b2431.

32. Shane AL, Mody RK, Crump JA, et al. 2017 Infectious Diseases Society of America Clinical Practice Guidelines for the Diagnosis and Management of Infectious Diarrhea. Clin Infect Dis 2017;65(12):e45–80.

33. McDonald LC, Gerding DN, Johnson S, et al. Clinical Practice Guidelines for Clostridium difficile Infection in Adults and Children: 2017 Update by the Infectious Diseases Society of America (IDSA) and Society for Healthcare Epidemiology of America (SHEA). Clin Infect Dis 2018;66(7):e1–48.

34. Davenport MS, Perazella MA, Yee J, et al. Use of Intravenous Iodinated Contrast Media in Patients with Kidney Disease: Consensus Statements from the American College of Radiology and the National Kidney Foundation. Radiology 2020; 294(3):660–8.

35. Qaseem A, Etxeandia-Ikobaltzeta I, Lin JS, et al. Clinical Guidelines Committee of the American College of Physicians. Colonoscopy for Diagnostic Evaluation and Interventions to Prevent Recurrence After Acute Left-Sided Colonic Diverticulitis: A Clinical Guideline From the American College of Physicians. Ann Intern Med 2022;175(3):416–31.

36. Sartelli M, Weber DG, Kluger Y, et al. 2020 update of the WSES guidelines for the management of acute colonic diverticulitis in the emergency setting. World J Emerg Surg 2020;15(1):32.

37. Moore CL, Carpenter CR, Heilbrun ME, et al. Imaging in Suspected Renal Colic: Systematic Review of the Literature and Multispecialty Consensus. J Am Coll Radiol 2019;16(9):1132–43.

38. Smith-Bindman R, Aubin C, Bailitz J, et al. Ultrasonography versus computed tomography for suspected nephrolithiasis. N Engl J Med 2014;371(12): 1100–10.

39. Fink HA, Lederle FA, Roth CS, et al. The accuracy of physical examination to detect abdominal aortic aneurysm. Arch Intern Med 2000;160(6):833–6.

40. Miura F, Okamoto K, Takada T, et al. Tokyo Guidelines 2018: initial management of acute biliary infection and flowchart for acute cholangitis. J Hepatobiliary Pancreat Sci 2018;25(1):31–40.

41. Buxbaum JL, Buitrago C, Lee A, et al. ASGE guideline on the management of cholangitis. Gastrointest Endosc 2021;94(2):207–21.

42. Sekimoto R, Iwata K. Sensitivity of murphy's sign on the diagnosis of acute cholecystitis: is it really so insensitive. J Hepatobiliary Pancreat Sci 2019;26:E10.

43. Padda M, Singh S, Tang S, et al. Liver test patterns with acute calculous cholecysitis and/or choledocholithiasis. Aliment Pharmacol Ther 2009;29:1011–8.

44. Pisano M, Allievi N, Gurusamy K, et al. 2020 World Society of Emergency Surgery updated guidelines for the diagnosis and treatment of acute calculus cholecystitis. World J Emerg Surg 2020;15(1):61.

45. De Simone B, Davies J, Chouillard E, et al. WSES-AAST guidelines: management of inflammatory bowel disease in the emergency setting. World J Emerg Surg 2021;16(1):23.

46. Bala M, Kashuk J, Moore EE, et al. Acute mesenteric ischemia: guidelines of the World Society of Emergency Surgery. World J Emerg Surg 2017;12:38.

47. Crockett SD, Wani S, Gardner TB, et al. American Gastroenterological Association Institute Clinical Guidelines Committee. American Gastroenterological Association Institute Guideline on Initial Management of Acute Pancreatitis. Gastroenterology 2018;154(4):1096–101.
48. Chappell CA, Wiesenfeld HC. Pathogenesis, diagnosis, and management of severe pelvic inflammatory disease and tuboovarian abscess. Clin Obstet Gynecol 2012;55(4):893–903.

Stroke: Act FAST, Time Is Brain

Vidya Paray, MS, PA-C

KEYWORDS

- Ischemic • Hemorrhagic • Stroke • NIHSS • Thrombectomy • Alteplase • AHA
- ENLS

KEY POINTS

- The use of stroke severity rating scaling, preferably the National Institute of Health Stroke Scale is recommended.
- Do not delay administration of intravenous (IV) thrombolytics for advanced imaging.
- Alberta Stroke Program Early CT score can be used to quickly determine if a patient is a good thrombectomy candidate when advanced imaging is not available.
- For patients with hemorrhagic strokes on anticoagulation, consider reversal agents.

CASE STUDY

Mr. Smith is a 60-year-old man with a past medical history significant for hypertension, hyperlipidemia, and atrial fibrillation on rate control but not started on anticoagulation due to a previous gastrointestinal (GI) bleed who was last seen in his normal state of health by his family at 3 PM. Around 5 PM, he tries to make a phone call when he has acute onset of left side weakness, right gaze deviation, slurring speech with noticeable left side facial droop. His partner quickly identifies the warning signs of a possible stroke and calls emergency medical services (EMS). On arrival to the emergency room, the patient is scored a 13 on the National Institute of Health Stroke Scale (NIHSS),[1] has a measured glucose finger stick of 120, BP 140/80, HR 130s with irregularly irregular rhythm, SpO$_2$ 94%. A stroke code is called, and the patient is taken to CT/CT angiography (CTA) stat. Imaging shows no hemorrhage, however, a dense spot sign (which can be an early indicator of thromboembolic occlusion) is seen within the left middle cerebral artery (MCA). As the last known well time was within the acceptable time limit[a] and the patient did not have any contraindications,[2] the patient was given alteplase. (See contraindications to receiving intravenous thrombolytics in Treatment section.) CT perfusion (CTP) scan performed showed large penumbra but no established core. Patient was then sent for thrombectomy with thrombolysis in

Yale New Haven Hospital, 20 York Street, Neurosciences ICU 6-2, New Haven, CT 06510, USA
E-mail address: vidyaparay@gmail.com

[a] for patients with mild disabling stroke symptoms IV alteplase is recommended for those who could be treated within 3 hours of symptoms, for otherwise eligible patients with mild disabling stroke symptoms, alteplase may be reasonable for patients who can be treated within 3 hours and 4.5 hours of onset of symptoms

Physician Assist Clin 8 (2023) 49–66
https://doi.org/10.1016/j.cpha.2022.09.002
2405-7991/23/Published by Elsevier Inc.

physicianassistant.theclinics.com

cerebral infarction (TICI 3) reperfusion. **Table 1**. Ultimately transferred to the neurocritical care ICU for post stroke care and workup.

INTRODUCTION TO ISCHEMIC STROKE

According to Harrison's Manual of Medicine, an ischemic stroke is caused from a sudden onset of neurologic deficit from a vascular mechanism. Two ways a vessel can become occluded are from thrombotic or embolic mechanism. Thrombotic strokes are from clots that are formed in arteries traveling to the brain while embolic strokes are stemmed from clots formed in different parts of the body (usually heart or neck) that break off and travel up to the brain and occlude a vessel. About 85% of strokes are ischemic versus about 15% are hemorrhagic.[3]

Differential Diagnosis

Bell's Palsy: peripheral nerve injury (ipsilateral side of injury and forehead, eyes, and nasolabial fold are all affected) versus in stroke, the forehead will be spared when checking cranial nerve 7.[4]

TIA: temporary blockage which clears, symptoms are short-lived.

Seizure: may have postictal symptoms (Todd's paralysis) which mimics ischemic stroke.

Migraine Aura: somatosensory symptoms can occur in migraines (tingling, pins-needles, and numbness).

Syncope: sudden reduction in perfusion to brain (vasovagal, orthostatic, and cardiac causes).

Hypoglycemia: can present with weakness and paresthesias.

RISK FACTORS OF ISCHEMIC STROKE
Non-Modifiable

- Age: risk increases as you get older, risk doubles every 10 years after age 55[5-7]
- Sex: men are at greater risk at a younger age but the risk of death is higher in women
- Race: higher risk in African American, Hispanics, and Native Americans versus White

Modifiable Risk Factors

- Cardiac: hypertension, hyperlipidemia, cardiomyopathy, atrial fibrillation

Table 1 Thrombolysis in cerebral infarction scoring (also known as TICI score)	
Grade	Appearance on Final Angiographic Image
0	No perfusion
1	Penetration with minimal perfusion
2A	Partial perfusion with <2/3 of entire vascular territory visualized
2B	Partial perfusion with complete filling of vascular territory but filling is slower than normal
3	Complete reperfusion

Data from Heit JJ, Wintermark M. Perfusion computed tomography for the evaluation of acute ischemic stroke. Stroke. 2016;24(2):293-304.

- Endocrine: diabetes
- Lifestyle: smoking/alcohol use, obesity, diet, and poor physical activity

CLINICAL SYMPTOMS

Clinical symptoms of a stroke are dependent on which vascular territory has been affected.[8] A clot (thrombotic or embolic) is usually lodged in a vessel causing obstruction of flow to that area and subsequently causes ischemic damage. Below are the major vascular territories and some associated symptoms. This can help guide differential diagnosis to help quickly identify which area of the brain is most likely affected when a patient comes in based on their specific symptoms. This is helpful because if someone is showing evidence of dense MCA syndrome, they may be a candidate for thrombectomy which is not available in all hospitals; this will prompt reaching out to appropriate hospitals that are approved by the Joint Commission to be Comprehensive Stroke Centers. See more in Treatments section.

Middle Cerebral Artery Occlusion

- Contralateral hemiparesis: paralysis on opposite side of occlusion
- Contralateral hypesthesia: loss of pain and heat sensation on the ipsilateral side of the face and the lower part of the body on the contralateral side
- Ipsilateral hemianopsia: loss of vision in half of visual field, on the side of occlusion
- Gaze preference toward side of occlusion
- Agnosia: unable to recognize and identify objects, persons, or sounds
- Receptive or expressive aphasia
- Neglect, inattention, and extinction of double simultaneous stimulation, with some nondominant hemisphere lesions

The MCA supplies the upper extremity motor strip. Consequently, weakness of the arm and face is usually worse than that of the lower limb.

Anterior Cerebral Artery Occlusion

Anterior cerebral artery occlusions affect frontal lobe functions, symptoms include:

- Altered mental status, impaired judgment, disinhibition
- Primitive reflexes (grasping/sucking reflex)
- Contralateral weakness legs greater than arms
- Contralateral cortical sensory deficits
- Gait apraxia: broad-based gait with short stride, freezing, falls, and an inability to "walk and talk"[9]
- Urinary incontinence

Posterior Cerebral Artery Occlusion

Posterior cerebral artery occlusions affect vision and thought, symptoms include:

- Altered mental status, impaired memory
- Contralateral homonymous hemianopsia: visual field loss on the same side of both eyes
- Cortical blindness: loss of vision secondary to damage to the visual pathways posterior to the lateral geniculate nuclei[10]
- Visual agnosia: unable to recognize and identify objects, persons, or sounds

Vertebrobasilar artery occlusions: may cause a wide variety of cranial nerve, cerebellar, and brainstem deficits, and may be vague in nature. These include the following:

- Vertigo: sensation of feeling off balance
- Nystagmus: eyes make repetitive uncontrolled movement which can cause decreased vision, dizziness, decrease depth perception and can affect coordination
- Diplopia: perception of one object as two images displaced either horizontal or vertically
- Visual field deficits
- Dysphagia: difficulty swallowing
- Dysarthria: muscles that are used to produce speech are damaged, paralyzed, or weakened
- Facial hypesthesia: reduced sense of touch/numbness
- Syncope: temporary loss of consciousness
- Ataxia: lack of muscle control or coordination of voluntary movements

Posterior circulation stroke is known for the presence of crossed findings: ipsilateral cranial nerve deficits and contralateral motor deficits. This contrasts with anterior stroke, which produces only unilateral findings.

Lacunar Stroke

Lacunar strokes occur from occlusion of small perforating arteries of deep subcortical areas of the brain.[11] The infarcts are generally from 2 to 20 mm in diameter. The most common lacunar syndromes include pure motor, pure sensory, and ataxic hemiparetic strokes. Presenting complaints would not generally include cortical signs which require high-level processing such as aphasia (language impairment), alexia (inability to comprehend written material), agraphia (inability to write), acalculia (inability to perform simple calculations), and memory impairment.

The clinical features and physical examination findings of lacunar syndromes are characteristic of the type of lacunar syndrome. In each type of lacunar stroke, there are no cortical signs.

Pure motor hemiparesis: Patient presents with weakness on one side of the body (face, arm, and leg) without cortical signs and sensory symptoms.

Pure sensory stroke: Patient presents with unilateral numbness of the face, arm, and leg without cortical signs or motor deficits. All sensory modalities will be impaired.

Ataxic hemiparesis: These patients present with unilateral limb ataxia and weakness that is out of proportion to the strength/motor deficit. Patients may also exhibit other ipsilateral cerebellar signs such as dysarthria, dysmetria, and nystagmus without exhibiting cortical signs.

Sensorimotor stroke: Patients present with weakness and numbness of the face, arm, and leg without cortical signs.

Dysarthria: clumsy hand syndrome: This is the least common of all lacunar syndromes. Patients present with facial weakness, dysarthria, dysphagia, and dysmetria/clumsiness of one upper extremity.

Focused neurologic examination: NIHSS is a very widely used subjective way to get examination on a stroke patient and be able to trend improvement versus worsening of condition after therapy. The NIH score for each section is rated between 0 and 4: 0 being normal functioning and 4 being completely impaired. The NIHSS score is then calculated by adding all of the numbers for each section together. A score of 0 shows no deficit, whereas the highest score (worse impairments) is up to 42.

NIHSS scoring chart with scale definition included in **Table 2**

Table 2
Official National Institute of Health Stroke Scale

Instructions	Scale Definition	Score
1a. Level of consciousness: The investigator must choose a response if a full evaluation is prevented by such obstacles as an endotracheal tube, language barrier, orotracheal trauma/bandages. A 3 is scored only if the patient makes no movement (other than reflexive posturing) in response to noxious stimulation.	0 = Alert; keenly responsive. 1 = Not alert; but arousable by minor stimulation to obey, answer, or respond. 2 = Not alert; requires repeated stimulation to attend, or is obtunded and requires strong or painful stimulation to make movements (not stereotyped). 3 = Responds only with reflex motor or autonomic effects or totally unresponsive, flaccid, and areflexic.	_____
1b. Level of consciousness questions: The patient is asked the month and his/her age. The answer must be correct: there is no partial credit for being close. Aphasic and stuporous patients who do not comprehend the questions will score 2. Patients unable to speak because of endotracheal intubation, orotracheal trauma, severe dysarthria from any cause, language barrier, or any other problem not secondary to aphasia are given a 1. It is important that only the initial answer be graded and that the examiner not "helps" the patient with verbal or nonverbal cues.	0 = Answers both questions correctly. 1 = Answers one question correctly. 2 = Answers neither question correctly.	_____
1c. Level of consciousness commands: The patient is asked to open and close the eyes and then to grip and release the non-paretic hand. Substitute another one step command if the hands cannot be used. Credit is given if an unequivocal attempt is made but not completed due to weakness. If the patient does not respond to command, the task should be demonstrated to him or her (pantomime), and the result scored (ie, follows none, one or two commands). Patients with trauma, amputation, or other physical impediments should be given suitable one-step commands. Only the first attempt is scored.	0 = Performs both tasks correctly. 1 = Performs one task correctly. 2 = Performs neither task correctly.	_____
2. Best gaze: Only horizontal eye movements will be tested. Voluntary or reflexive	0 = Normal. 1 = Partial gaze palsy; gaze is abnormal in one or both eyes, but	_____

(continued on next page)

Table 2
(continued)

Instructions	Scale Definition	Score
(oculocephalic) eye movements will be scored, but caloric testing is not done. If the patient has a conjugate deviation of the eyes that can be overcome by voluntary or reflexive activity, the score will be 1. If a patient has an isolated peripheral nerve paresis (cranial nerves III, IV, or VI), score a 1. Gaze is testable in all aphasic patients. Patients with ocular trauma, bandages, preexisting blindness, or other disorder of visual acuity or fields should be tested with reflexive movements, and a choice made by the investigator. Establishing eye contact and then moving about the patient from side to side will occasionally clarify the presence of a partial gaze palsy.	forced deviation or total gaze paresis is not present. 2 = Forced deviation or total gaze paresis not overcome by the oculocephalic maneuver.	
3. Visual: Visual fields (upper and lower quadrants) are tested by confrontation, using finger counting or visual threat, as appropriate. Patients may be encouraged, but if they look at the side of the moving fingers appropriately, this can be scored as normal. If there is unilateral blindness or enucleation, visual fields in the remaining eye are scored. Score 1 only if a clear-cut asymmetry, including quadrantanopia, is found. If patient is blind from any cause, score 3. Double simultaneous stimulation is performed at this point. If there is extinction, patient receives a 1, and the results are used to respond to item 11.	0 = No visual loss. 1 = Partial hemianopia. 2 = Complete hemianopia. 3 = Bilateral hemianopia (blind including cortical blindness).	_____
4. Facial palsy: Ask—or use pantomime to encourage—the patient to show teeth or raise eyebrows and close eyes. Score symmetry of grimace in response to noxious stimuli in the poorly responsive or non-comprehending patient. If facial trauma/bandages, orotracheal tube, tape, or other physical barriers obscure the face, these should be removed to the extent possible.	0 = Normal symmetric movements. 1 = Minor paralysis (flattened nasolabial fold, asymmetry on smiling). 2 = Partial paralysis (total or near-total paralysis of lower face). 3 = Complete paralysis of one or both sides (absence of facial movement in the upper and lower face).	_____

(continued on next page)

Table 2
(continued)

Instructions	Scale Definition	Score
5. Motor arm: The limb is placed in the appropriate position: extend the arms (palms down) 90° (if sitting) or 45° (if supine). Drift is scored if the arm falls before 10 s. The aphasic patient is encouraged using urgency in the voice and pantomime, but not noxious stimulation. Each limb is tested in turn, beginning with the non-paretic arm. Only in the case of amputation or joint fusion at the shoulder, the examiner should record the score as untestable (UN), and clearly write the explanation for this choice.	0 = No drift; limb holds 90° (or 45°) for full 10 s. 1 = Drift; limb holds 90° (or 45°), but drifts down before full 10 s; does not hit bed or other support. 2 = Some effort against gravity; limb cannot get to or maintain (if cued) 90° (or 45°) degrees, drifts down to bed, but has some effort against gravity. 3 = No effort against gravity; limb falls. 4 = No movement. UN = Amputation or joint fusion, explain:_____ 5a. Left arm 5b. Right arm	_____
6. Motor leg: The limb is placed in the appropriate position: hold the leg at 30° (always tested supine). Drift is scored if the leg falls before 5 s. The aphasic patient is encouraged using urgency in the voice and pantomime, but not noxious stimulation. Each limb is tested in turn, beginning with the non-paretic leg. Only in the case of amputation or joint fusion at the hip, the examiner should record the score as untestable (UN), and clearly write the explanation for this choice.	0 = No drift; leg holds 30° position for full 5 s. 1 = Drift; leg falls by the end of the 5-s period but does not hit bed. 2 = Some effort against gravity; leg falls to bed by 5 s, but has some effort against gravity. 3 = No effort against gravity; leg falls to bed immediately. 4 = No movement. UN = Amputation or joint fusion, explain:_____ 6a. Left leg 6b. Right leg	_____
7. Limb ataxia: This item is aimed at finding evidence of a unilateral cerebellar lesion. Test with eyes open. In case of visual defect, ensure testing is done in intact visual field. The finger-nose-finger and heel-shin tests are performed on both sides, and ataxia is scored only if present out of proportion to weakness. Ataxia is absent in the patient who cannot understand or is paralyzed. Only in the case of amputation or joint fusion, the examiner should record the score as untestable (UN), and clearly write the explanation for this choice. In case of blindness, test by having the patient touch nose from extended arm position.	0 = Absent. 1 = Present in one limb. 2 = Present in two limbs. UN = Amputation or joint fusion, explain:_____	_____

(continued on next page)

Table 2 (continued)		
Instructions	**Scale Definition**	**Score**
8. Sensory: Sensation or grimace to pinprick when tested, or withdrawal from noxious stimulus in the obtunded or aphasic patient. Only sensory loss attributed to stroke is scored as abnormal and the examiner should test as many body areas (arms [not hands], legs, trunk, face) as needed to accurately check for hemisensory loss. A score of 2, "severe or total sensory loss," should only be given when a severe or total loss of sensation can be clearly demonstrated. Stuporous and aphasic patients will, therefore, probably score 1 or 0. The patient with brainstem stroke who has bilateral loss of sensation is scored 2. If the patient does not respond and is quadriplegic, score 2. Patients in a coma (item 1a = 3) are automatically given a 2 on this item.	0 = Normal; no sensory loss. 1 = Mild-to-moderate sensory loss; patient feels pinprick is less sharp or is dull on the affected side; or there is a loss of superficial pain with pinprick, but patient is aware of being touched. 2 = Severe to total sensory loss; patient is not aware of being touched in the face, arm, and leg.	_____
9. Best language: A great deal of information about comprehension will be obtained during the preceding sections of the examination. For this scale item, the patient is asked to describe what is happening in the attached picture, to name the items on the attached naming sheet and to read from the attached list of sentences. Comprehension is judged from responses here, as well as to all of the commands in the preceding general neurologic examination. If visual loss interferes with the tests, ask the patient to identify objects placed in the hand, repeat, and produce speech. The intubated patient should be asked to write. The patient in a coma (item 1a = 3) will automatically score 3 on this item. The examiner must choose a score for the patient with stupor or limited cooperation, but a score of 3 should be used only if the patient is mute and follows no one-step commands.	0 = No aphasia; normal. 1 = Mild-to-moderate aphasia; some obvious loss of fluency or facility of comprehension, without significant limitation on ideas expressed or form of expression. Reduction of speech and/or comprehension, however, makes conversation about provided materials difficult or impossible. For example, in conversation about provided materials, examiner can identify picture or naming card content from patient's response. 2 = Severe aphasia; all communication is through fragmentary expression; great need for inference, questioning, and guessing by the listener. Range of information that can be exchanged is limited; listener carries burden of communication. Examiner cannot identify materials provided from patient response. 3 = Mute, global aphasia; no useable speech or auditory comprehension.	_____
10. Dysarthria: If patient is thought to be normal, an adequate sample of speech must be obtained by asking	0 = Normal. 1 = Mild-to-moderate dysarthria; patient slurs at least some words	_____

(continued on next page)

Table 2 *(continued)*		
Instructions	**Scale Definition**	**Score**
patient to read or repeat words from the attached list. If the patient has severe aphasia, the clarity of articulation of spontaneous speech can be rated. Only if the patient is intubated or has other physical barriers to producing speech, the examiner should record the score as untestable (UN), and clearly write an explanation for this choice. Do not tell the patient why he or she is being tested.	and, at worst, can be understood with some difficulty. 2 = Severe dysarthria; patient's speech is so slurred as to be unintelligible in the absence of or out of proportion to any dysphasia, or is mute/ anarthric. UN = Intubated or other physical barrier, explain:_____	
11. Extinction and inattention (formerly neglect): Sufficient information to identify neglect may be obtained during the prior testing. If the patient has a severe visual loss preventing visual double simultaneous stimulation, and the cutaneous stimuli are normal, the score is normal. If the patient has aphasia but appears to attend to both sides, the score is normal. The presence of visual spatial neglect or anosognosia may also be taken as evidence of abnormality. As the abnormality is scored only if present, the item is never untestable.		

Goldstein LB, Samsa GP. Reliability of the National Institutes of Health Stroke Scale. Extension to non-neurologists in the context of a clinical trial. Stroke 1997; 28:307.

Imaging

On arrival to the emergency department, if a stroke is suspected, the patient will immediately be routed to get a non-contrast CT head. This is to rule out any hemorrhage or any other contraindications of getting alteplase. Usually, a CTA head and neck is also performed simultaneously to visualize any large vessel occlusions and to evaluate for any carotid stenosis and atherosclerosis. A CT perfusion scan is performed to determine at-risk brain tissue (also known as the penumbra) versus the already damaged infarcted brain (also known as the infarcted core). On MRI, diffusion-weighted imaging (DWI) and apparent diffusion coefficient (ADC) are sequences that are more sensitive to early ischemic changes. Recent data show that for many people with restricted diffusion and no change on fluid-attenuated inversion recovery (FLAIR sequence on MRI), it is more likely that the stroke is less than 6 hours old. However, MRI may be harder to physically access in lower staffed hospitals or smaller health centers, and also takes longer to perform especially when treatments are time sensitive. If a hyperacute MRI is available, this would be preferred to identify the ischemic core, since it does have higher sensitivity and specificity for detecting hyperacute ischemia versus a CTP.[12] Note that any additional imaging other than non-contrast CTH should not delay administration of alteplase.

In some hospitals, CT perfusion scans are also not available. In this case, using the Alberta Stroke Program Early CT Score (ASPECTS) can help to identify if a patient is a good candidate for thrombectomy.

The ASPECT score requires a non-contrast CTH to calculate, which may be the only accessible resource in smaller community hospitals. This score ranges from 0 to 10 with higher numbers indicating less ischemia. One point is subtracted for each area of infarct (see attached depiction from MDCalc). Patients with score of greater than or equal to 7 usually benefit from thrombectomy[13,14] Scores less than 7 usually indicate larger areas of infarct which would indicated that the patient is a poor candidate for thrombectomy as these patients have worse functional outcome at 3 months follow-up as well as increased risk of hemorrhage (**Fig. 1**).

Stroke Workup

On arrival to the hospital if a stroke is suspected a basic workup is conducted. The point in this basic workup is to try to rule in/out causes of the stroke.

Laboratory work includes:

- Complete blood count (CBC)/Comprehensive metabolic panel (CMP)/Coags
- High-sensitivity troponin
- Hemoglobin A1C (uncontrolled glucose levels can cause damage to vessels leading to stroke)
- Lipid panel—(high levels can give indication to atherosclerosis, fatty plaques that can build up in vessels leading to blocked arteries and eventually ischemia)
- Thyroid stimulating hormone (TSH)—elevated levels are associated with atrial fibrillation and cardioembolic strokes

Cardiac workup

- Electrocardiogram (EKG) to check for arrhythmias or areas of ischemia
- Attach patient to telemetry to monitor for atrial fibrillation or any arrhythmia

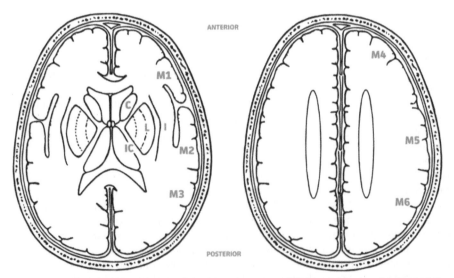

Fig. 1. Ref.—Calculate ASPECT score by subtracting one point for every area of infarcted tissue on non-contrast CTH. Scores below 7 indicate poor thrombectomy candidate as there is a significant infarct burden.

- Obtain ECHO to monitor for any shunts, thrombi, monitor ejection fraction (EF), monitor chamber sizes, and functioning

For patients (usually <40) with unclear cause of stroke: consider sending hypercoagulability workup.

Treatments

- Alteplase: According to the American Heart Association (AHA), alteplase is recommended for patients who can be treated within 3 hours of onset of symptoms, although for patients with mild disabling stroke symptoms alteplase may be reasonable for patients who can be treated within 3 and 4.5 hours of onset of symptoms. Beyond this time, alteplase has been known to be less effective and risks now outweigh benefits.[13–20]
- Absolute contraindications per Neurocritical Care Society (NCS) Emergency Neurologic Life Support:
  - No evidence of intracranial hemorrhage or acute trauma on examination
  - No major head trauma in previous 3 months
  - No intracranial or intraspinal surgery in previous 3 months
  - No arterial puncture at noncompressible site or lumbar puncture in previous 7 days
  - BP greater than 185/110 (should be lowered before administering alteplase, try IV push (IVP) beta blocker/calcium channel blocker or continuous drip with cardene before alteplase administration)
  - Anticoagulation use with international normalized ratio (INR) greater than 1.7 or PT greater than 15 seconds
  - Direct thrombin inhibitor use
  - Platelets less than 100,000

If patient improves over the first hour of receiving alteplase or has suspicion of having large vessel occlusion, arrangements should be made to get patient over to an endovascular center for thrombectomy consideration.

Thrombectomy, also known as Tier 2: accessing arterial site (usually radial or femoral artery) and manually removing a clot or obstruction from a large vessel. Thrombectomy was initially considered if the patient presented within 6 hours but recent studies show success rates within 24 hours of onset of symptoms. Careful consideration must go into determining if a patient is a thrombectomy candidate and weigh risks versus benefits. Some risks include propagation of clot to a more distal area that is not accessible for removal, vessel injury including but not limited to rupture of artery, hematoma or pseudoaneurysm at access site post-procedure.[21–23]

Once a patient undergoes thrombectomy, the reperfusion obtained is scored on the TICI or Thrombolysis in Cerebral Infarction Scale. As we see from the chart below, our patient Mr Smith from the case study obtained complete reperfusion after his thrombectomy (**Fig. 2**).

Intracranial Hemorrhagic

Case study #2

Mr Patel is a 68-year-old man with history of poorly controlled hypertension, Diabetes mellitus (DM) II, hyperlipidemia, atrial fibrillation on coumadin, and obesity with BMI 31 who presents after having witnessed acute onset dizziness, nausea, and gait instability including left leg weakness while walking. He was brought to the emergency room and initially found to be oxygenating at 98% on room air, glasgow coma scale (GCS) of 15, BP 218/100, Glucose 140, and INR 3.5. CTH showed right side cerebellar

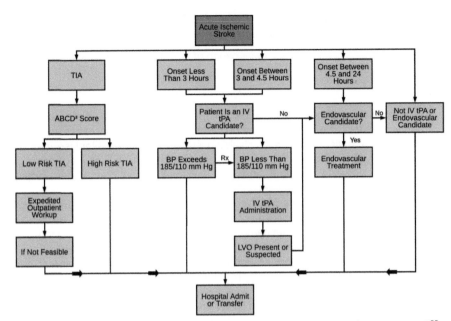

Fig. 2. To summarize: treatment algorithm per Emergency Neurologic Life Support. Ref.[23]—pathway for acute ischemic stroke per ENLS.

intracranial hemorrhage with IVH in the fourth ventricle. Intracranial hemorrhage (ICH) score calculated to 3 (ICH >30 mL, intraventricular hemorrhage (IVH), and location is infratentorial). He was immediately treated with vitamin K and prothrombin complex concentrates (PCC). Cardene infusion started for BP control.

Although in the ER, Mr Patel unfortunately had a continuous decline in mental status with new GCS of 8 (now very somnolent opening eyes only to pain, verbalizing in incomprehensible sounds, and withdrawing to noxious × 4). Airway was reassessed and he was intubated for airway protection and to prevent aspiration. Repeat imaging showed an expansion of hematoma with worsening IVH and a component of hydrocephalus. Decision was made to quickly initiate transfer to a neurocritical care center to undergo surgical evaluation.

INTRODUCTION TO INTRACRANIAL HEMORRHAGE

ICH is a subtype of stroke which occurs when a hematoma is formed within brain parenchyma with or without blood extension into the ventricles. In the United States, ICH only counts for 10% to 15% of all strokes (85% stemming from ischemic strokes), but ICH carries a high risk of morbidity and mortality.[24]

Location

ICH from different etiologies tends to occur in certain locations of the brain. Hypertensive ICH is more frequently located in basal ganglia, thalamus, pons (brainstem), and cerebellum. ICH from cerebral amyloid angiopathy (CAA), arteriovenous malformation (AVM), or sympathomimetic drugs such as cocaine or methamphetamine tends to have lobar locations.[21] The location of these hematomas is important to quickly identify as it can influence outcome and treatment plans. ICH can further be delineated as supratentorial versus infratentorial. A supratentorial ICH would be considered cerebrum (basal ganglia, thalamic, or lobar), whereas infratentorial ICH would be cerebellum, midbrain, pons, medulla.

Size

Although the location of ICH is important, the volume of hemorrhage is a stronger predictor of patient outcome.[25–29] To calculate hemorrhage volume, a plain CTH and the equation ABC/2 is used. Start by selecting an axial CT image with the largest cross-sectional area of hemorrhage and use this as the reference slice.

A. Largest diameter across
B. Length perpendicular to (A)
C. Calculated based on the number of slices the hemorrhage is seen on, multiplied by the thickness of each slice.

Finally, multiply all numbers (An $\times$ B $\times$ C) then divide by 2.

ICH Score: predicts mortality based on GCS, ICH volume, presence of IVH, supratentorial versus infratentorial origin, and age. **Table 3** for scores and mortality rate.[30,31]

Risk of Expansion

Up to 40% of ICH patients experience hematoma expansion after initial presentation. These patients usually have worse clinical outcome and requiring high level of monitoring.[32]

On arrival, if CTA is able to be obtained, it can show a "spot sign" which indicates active extravasation from hematoma. Unfortunately, CTA is not always routinely available. Recently, the BAT score (predictor of hematoma expansion) has been used more which only requires a non-contrast CTH. It is reported to have 50% sensitivity, 89% specificity, and 82% accuracy to predict hematoma expansion when the ICH score is greater than 3.[33] (See **Tables 3** and **4**)

Common Causes of Intracranial Hemorrhage

Chronic hypertension in 60% of cases: rupture of small arterioles
CAA: amyloid plaques replace muscle/elastic fibers that give blood vessels flexibility causing them to become weak and prone to rupture
Coagulopathy: medications (antiplatelets/anticoagulation) kidney (uremia related platelet dysfunction, liver (impaired synthesis of clotting factors)
Sympathomimetic drugs: cocaine, methamphetamine
Vascular: malformation: AVM/cavernous malformations
Transformation of arterial or venous infarct

Management

Prehospital/Emergency room (ER)

- ABCs, glucose check, urine tox screen, obtain peripheral IVs
- Obtain laboratories including CBC, CMP, partial thromboplastin time (PTT)/INR, type, and screen
- Obtain history including past medical hx, medication lists (specifically anticoagulation/antiplatelets)
- Perform focused neuro examination (GCS, NIHSS)
- Continuously monitor airway. Patients may arrive at their baseline but can rapidly decline.
  ○ Consider intubation if GCS less than 9

Table 3
ICH scoring

Intracranial Hemorrhage Scoring[9]	
Component	ICH Score
Glasgow Coma Scale	
3–4	2
5–12	1
13–15	0
ICH Volume (mL)	
> 30	1
< 30	0
Presence of IVH	
Yes	1
No	0
Infratentorial Origin of ICH	
Yes	1
No	0
Age (Years)	
> 80	1
< 80	0
Toayal ICH Score	0–6

30-d Morality: ICH score: 0, 0%; 1, 13%; 2, 26%; 3, 72%; 4, 97%; 5, 100%.
Data from https://enls.neurocriticalcare.org/courses/enls-certification.

Table 4
Individual components of the BAT score

BAT Scoring	
Variable	Point
Blend sign	
Present	1
Absent	0
Any hypodensity	
Present	2
Absent	0
Time from onset on NCCT	
<2.5 h	2
≥ 2.5 h or unknown	0

The blend sign is defined as a hypoattenuating area next to a hyperattenuating area of the hematoma, with sharp separation between the two regions and a density difference of at least 18 Hounsfield units. Intrahematomahypodensity is defined as a hypodense region inside the hemorrhage with any shape and dimension and lack of connection with the surrounding brain parenchyma.
Abbreviation: NCCT, noncontract computed tomography.
Data from https://enls.neurocriticalcare.org/courses/enls-certification.

Inpatient

- Obtain *imaging* ASAP. Can obtain CT/CTA at the same time but do not delay non-contrast CTH if further imaging is not immediately available.
- *Characterize* ICH once visualized on imaging
  - Quantify volume (ABC/2 calculation)
  - Perform ICH score (0–6)
- Plan to get *stability imaging* in 4 to 6 hours or sooner if there is an acute examination change, keep in mind risk for hematoma expansion.
- Maintain *BP control* less than 140 to 180[34–38]
  - Start with shorter acting agents (beta blocker [BB] or calcium channel blocker [CCB]) but low threshold to start continuous infusion for BP control. Avoid using nitroprusside or nitroglycerin as this can cause vasodilation which can increase ICP.
  - AHA/American Stroke Association (ASA) guidelines from 2015 for management of ICH recommends if patient presents with SBP between 150 and 220, it is reasonable to acutely lower systolic blood pressure (SBP) to less than 140. For those presenting with SBP greater than 220, it is reasonable to target SBP 140 to 180 based on comorbidities and level of chronic hypertension.
  - Two clinical trials INTERACT and ATACH suggest SBP less than 140 acutely is safe
  - Clinical trial INTERACT2 showed patients with goal less than 140 versus goal less than 180 had 3% fewer death/severe disability, but there was no difference in hematoma expansion between the groups
- Correct coagulation concerns based on patient coagulation laboratories and past medical hx/current medications
  - As our patient Mr Patel was taking coumadin for atrial fibrillation with an INR 3.5 on arrival, this needs to be quickly corrected and have coags rechecked.
  - Aim for goal INR less than 1.4 ideally within minutes
  - Warfarin reversal agents:
    - Vitamin K: takes longer to act but lasts longer
    - PCC recommended: higher concentration of clotting factors in smaller volume
    - FFP: (10–15 mg/kg) usually required for full reversal, which can take longer because it has to thaw after cross-match by blood bank, you have to do type and screen, its larger volumes so may cause volume overload and pulmonary edema, can have transfusion reactions
      - The most recent NCS guidelines recommend weight-based dosing for PCC (or FFP only if PCC is not available) with the dose-adjusted based on INR
      - Recent study by Steiner and colleagues showed 4-factor PCC more likely to achieve reduction of INR less than 1.3 and associated with less hematoma expansion compared with fresh frozen plasma (FFP).[39–41]
- Anticoagulation with reversal options

Warfarin	Vitamin K Antagonist	Vitamin K 10 mg IV over 30 min 4-factor PCC
Dabigatran	Direct Thrombin Inhibitor	Idarucizumab Can consider emergent HD (can remove up to 68%) Weak evidence for FFP 15–20 mL/kg
Rivaroxaban/Apixaban	Factor Xa Inhibitor	Andexanet

- Other things to continuously monitor:
  - Monitor for worsening signs of hydrocephalus: worsening mental status, upward gaze restriction, radiological evidence on non-contrast CTH.
  - Glucose control: hyper or hypoglycemia may worsen outcomes of ICH
  - Temperature: high fevers worsen outcomes, shivering can increase metabolic demand
  - Seizures: more common in lobar hemorrhages compared with deep hemorrhages, can happen in both, do not need prophylaxis antiepileptic drugs, treat only if clinical or electrographic seizure.
  - Patient may be hospitalized for several days/weeks, make sure to keep sequential compression devices on when patient not ambulating to avoid deep vein thrombosis (DVTs)
- *Consult neurosurgery* for surgical options if necessary. Options include:
  - Consider external ventricular drain for hydrocephalus control and ICP monitoring.
    - ICP goal less than 22, CPP goal 50 to 70
  - Consider craniotomy if infratentorial ICH with size greater than 3 cm, compression of brain stem or hydrocephalus. Several case studies show patients who meet this criterion may benefit from surgical evacuation

CLINICS CARE POINTS

- Patients should be treated with alteplase within 3 hours of onset of symptoms but may be reasonable to treat within 3 and 4.5 hours of onset of symptoms based on eligible criteria.

DISCLOSURE

The author has nothing to disclose.

REFERENCES

1. National Institute of Neurological Disorders and Stroke (U.S.). NIH Stroke Scale. National Institute of neurological disorders and stroke. Bethesda, MD: Dept. of Health and Human Services; 2011.
2. Demaerschalk BM, Kleindorfer DO, Adeoye OM, et al. Scientific Rationale for the Inclusion and Exclusion Criteria for Intravenous Alteplase in Acute Ischemic Stroke: A Statement for Healthcare Professionals From the American Heart Association/American Stroke Association. Stroke 2016;47:581–641.
3. Kasper DL, Fauci AS, Hauser SL, et al. Stroke. In: Shanahan JF, Davis KJ, editors. Harrison's manual of medicine. 19th edition. NY, USA: McGraw Hill; 2016. Available at: https://accessmedicine.mhmedical.com/content.aspx?bookid=1820&sectionid=127553981. Accessed February 8, 2022.
4. Mullen MT, By, Mullen MT, et al. Differentiating facial weakness caused by Bell's Palsy vs. acute stroke - JEMS: EMS, emergency medical services - training, paramedic, EMT News. JEMS. Available at: https://www.jems.com/patient-care/differentiating-facial-weakness-caused-b/. Accessed February 10, 2022.
5. UpToDate. Uptodate.com. Available from: https://www.uptodate.com/contents/differential-diagnosis-of-transient-ischemic-attack-and-acute-stroke. Accessed February 10, 2022.

6. Nogles TE, Galuska MA. Middle cerebral artery stroke. In: StatPearls [Internet]. Treasure Island (FL): StatPearls Publishing; 2022. Available from: https://www.ncbi.nlm.nih.gov/books/NBK556132/.
7. Yousufuddin M, Young N. Aging and ischemic stroke. Aging (Albany NY) 2019; 11(9):2542–4. https://doi.org/10.18632/aging.101931.
8. Ischemic Stroke Clinical Presentation: History, Physical Examination." Medscape.com. 2019. http://emedicine.medscape.com/article/1916852-clinical#b3. Accessed 10 February 2022.
9. Walsh R, de Bie R, Fox S. (2013-07). Frontal Lobe Gait Apraxia. In Movement disorders. Oxford, UK: Oxford University Press. Retrieved 9 April, 2022, Available at: https://oxfordmedicine.com/view/10.1093/med/9780199927524.001.0001/med-9780199927524-chapter-11.
10. Sarkar S, Tripathy K. Cortical blindness. In: StatPearls [Internet]. Treasure Island (FL): StatPearls Publishing; 2022. Available at: https://www.ncbi.nlm.nih.gov/books/NBK560626/.
11. Lacunar stroke: overview of lacunes, classification of ischemic strokes. Formation of Lacunes." Medscape.com; 2019. Available at: emedicine.medscape.com/article/322992-overview.
12. Nael K, Kubal W. Magnetic resonance imaging of acute stroke. Magn Reson Imaging Clin N Am 2016;24(2):293–304.
13. Saver JL. Intra-arterial thrombolysis. Neurology 2001;57(5 Suppl 2):S58–60.
14. Goyal M, Demchuk AM, Menon BK, et al. Randomized assessment of rapid endovascular treatment of ischemic stroke. N Engl J Med 2015;372:1019–30.
15. AHA. Current Treatment Approaches for Acute Ischemic Stroke.
16. O'Carroll CB, Rubin MN, Chong BW. What is the Role for Intra-Arterial Therapy in Acute Stroke Intervention? Neurohospitalist 2015;5(3):122–32.
17. Ma Q, Chu C, Song H. Intravenous versus Intra-Arterial Thrombolysis in Ischemic Stroke: A Systematic Review and Meta-Analysis. PLoS One 2015;10(1):e0116120.
18. Diagnosis and initial treatment of ischemic stroke. Institute for Clinical Systems Improvement; 2016. https://www.icsi.org/wp-content/uploads/2019/01/Stroke.pdf.
19. Jovin TG, Chamorro A, Cobo E, et al. Thrombectomy within 8 hours after symptom onset in ischemic stroke. N Engl J Med 2015;372(24):2296–306.
20. Gaillard, F., Murphy, A. CT perfusion in ischemic stroke. Reference article, Radiopaedia.org. (Accessed on 19 February, 2022) https://doi.org/10.53347/rID-24526
21. Hinduja A, Grose N, Tran D, et al. Emergency Neurological Life Support Acute Ischemic Stroke Protocol Version 4.0. Neurocrit Care Soc 2019;2.
22. Beckhauser MT, Castro-Afonso LH, Dias FA, et al. Extended Time Window Mechanical Thrombectomy for Acute Stroke in Brazil. J Stroke Cerebrovasc Dis 2020 Oct;29(10):105134.
23. Heit JJ, Wintermark M. Perfusion computed tomography for the evaluation of acute ischemic stroke. Stroke 2016;24(2):293–304.
24. Rajashekar D, Liang JW. Intracerebral Hemorrhage. In: StatPearls [Internet]. Treasure Island (FL): StatPearls Publishing; 2022. Available at: https://www.ncbi.nlm.nih.gov/books/NBK553103/.
25. Kothari R, Brott T, Broderick J, et al. The ABCs of measuring intracerebral hemorrhage volume. Stroke 1996;27:1304–5.
26. Hemphill JC 3rd, Bonovich DC, Besmertis L, et al. The ICH score: a simple, reliable grading scale for intracerebral hemorrhage. Stroke 2001;32(4):891–7.

27. Broderick JP, Brott TG, Duldner JE, et al. Volume of intracerebral hemorrhage. A powerful and easy-to-use predictor of 30-day mortality. Stroke 1993;24(7): 987–93.
28. Rost NS, Smith EE, Chang Y, et al. Prediction of functional outcome in patients with primary intracerebral hemorrhage: the FUNC score. Stroke 2008;39(8): 2304–9.
29. Tuhrim S, Horowitz DR, Sacher M, et al. Validation and comparison of models predicting survival following intracerebral hemorrhage. Crit Care Med 1995;23(5): 950–4.
30. The ICH score: a simple, reliable grading scale for intracerebral hemorrhage. Stroke 2001;32(4):891–7.
31. Score for 12-month functional outcome. Neurology 2009;73(14):1088–94.
32. Brott T, Broderick J, Kothari R, et al. Early hemorrhage growth in patients with intracerebral hemorrhage. Stroke 1997;28:1–5.
33. Morotti A, Dowlatshahi D, Boulouis G, et al. Predicting Intracerebral Hemorrhage Expansion With Noncontrast Computed Tomography: The BAT Score. Stroke 2018;49(5):1163–9.
34. Antihypertensive treatment of acute cerebral hemorrhage. Crit Care Med 2010; 38(2):637–48.
35. Anderson CS, Huang Y, Wang JG, et al. Intensive blood pressure reduction in acute cerebral haemorrhage trial (INTERACT): a randomised pilot trial. Lancet Neurol 2008;7(5):391–9.
36. Anderson CS, Heeley E, Huang Y, et al. Rapid blood-pressure lowering in patients with acute intracerebral hemorrhage. N Engl J Med 2013;368(25):2355–65.
37. Qureshi AI, Palesch YY, Barsan WG, et al. Intensive Blood-Pressure Lowering in Patients with Acute Cerebral Hemorrhage. N Engl J Med 2016;375(11):1033–43.
38. Frontera JA, Lewin JJ 3rd, Rabinstein AA, et al. Guideline for Reversal of Antithrombotics in Intracranial Hemorrhage: A Statement for Healthcare Professionals from the Neurocritical Care Society and Society of Critical Care Medicine. Neurocrit Care 2016;24(1):6–46.
39. Steiner T, Poli S, Griebe M, et al. Fresh frozen plasma versus prothrombin complex concentrate in patients with intracranial haemorrhage related to vitamin K antagonists (INCH): a randomised trial. Lancet Neurol 2016;15(6):566–73.
40. Firsching R, Huber M, Frowein RA. Cerebellar haemorrhage: management and prognosis. Neurosurg Rev 1991;14(3):191–4.
41. Kirollos RW, Tyagi AK, Ross SA, et al. Management of spontaneous cerebellar hematomas: a prospective treatment protocol. Neurosurgery 2001;49(6): 1378–2194, discussion 86-7.

Burns

An Introduction to Burns and Basic Wound Care

Jennine McAuley, PA-C

KEYWORDS

- Epidermis • Dermis • Thermal burn • Chemical burns • Superficial thickness
- Partial thickness • Deep partial thickness • Full thickness

KEY POINTS

- Burns are a traumatic injury and you need to address the patient as you would any acute trauma.
- First aid across burn organizations is universal; the goal is to cease burning, decrease injury, and increase burn healing.
- Wound dressing designs are based on a few key concepts.
- Good wound healing is based on an optimal environment.
- If there is concern for airway involvement intubate early before it become too difficult.

INTRODUCTION

Burns can be a minor inconvenience or the most devastating event in a person's life. Burn injuries are one of the leading causes of injury and accidental death in the world. They are an insult to the body's first line of defense. Although these patients are often perceived to be a person with an isolated skin injury, other systemic reactions and injuries can occur. Burn victims are considered trauma patients and, therefore, when a provider assesses a burn victim, they must follow the same algorithm as any trauma, with a primary and secondary survey. The systemic response of the body to a burn is complex and will include the release of inflammatory and vasoactive mediators. In the case of severe burns, it can lead to systemic fluid losses and hypovolemic states including hypovolemic shock. These patients are at risk of rhabdomyolysis and renal failure. The loss of that initial defense leads to high incidence of infections which can become severe and life-threatening, for example, septic shock or multisystem organ failure. This article focuses on burn care. The initial first aid, wound care, and systemic management will be discussed. This will allow providers to stabilize a patient in the emergency room and to know when to transfer to a higher level of care.

Department of Emergency Medicine, Weill Cornell Medicine, 525 East 68th Street, New York, NY 10065, USA
E-mail address: jev9040@med.cornell.edu

Physician Assist Clin 8 (2023) 67–77
https://doi.org/10.1016/j.cpha.2022.09.001
2405-7991/23/© 2022 Elsevier Inc. All rights reserved.

physicianassistant.theclinics.com

Clinical Features

General clinical presentation and considerations
Patients will present to the emergency department for an evaluation of a burn because they are in pain, have loss of function, or they are concerned about possible infections. The catecholamine response of a burn may cause mild sinus tachycardia in the 100 to 120 bpm range. Burns are also a cause for psychological injury due to the risk of possible scarring and deformity. Treatment is based on its classification and is determined by its depth, location, and wound size. There are some special considerations for all burns regardless of type. Does the burn cross a joint impeding function? Does it involve the face, with the potential for lifetime scarring or worse threaten airway function? Does it involve the genitalia? Is the burn circumferential, leading to the increased risk of compartment syndrome and functional deficits?

Special considerations in thermal, chemical, and electrical burns
Thermal burns occur commonly and often due to accidental direct contact to a heat source. This can manifest as a kitchen spill of hot water, a splash of frying oil, touching direct flame, or radiant heat from a heater. The astute clinician should always be looking at the pattern of the burn as well as the location as this can be a presentation of abuse. Red flag injuries such as scald burns where extremities or genitalia are dipped into hot liquids, specific branding patterns, or splatter patterns that do not coincide with the patient history should trigger the investigation of home safety and to contact the authorities when indicated. Burns can also be the result of electrical shock. In the patient with an electrical injury, consideration should be given to the injuries caused by the current and their effects on the physiology of the patient. Always look for an exit wound and immobilize the spine until internal injury has been ruled out. Last, in the case of chemical burns, consider the effects on the cellular and systemic level during wound management and the resultant corrosive or liquefactive effects. Monitoring and management of electrolyte disturbances is essential. The classic example of a direct electrolyte abnormality caused by a chemical burn is hydrofluoric acid exposure which leads to profound hypocalcemia and possibly resulting in arrhythmias.[1]

Considerations of the initial examination
A burn patient is a trauma patient and, as such, the primary survey should begin with airway, breathing, circulation (ABCs). It is important to confirm the airway is patent and not at risk of impending airway compromise due to inhalation, perioral, and/or neck burns. Inhalation burns, due to heated gases, can cause thermal burns and ulcerations to the oropharynx and local edema in the airway that can precipitate rapid narrowing of the airway via laryngeal edema. Singed nares and soot in the oropharynx are key physical examination findings which may be a clue to more extensive airway involvement. The combination of local edema and the presence of soot in the oropharynx can make locating anatomic landmarks and endotracheal intubation challenging. The provider should approach this airway ready with alternatives and adjuncts to direct laryngoscopy, such as alternate size endotracheal tubes, a bougie video laryngoscopy, and a cricothyroidotomy kit at the ready. The environment in which burns take place increases the risk of hypoxemia due to chemical inhalants and the risk of carbon monoxide exposure and/or toxicity. Details of the scene relayed by emergency medical services are important clues. Consider the potential of blast injuries. Your laboratory evaluation should include a complete blood cell count, complete metabolic panel, prothrombin time, partial thromboplastin time, international normalized ratio, type and screen, and a carboxyhemoglobin level. The patient who was in a smoke-filled environment may have significantly elevated carboxyhemoglobin levels and should be

placed on oxygen therapy via a non-rebreather mask. An electrocardiogram should be obtained to screen for arrhythmias from electrolyte disturbances. Last, expert consultation should be considered for potential hyperbaric management in severe cases.

Initial pharmacologic management

Pain management in the acute setting is important and can be as simple as cooling the affected area and nonnarcotic interventions such as acetaminophen and nonsteroidal anti-inflammatory drugs. The perception of pain is differential and depends on patient factors and extent of injury, and as a result, pain management may need to be escalated accordingly. The patient may require temporary narcotic pain medication via oral or parenteral routes. Some patients may require anxiolytics as well to allow for cooperation of the examination and wound care management. Tetanus immunization should be updated in all burn patients even in the case of minor burns.

Considerations in cooling and cleansing

Consensus across all burn organizations indicates that the initial first aid is "stop the burning." Cooling is an early intervention of burn first aid and is often completed by the patient or the prehospital care team before their arrival to the emergency department (see below). This should be done during the primary survey after confirmation of airway patency and the determination that no immediate, definitive airway management is required. The wound should be cleaned and any clothing or jewelry that can continue to conduct heat or potentially create a tourniquet, cause ischemia if the swelling becomes severe, should be removed. Although universal burn wound treatment guidelines do not currently exist, each burn organization has individual management guidelines. Although there are minor differences, many basic wound care tenets are universal. Personal safety is a priority. Never risk exposure to a caustic agent or other risk of burn. To stop the burning, expose the patient while maintaining body temperature and preventing hypothermia. Cooling is critical and often accomplished with cool tap water, sterile water, or saline soaked gauze. However, be mindful of the total body surface area (TBSA) being cooled and caution not to cause hypothermia. By including appropriate warming to the non-affected area can forestall this. The recommended amount of cooling varies across international burn organizations. The German Society of Burn Treatment (DGV) recommends only cooling of small burn injuries and does not recommend any cooling for burns greater than 5% TBSA. The American Burn Association (ABA) recommends cooling of first-degree burns for greater than 5 minutes. However, the British Burn Association (BBA), European Burns Association (EBA), Australian and New Zealand Burn Association (ANZBA), and the International Society for Burn Injuries (IBSI) recommend up to 20 minutes of cooling. The dressing options will be discussed later in the section on wound care. Wound need to be cleaned. Hydrotherapy has been recommended for patients with minor burns and who can be managed outpatient. However, it is not recommended for those who will be inpatient unless bedside lavage is the method of choice. Avoid the use of shared equipment in which the burns are immersed and can lead to bacterial infections including methicillin-resistant staphylococcus aureus (MRSA) and Pseudomonas.[2]

Pathophysiology and Burn Classification

Burns, as has been established, are an insult to the skin. What does that mean? Understanding of the skin anatomy is critical to assessing the severity and prognosis of burns. The inner most layer of the skin is the hypodermis. Immediately above the hypodermis is the thick layer known as the dermis. The dermis, on a cellular level, consists of fibroblasts, mast cells, and vascular smooth muscle cells. Structurally, the dermis contains vasculature, nerve endings, hair follicles, and sebaceous glands. The top layer of skin is the epidermis which consists of stratified squamous epithelial cells. The epidermis is the thinnest layer consisting of the sublayers stratum germinativum, stratum spinosum, stratum granulosum, and stratum corneum. The skin anatomy plays an integral role in developing a model to assist in understanding the pathophysiology and prognosis of thermal burns. The name of one such model is the Jackson Burn Model (**Fig. 1**). According to this model, the injured area is composed of three zones, with the outermost zone being the *zone of hyperemia*. The zone of hyperemia is the area in which the inflammatory response occurs, whether it is a burn or blunt traumatic injury to the skin, and will heal in a few hours often without intervention. The innermost zone is the *zone of coagulation* which represents the area that has very little chance of tissue recovery despite all medical interventions. Between these two zones is the *zone of stasis*. Proper care of the zone of stasis can decrease the total amount of tissue lost and increase growth in the zone of coagulation.[3] Histamine, prostaglandins, thromboxane, and nitric oxide are released within the zone of stasis and contribute to local edema in the first minutes to hours. Subsequently, highly reactive oxygen species are produced during reperfusion of ischemic tissues in this zone causing further damage.[4] All burns evolve, especially in the first 48 hours, and reassessment is key.

Burn Classification

Historically, burns have been classified by depth of injury, which is described as the degree of burn (**Fig. 2**). *First degree* is superficial often noted to be erythematous and will most likely heal on its own without treatment. Superficial sunburns often are used as an example of a first-degree burn. These will heal without scar formation in several days as they only involve the most superficial layers of the epidermis. *Second-degree* burns are slightly deeper burns and will reach down into the layers of the dermis. These burns can be subclassified as a superficial dermal burn or a deep dermal burn. Second-degree burns will likely present as a blister. Superficial dermal burns will have erythematous dermis at the base of the blister. Deep dermal burns as the name suggests go deeper into the dermis and will present with the base of the blister appearing white or hypopigmented. All second-degree burns can result in a scar but the deep dermal burns are more likely to scar but typically not resulting in a hypertrophic scar. Superficial dermal burns usually take 1 to 2 weeks to heal and closer to 3 to 4 weeks for a deep dermal burn. Comorbidities, such as diabetes

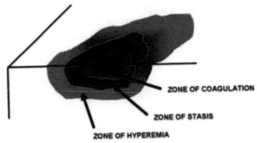

ZONE OF COAGULATION

ZONE OF STASIS

ZONE OF HYPEREMIA

Fig. 1. Jackson's burn model. (*From* Gomez et al: Management of burn wounds in the emergency department. Emerg Med Clin North Am. 25 (1):135-46, 2007, Figure 1. Thermal Burns. Elsevier Point of Care (see details) Updated January 31, 2020. Copyright Elsevier BV. All rights reserved.)

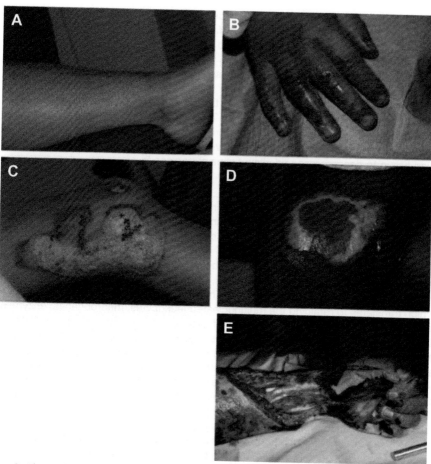

Fig. 2. Thermal burn wounds. (*A*) Superficial sun burn first-degree burn. (*B*) Superficial second-degree burn. (*C*) Deep second-degree burn. (*D*) Third-degree burn. (*E*) Fourth-degree burn. (*From* Romanelli T: Anesthesia for burn injuries. In: Davis PJ et al, eds:Smith's Anesthesia for infantsand Children. 8th Ed.Philadelphia PA: Mosby: 2011, 1003-22, Figure 31-1. Thermal Burns. Elsevier Point of Care (see details). Updated January 31, 2020. Copyright Elsevier BV. All rights reserved.)

and peripheral vascular disease, can lengthen healing time and complicate the clinical course. Classically, a second-degree burn is tender and the patient is often in extreme pain. *Third-degree burns* are deeper through the epidermis and all the layers of the dermis. As a full thickness burn, this will ultimately injure the structures found in this layer such as capillaries, nerves, hair follicles, and sebaceous glands. Therefore, third-degree burns do not present in as much pain if the nerves have been damaged. This can lead to hypertrophic scar formation and often take 1 to 3 months to heal.[12] Some experts believe that once a burn is healed the new epidermis may have increased melanocyte activity and with exposure to sunlight this can cause hyperpigmentation thus, some groups recommend avoidance of sun exposure for up to 2 years.[5] *Fourth-degree burns* extend even deeper into the underlying, tissues, muscles, and even bones creating further complications that require extensive surgical debridement and even amputation. Deep burns that invade the dermis and beyond are high risk for complications due to the loss of elasticity, capillary leakage, and fluid expansion, especially if these are circumferential burns. Circumferential burns can become life- or limb-threatening and lead to compartment syndrome. In some instances, an emergent escharotomy can be lifesaving. The burn is evolving as mentioned previously and continuous reassessment to monitor for signs of neurovascular compromise is important. If there is concern for tense compartments or decreased profusion or inability to expand the chest leading to decreased ventilation, an escharotomy or fasciotomy is required. These procedures are typically performed by surgeons. An escharotomy can be performed by any trained emergency provider in rare emergent cases. The procedure involves incising the eschar down to the underlying tissue to decompress and allow tissue expansion.[6]

Wound Care

The universally accepted management of first-degree burns involves first aid, cooling, pain control, and topical ointments to maintain moisture and promote healing. Second- and third-degree burns have a more complex management. The literature illustrates basic tenets for optimizing wound healing. A moist environment promotes good wound healing. The wound needs to be covered to decrease the risk of bacterial colonization leading to infection. A covered, moist environment can lead to the wound becoming oversaturated and macerated. The main focus is on "moist wound healing" which translates to retaining the multinucleated leukocytes, macrophages, enzymes, and cell growth factors maintained in the effusion on the wounds surface.[2] As stated in the IBSI practice guidelines, current studies have not discovered the perfect dressing but the characteristics of such a dressing would be: (1) available in all settings, (2) allow wound monitoring with infrequent changes, (3) provide a moist environment, (4) allow oxygen, carbon dioxide, and water vapor exchange, (5) offer thermal insulation, block out microorganisms and particulates, (6) non-adherent and nonflammable, (7) sterile, (8) safe to the tissue, (9) easy for the patient to use, (10) cost-effective, (11) have high absorption properties, and (12) allow mobility.[7] A less daunting wish list includes an absorbent dressing that promotes wound healing, prevents conversion to a deeper burn by adequately treating the zone of stasis, allowing mobility and pain relief and decreasing swelling.[5] The modern dressings available today meet many, but not all, of these criteria and it is the duty of the clinician to choose the appropriate dressing.

Silver sulfadiazine (SSD) has been the gold standard of partial thickness and mid-dermal burns; however, moisture retention dressings have now been shown to have certain advantages. SSD should be applied directly to the burned area 1/16 of an inch thick and dressed once daily (not to be used on the face due to the potential of staining). Moisture retention dressings such as hydrocolloid are changed less frequently, once every 3 days to once a week. The benefit of more infrequent dressing changes is less pain and ease of compliance.[8]

Superficial dermal burn and deep dermal burn often present as an intact or unroofed blister. There is controversy in the literature concerning the removal of intact blisters. Although there are limited studies on blister removal, hence some controversy, it is accepted practice among most burn organizations to excise the blister.[7] The Royal Australian College of General practitioners clearly lay out the benefits of blister debridement. The fluid that collects under the blister can increase pressure on the underlying dermis. Further, the fluid contains thromboxane B2 which is a vasoconstrictor. Both of these factors can decrease perfusion to the tissue and increase the zone of coagulation. The blister skin is dead and can be a source of infection. The purpose of the dressings as we have established is to create an optimal environment for healthy skin regrowth and to prevent bacterial infection. Dressings need to be in direct contact with the injured tissue and the intact blister would prevent this. Last, but not of any less importance, intact blisters are painful and could reduce movement which can increase swelling and decrease perfusion.[5] Resource-limited areas may not have modern dressings, and the recommendation is often to at least snip the blister with a sterile scissor and then add a bulky standard dressing in place to absorb the drainage while trying to maintain a clean moist environment. The initial dressing is often left in place for 3 to 5 days leaving the surface uninterrupted and limiting risk of bacterial exposure while allowing the bandage to be removed once it is fully soaked. Subsequent dressing changes, in theory, should have less drainage and can be done more infrequently.[7] Superficial or partial thickness burns can be managed with a variety of appropriate antibiotic ointments such as bacitracin, polymyxin, or Silvadene, or any silver-based dressing.

Hydrocolloids, foams, alginates, and hydrogels are the more common modern dressings. Some resource-limited areas may not have access to these dressings and must also be taken into account when dealing with wound care.[2] These dressings can be used for different types of wounds, like decubitus ulcers, surgical excision sites or any other open wounds with slow healing.

Hydrocolloid dressings are manufactured adhesive dressings that are cross-linked polymers of gelatin, pectin, and carboxymethylcellulose. They contact and hold exudate as a gel in the dressing and are good for low to moderate exudating burns and can be used on all burn depths. Foams, on the other hand, are useful in wounds with large amounts of exudates as they are very absorbent. Another benefit of foams is that they are available in plain or sliver, thus they absorb the exudate and help manage and prevent hypergranulation and maceration, whereas the silver provides additional antimicrobial benefits. Alginates can be used on moist granulating tissue or small superficial dermal areas of burn. Alginates are highly absorbent biodegradable dressings derived from seaweed and contain calcium. These are good when hemostasis has not been achieved and there is some superficial bleeding. Hydrogels are good for dry wounds that are sloughing as they are hydrophilic interactive dressings and will donate water to the wound and rehydrate a dry eschar or necrotic slough and absorb exudate.[5]

All wounds should be cleansed before dressing. There is no definitively superior solution for wound irrigation; however, the modality of irrigation is the key. Mechanical cleansing by irrigation has been shown to significantly decrease bacteria present on the surface of the wound. Tap water which meets the World Health Organization standards for non-contaminated water, under pressure, with any available means (whether a syringe, commercial irrigation equipment, or even a hand-held shower), will sufficiently clean the wound. "Clean" wounds should be gently cleansed to avoid injury to the underlying layers of the epidermis and dermis. "Contaminated" wounds of any kind require more aggressive cleansing to remove all necrotic tissue and bacteria that may be present.[7]

The acronym "TIME," as described in the Wound/Burn Guidelines-6 in the Journal of Dermatology, help illustrate the basic concepts in all wound preparation, burn, or otherwise. These concepts are based on improved wound healing by focusing on the (T) factors that prevent healing from the perspective of tissue, (I) infection or inflammation, (M) moisture, and (E) wound edge.[2] Once taken into consideration when choosing debridement, irrigation, and dressing, the patient's outcome will be optimized via improved healing, decreased risk of infection and possibly prevent further evolution of the wound and improve cosmetic outcomes.

For deep burns such as full thickness and fourth degree burns will not heal within 14 to 21 days and surgical intervention is critical. This is the patient who needs a higher level of care provided by a burn center. The goal is to prevent spread of tissue destruction and infection that can lead to sepsis and increased mortality. Excision should be within the first 48 to 72 hours; this will also diminish the risk for other complications such as blood loss. Surgeons will do an allograft or autograft transfer to close the wound. Early excision and grafting have been standard of care for this type of burn since the 1970s.[9]

Burn Size and Fluid Management

Burn size is described as the total percent of the body surface area involved. The most widely used tool for measurement of TBSA to determine the size of a burn is the Rule of Nines (**Fig. 3**). The Rule of Fives and the Lund and Browder Chart are also acceptable. The Palm method where the patient's palm is 1% of their body surface area in an adult can also be useful.[2] The apportionment of affected TBSA using the Rule of Nines system is yielded using the following values: (1) the whole head and neck is 9% TBSA, (2) each upper extremity, from shoulder to the hand is 9% TBSA, (3) each lower extremity, from the hip to knee circumferentially is 9% TBSA and 9% TBSA knee to foot circumferentially, (4) the chest is 9% TBSA for anterior and 9% for posterior, (5) the abdomen measured as 9% TBSA for the anterior aspect and 9% TBSA for posterior, and (6) the genitalia are 1% TBSA. The infant is proportionally different than the average adult, with their head being the largest part of their body therefore for the infant the head is 18% TBSA and the entire torso 18% TBSA and each lower extremity is only 14% TBSA. See **Fig. 3**, for a comparison of the adult and infant Rule of Nines and the Lund and Browder Chart. The rule of fives becomes helpful in patients who are obese 5% TBSA for each arm, 5 × 4 or 20% TBSA for each leg, 10 × 5 or 50% TBSA for the trunk, and 2% TBSA for the head.[10]

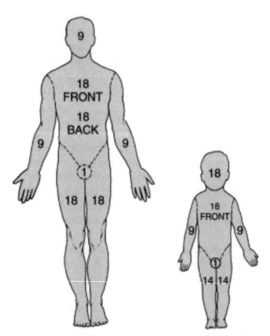

Fig. 3. Rule of nines. (*From* Mazzeo AS: Burn care procedures. In: Roberts JR et al, eds: Roberts and Hedges Clinical Procedures in Emergency Medicine and Acute Care 7th ed. Philadelphia, PA: Elsevier, 2019:774-805e2 Figure 38-5. Thermal Burns. Elsevier Point of Care (see details). Updated January 31, 2020. Copyright Elsevier BV. All rights reserved.)

The calculated TBSA burned is used to determine the severity of the injury and potential need for higher level of care and transfer to a specialized burn center. It is also useful in calculating the fluid management of the patient.

The DGV, ABA, ANZBA, and ISBI recommend transfer to a burn center if second-degree burn is greater than 10% TBSA. The EBA recommends transfer of any degree burn greater than 5% in children under 2 years old, greater than 10% TBSA in children 3 to 10 year old, greater than 15% TBSA in children 10 to 15 year old, greater than 20% TBSA in adults greater than 10% TBSA in adults over 65 year old; therefore, they have a lower threshold of criteria to transfer special populations to a higher echelon of care. All of the burn organizations, with the exception of the BBA, also recommend transfer to a burn center for mechanisms of injury such as chemical burns and electrical burns or for high-risk burns such as hands, face, genitals, major joints, or inhalation injury.[3]

Burns of significant size can lead to hypoperfusion and hypovolemic shock due to fluid loss. The objective of rehydration is to prevent hypoperfusion of end organs. Fluid resuscitation is vital in the survival of major burns.[4] Urine output is often used as a marker to determine whether fluid maintenance is appropriate.[7] Fluid resuscitation should be considered with TBSA of greater than or equal to 20% in adults and greater than or equal to 10% in children. Once a percent of TBSA is between 15% and 20% in the adult patient the systemic inflammatory response syndrome is initiated and massive fluid shifts can occur.[4] Acute renal failure occurs in 15% of patients with a large burn due to rhabdomyolysis and should be managed early. With respect to the type of fluids given there are no clear data that indicate which isotonic crystalloid is empirically better. However, patients with hypoalbuminemia benefit from colloid fluids. The use of isotonic crystalloid can create edema in non-burned areas. Similarly, the data do not clearly state that hypertonic lactated saline will have increased survival rates as compared with those given isotonic crystalloid. The benefit of the hypertonic fluids is that less volume can be used, therefore less fluid and reduce intra-abdominal pressure. Decreased intra-abdominal pressure encourages improved urine output and decreased maximum inspiratory pressure.[2] It should be said that although there are no clear data supporting the practice, Lactated Ringers is typically the fluid of choice in most clinical practices for initial fluid resuscitation.

The amount of fluid to administer is a calculated but the patient's clinical course should ultimately dictate the ideal amount. If given insufficient amounts of fluid it can worsen shock and if a patient is over hydrated, they can become fluid overload and suffer from acute pulmonary edema, anasarca, or local edema. Formal fluid resuscitation formulas were created in the 1960s and 1970s.[4] The Parkland formula is widely used in most burn facilities today. Some will vary and use the modified Parkland formula or the Brooke formula. The Parkland formula uses the TBSA burned to determine the fluid resuscitation in the first 24 hours. The Parkland formula is 4 mL × % TBSA × weight (kg) that number is then divided in half with the first half to be given in the first 8 hours and the second half over the next 16 hours.

Parkland Formula:

4ml x % TBSA x weight (kg)

½ total ml in first 8 hours   ½ total ml in next 16 hours

The modified Parkland formula uses Ringer's lactate 4 mL/kg/% burn for the initial 24 hours and hour then 0.3 to 1 mL/kg/% burn/16 per colloid infusion 5% albumin for the next 24 hours.

The Brooke formula is Ringer's lactate 1.5 mL/kg/% burn plus colloids 0.5 mL/kg/% burn plus 2000 mL glucose in water for the initial 24 hours and then Ringer's lactate 0.5 mL/kg/% burn, colloids 0.25 mL/kg/%burn and the same amount of glucose in water as in the first 24 hours. In clinical practice, urinary output and cardiorespiratory response is often considered rather than strict adherence to any of the above formulas after the initial 24-hour bolus, typically with a urine output goal of 0.5 mg/kg/h.

SUMMARY

Burns can be fatal if not managed appropriately and in a timely fashion. Complications can include airway compromise, respiratory failure, dysrhythmias, compartment syndrome, rhabdomyolysis, dehydration, acute renal failure, septic shock, and multisystem organ failure. Approach every burn victim as a trauma patient and perform a detailed primary and secondary survey. Frequent reassessments of the burn in early stages are critical as they can evolve dramatically within the first 72 hours. Stop the burning process, remove the insulting agent, perform debridement, or conduct surgical excision early to preserve underlying tissue. One can prevent infectious complications by updating tetanus immunization, using topical and/or systemic antibiotics as needed, and by covering the wound to promote healing and decrease bacterial growth. For definitive burn management, use either a standard dressing in a resource limited area or a biologic dressing when available. For severe burns, skin grafting and surgical intervention may be warranted.

CLINICS CARE POINTS

- If a burn wound is not managed appropriately in a timely manner, it can lead to disfigurement, loss of limb, or life.
- When treating a burn patient, wound care is a priority to prevent complications and poor outcomes, but a key part of the assessment of a burn patient also includes identifying if the pattern of injury is indicative of foul play or abuse.
- It is imperative to identify the need for transfer to a higher level of care in the setting of a traumatic injury such as burns to either a designated burn center or a trauma center early.
- When performing burn wound care do not forget to update tetanus vaccincation status, to avoid infection.

DISCLOSURE

The author has nothing to disclose.

REFERENCES

1. Fang H, Wang GY, Wang X, et al. Potentially fatal electrolyte imbalance caused by severe hydrofluoric acid burns combined with inhalation injury: A case report. World J Clin cases 2019;7(20):3341–6.
2. Yoshino Y, Ohtsuka M, Kawaguchi M, et al. Wound/Burn Guidelines Committee. The wound/burn guidelines - 6: Guidelines for the management of burns. J Dermatol 2016;43(9):989–1010. Epub 2016 Mar 12. PMID: 26971391.
3. Koyro KI, Bingoel AS, Bucher F, et al. Burn Guidelines—An International Comparison. Eur Burn J 2021;2(3):125–39.

4. Haberal M, Sakallioglu Abali AE, Karakayali H. Fluid management in major burn injuries. Indian J Plast Surg 2010;43(Suppl):S29–36.

5. Douglas HE, Wood F. Burns dressings. Aust Fam Physician 2017;46(3):94–7. PMID: 28260266.

6. Sherman SC, Christopher R, et al. Atlas of clinical emergency medicine. Wolters Kluwer Health; 2016.

7. ISBI Practice Guidelines Committee, Ahuja RB, Gibran N, et al. ISBI Practice Guidelines for Burn Care. Burns 2016;42(5):953–1021.

8. Muangman P, Muangman S, Opasanon S, et al. Benefit of hydrocolloid SSD dressing in the outpatient management of partial thickness burns. J Med Assoc Thai 2009;92(10):1300–5. PMID: 19845237.

9. Jeschke MG, Shahrokhi S, Finnerty CC, et al. ABA Organization & Delivery of Burn Care Committee. Wound Coverage Technologies in Burn Care: Established Techniques. J Burn Care Res 2018;39(3):313–8.

10. Livingston EH, Lee S. Percentage of burned body surface area determination in obese and nonobese patients. J Surg Res 2000;91(2):106–10.

Traumatic Injuries of the Eye, Ear, Nose, and Throat

Loryn Fridie, MPAS, PA-C[a],*, Dan Michael Tzizik, MPAS, MPH, PA-C[b]

KEYWORDS

- Orbital trauma • Auricular trauma • Nasal trauma • Esophageal trauma

KEY POINTS

- Vision-threatening injuries require rapid recognition and management by emergency providers.
- The ears' vascular anatomy results in unique challenges when repairing auricular injuries to avoid disfiguring outcomes.
- Clinicians must have a high degree of suspicion of esophageal injury based on the mechanism and location secondary to varied clinical presentations.

TRAUMATIC EYE INJURIES
Introduction

Frequently seen in the emergency department, traumatic injuries to the eye are one of the most common causes of preventable visual impairment worldwide.[1] In the United States alone, an estimated 2.0 to 2.4 million cases of eye trauma occur each year, and nearly 1 million individuals have permanent significant visual impairment as a result.[1] It is essential for emergency medicine providers to be able to rapidly recognize and manage vision-threatening injuries.

In all trauma patients, the initial evaluation must first address life-threatening injuries prior to assessing periocular and ocular damage.[2] Once life-threatening injuries are addressed, an ocular assessment should include a focused history and physical examination.[3] This section will focus on the diagnosis and management of four vision-threatening injuries including orbital compartment syndrome, open globe injuries, traumatic hyphema, and orbital fractures.

Orbital compartment syndrome

The orbit's confined space and limited ability to expand makes it particularly susceptible to developing compartment syndrome.[4] Trauma resulting in the sudden development of an intraorbital hematoma can cause rapidly elevated intraorbital pressure.[5]

[a] Emergency Department, 525 E 68th St, New York, NY 10065, USA; [b] Boston University School of Medicine, Physician Assistant Program, 72 East Concord Street, Boston, MA 02118, USA
* Corresponding author. Emergency Department, 525 E 68th St, New York, NY 10065, USA
E-mail address: lof9026@med.cornell.edu

Physician Assist Clin 8 (2023) 79–93
https://doi.org/10.1016/j.cpha.2022.08.011
2405-7991/23/© 2022 Elsevier Inc. All rights reserved.

physicianassistant.theclinics.com

This pressure can cause ischemia to the eye and optic nerve.[5] If not treated promptly this can lead to irreversible blindness.

Evaluation

Orbital compartment syndrome is a *clinical diagnosis* . Patients will often present with the acute onset of decreased vision, diplopia, eye pain, and or periorbital swelling.[6] On physical examination patients present with markedly decreased visual acuity, an afferent pupillary defect, proptosis, diffuse subconjunctival hemorrhage and evidence of increased intraorbital pressure including "Rockhard" eyelids and decreased retro-pulsion (**Fig. 1**).[6]

An afferent pupillary defect is the result of unilateral damage to the retina or optic nerve and causes pupils to respond differently to light stimuli shone in one eye at a time.[7] This is often tested with the swinging flashlight test by observing the pupillary response to consensual light looking for differing responses which should normally be equal.[8]

Imaging

In patients with evidence of orbital compartment syndrome on history and physical exam emergent orbital decompression should not be delayed by further imaging or testing.[6] This is a clinical diagnosis and treatment should be initiated immediately because of the risk of irreversible vision loss.[9]

Management

Orbital compartment syndrome once suspected requires orbital decompression with an emergent lateral canthotomy and inferior cantholysis as depicted later in discussion (**Fig. 2**).[6] The procedure should be performed by an ophthalmologist or other experienced provider whenever possible.

OPEN GLOBE INJURIES

Open globe injuries are defined as full-thickness wounds of the eye wall.[10] These injuries are further classified into lacerations and ruptures based on the mechanism of injury. Lacerations are caused by the penetration of sharp objects or projectiles, whereas ruptures are caused by blunt trauma.[9]

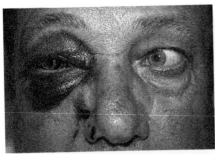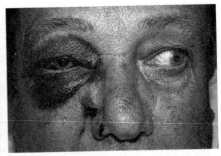

Fig. 1. Clinical photograph of a patient with orbital compartment syndrome after blunt trauma who had right periocular edema, ecchymosis, proptosis, and limitation in right gaze (*left*) and left gaze (*right*). (*From* [Lima V, Burt B, Leibovitch I, Prabhakaran V, Goldberg RA, Selva D. Orbital compartment syndrome: the ophthalmic surgical emergency. *Surv Ophthalmol*. 2009 Jul;54(4):441-9.]; with permission.)

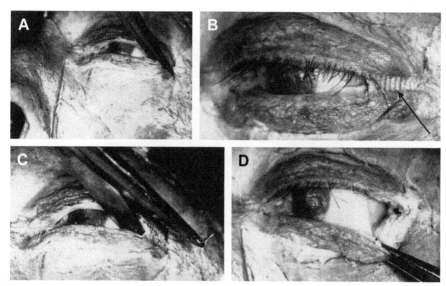

Fig. 2. (*A*). A clamp is placed across the lateral canthus to compress tissue and reduce bleeding. (*B*). Clamp removed leaving an impression on the soft tissue. (*C*). Sterile scissors are used to make a one centimeter incision into the tissue at the clamp site. (*D*). A 1 to 2 cm cut is made to lyse the inferior crus. (*From* [Vassallo S, Hartstein M, Howard D, Stetz J. Traumatic retrobulbar hemorrhage: emergent decompression by lateral canthotomy and cantholysis. *J Emerg Med.* 2002 Apr;22(3):251-6.] with permission.)

Evaluation

Patients presenting with a history of ocular injuries involving high-velocity projectiles, high impact blunt trauma, or sharp objects should raise suspicion for an open globe injury.[11]

On inspection of the eye common findings include obvious corneal or scleral laceration, volume loss to the eye, uveal prolapse, iris abnormalities as seen in **Fig. 3** 360-degree bullous subconjunctival hemorrhage or an intraocular or protruding foreign body (See **Fig. 3**).[11]

On physical examination markedly decreased visual acuity and a relative afferent pupillary defect are often seen.[11]

If an open globe is suspected on history and physical exam *emergent* consultation with ophthalmology is indicated.[12] A noncontrast CT of the orbits is often obtained for further evaluation.[13]

Management

Surgery is the definitive management of open globe injuries, ideally within 24 hours.[14] After initial examination place an eye shield, do not remove any protruding foreign bodies and avoid eye manipulation that could increase intraocular pressure.[14]

Patients are started on IV antibiotics to prevent the development of traumatic endophthalmitis which can lead to irreparable vision loss.[15] A typical regimen includes Vancomycin plus Ceftazidime.[16]

ORBITAL FLOOR FRACTURES

The orbital floor is composed of the zygoma and maxillary bone and is closely associated with the inferior oblique and rectus muscle, maxillary sinus, and infraorbital

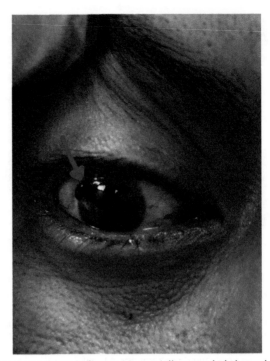

Fig. 3. Lacerated limbus. Arrow indicates iris partially extruded through laceration. (*From* [Zimmerman B, Ashburn N, Kelly E. (2020). Lacerated limbus: Management of an open globe injury. *Visual Journal of Emergency Medicine. 2020; 19*: 100710.] with permission.)

nerve.[17] Fractures of the floor of the orbit also known as "blowout fractures" typically occur when a small, round object strikes the eye.[18] A significant consequence of fractures of the orbital floor is the entrapment of the inferior rectus and/or orbital fat which can lead to ischemia and loss of muscle function.[19]

Evaluation

Patients typically present with bony tenderness and swelling, periocular ecchymosis, diplopia, and/or orbital emphysema.[20] There are several common complications seen with orbital fractures. Entrapment of the inferior rectus and/or orbital fat is suggested by the inability to look up in the affected eye on extraocular examination.[20] Injury to the infraorbital nerve is suggested by decreased sensation along the cheek, upper lip, or upper gingiva.[21] Prolapse of tissue into the maxillary sinus is suggested by enophthalmos or when the eye recedes into the orbit.[21] Thin-cut coronal CT of the orbits is the imaging modality of choice to diagnose orbital fractures.[21]

Management

Emergent ophthalmology consultation should occur when there is decreased visual acuity, disruption of medial canthal ligament, severe vagal symptoms, concern for orbital compartment syndrome or open globe.[20] Close outpatient ophthalmology follow-up within 24 hours should be ensured with patients with muscle entrapment or enophthalmos.[20] On discharge patients should be advised to use ice packs, sleep with the head of the bed elevated and avoid nose blowing and sniffing.[21] The evidence for prophylactic antibiotics and corticosteroids remain limited.[21]

TRAUMATIC HYPHEMA

Traumatic hyphema is the accumulation of blood in the anterior chamber of the eye due to damage to the vessels of the ciliary body and iris.[22] A common complication of blunt or penetrating injury which can result in permanent vision loss.

Evaluation

Hyphemas are typically caused by blunt trauma to the orbit and are often associated with head trauma, orbital fracture, posterior segment injury and rarely open globe injuries.[22] Patients typically present with pain, blurred vision, photosensitivity, and layering of blood in the anterior chamber.[23] Poor outcomes are associated with sickle cell disease or trait and bleeding tendencies such as von Willebrand disease or anticoagulation.[23]

On physical exam blood in the anterior chamber is grossly visible (**Fig. 4**). There are four grades of hyphema based on the volume of circulating red blood cells in the anterior chamber.[24]

Grade 3, greater than 50%, and Grade 4 or 100% are the most clinically significant and often result in decreased visual acuity.[24]

Management

Several observational studies suggest that most patients can safely receive outpatient treatment and close ophthalmology follow-up.[25] Emergent ophthalmology consultation and often hospitalization is indicated in patients with large hyphemas (Grade 3 or higher), severely elevated intraocular pressure (IOP), and patients with sickle hemoglobinopathy, bleeding tendency or coagulopathy.[25]

Treatment of traumatic hyphema focuses on the prevention of secondary hemorrhage and intraocular hypertension.[25] This often requires daily monitoring of IOP, limitation of activity, eye shield, and dilating and glucocorticoid eye drops.[25] It is recommended that patients elevate the head of the bed to 30 degrees to promote inferior settling of blood.[25] If conservative measures are unsuccessful surgical management may be required.

CLINICS CARE POINTS

- Orbital compartment syndrome is a *clinical diagnosis* that once suspected requires orbital decompression with an emergent lateral canthotomy and inferior cantholysis

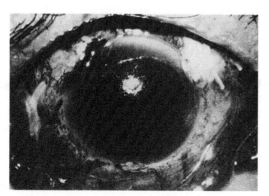

Fig. 4. "Black-ball" hyphema. Dark, clotted blood fills the anterior chamber and obscures the iris. (*From* [Wilson, F. (1980). Traumatic hyphema. Pathogenesis and management. *Ophthalmology. 1980; 87*(9): 910-919.] with permission.)

- Open globe injuries are full-thickness wounds of the eye wall which require emergent ophthalmology consultation and surgical management
- The common complications of orbital floor fractures include the entrapment of the inferior rectus and/or orbital fat, injury to infraorbital nerve, and prolapse of tissue into maxillary sinus
- Traumatic hyphema requires emergent ophthalmology consultation in patients with large hyphemas (Grade 3 or higher), severely elevated intraocular pressure, and patients with increased bleeding tendency.

TRAUMATIC EAR INJURIES
Introduction

The management of common ear injuries as a result of blunt or penetrating trauma will be reviewed here. The focus will be on the evaluation and management of injuries whose improper management could lead to poor cosmetic appearance or permanent hearing loss. These include auricle lacerations, auricular hematomas, tympanic membrane ruptures, and middle ear injuries.

AURICULAR LACERATIONS

Auricle lacerations can be complex and if improperly repaired can be disfiguring to patients. The external ear is composed of the auricle and the external auditory canal.[26] The auricle is made up of several elastic cartilage subunits which are avascular and receive nourishment from perichondrium.[26]

Cartilage exposure after auricular lacerations can cause infection, erosive chondritis, and necrosis.[27] Loss of auricular cartilage (notching) or replacement of health cartilage with fibrocartilage (cauliflower ear) is disfiguring and not easily reversed.[27] Therefore, ensuring tissue coverage of exposed cartilage is key during auricular laceration repair.

Evaluation

Most ear lacerations result from isolated trauma. During the patient's history a clinician should identify the causing traumatic force, associated symptoms of middle and inner ear injury (tinnitus, hearing loss, vertigo, vomiting), associated symptoms of head injury (altered mental status, vomiting, headache), age of wound, likelihood of wound contamination and the potential presence of foreign body.[28]

Wound assessment should focus on the location/depth of the injury, degree of cartilage involvement, extension of the laceration into the auditory canal, and the presence of tissue avulsion or auricular hematoma.[28]

Management

Primary closure is the preferred treatment of auricular lacerations, especially if the ear cartilage is exposed or the wound extends through the ear.[28] Wounds are anesthetized with the local infiltration of lidocaine without epinephrine, epinephrine should be avoided to prevent the vasoconstriction and disruption of the vascular supply to the ear.[29] A regional auricular block may be used for repair of extensive auricular lacerations or to avoid local tissue distortion when cosmetic alignment is important.[29]

Once anesthetized the wound should undergo thorough irrigation. The clinician should avoid excessive pressure or debridement to ensure exposed cartilage can be covered and to avoid notching.[28]

The surgical technique used for wound closure will depend on the complexity of the laceration.[3] Consultation with a surgical subspecialist is suggested for auricular avulsions and lacerations that extend into the external auditory canal.[28] Through and through lacerations of the auricle may also require a subspecialist depending on the capability of the clinician.[28]

AURICULAR HEMATOMA

An auricular hematoma is a collection of blood between the perichondrium and the cartilage.[30] This collection of blood acts as a mechanical barrier between the cartilage and its blood supply.[30] As a result the underlying cartilage can necrose and become infected resulting in cartilage loss. The formation of new cartilage can lead to fibrocartilaginous overgrowth commonly known as "cauliflower ear."[30] Early drainage of the hematoma and appropriate wound closure reduces the likelihood of this complication.

Evaluation

Most commonly seen among people playing contact sports including wrestling, rugby, and mixed martial arts.[31] Typically the result of an isolated blow to the ear and is associated with few other injuries.[31] An acute auricular hematoma, as demonstrated in **Fig. 5**, present as a tender, tense and fluctuant collection of blood (**Fig. 5**).[31]

Management

The cornerstones of management are prompt drainage and prevention of reaccumulation.[32]

A recent Cochrane review found no superior drainage method due to a lack of randomized, controlled trials.[32]

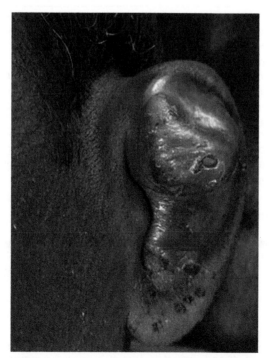

Fig. 5. Diffuse tense swelling of left pinna. (*From* [Bakshi S, Ramesh S. Auricular hematoma following trauma. *Visual Journal of Emergency Medicine.* 2021;*25*: 101199.] with permission.)

Some studies suggest that small hematomas < 2 cm in diameter and less than 48 hours old may undergo needle aspiration with an 18G needle rather than incision and drainage.[32] Larger hematomas should be drained with an open incision or intravenous catheter evacuation, as aspirations will not achieve adequate removal of the hematoma.[33]

Incision and drainage should be conducted along the anatomic fold and avoid the cartilage to minimize scarring.[34] Hematoma should be evacuated completely and irrigated.[34] Closure is then achieved with absorbable mattress sutures through and through the ear to ensure adherence of the skin to the cartilage and eliminate potential dead space.[34] Wounds should be dressed with ample antibiotic ointment and can otherwise be left open to the air. All patients need to have a close follow-up with an otolaryngologist.

An alternative to incision and drainage is intravenous catheter evacuation. The hematoma is first aspirated with an 18G catheter, the cannula is then left in the hematoma cavity and a compression dressing is applied.[35] Studies have shown this is a simple, cost-effective approach that provides rapid recovery, comparable to other methods.[35]

Traumatic tympanic membrane rupture

The tympanic membrane separates the outer ear and middle ear.[26] Rupture is typically the result of blunt blows to the head, penetrating trauma, and blast injuries.[36] Patients present with pain, hearing loss, tinnitus, or discharge from the ear.[36]

Management

In cases of minimal hearing loss (decreased perception of whisper, minor asymmetry to < 40 dB on formal audiometry), absence of vestibular findings (nystagmus, vomiting, ataxia) or facial nerve weakness outpatient follow-up with thorough discharge instructions and outpatient otolaryngology follow-up as needed[37]

Patients should be advised to avoid water in the ear and watchful waiting as most injuries will heal with time.[37] Traumatic perforations less than 25% of drum surface will often heal spontaneously within 4 weeks.[38] Risk factors for nonhealing include penetrating trauma, older age, and ear irrigation following rupture.[38]

Antibiotic ear drops are often prescribed for contaminated wounds and canals occluded with blood or drainage.[37] Patients with significant hearing loss associated with their injury may have middle ear damage and should have a prompt evaluation by an otolaryngologist.[37]

MIDDLE EAR TRAUMA

The middle ear is an air-filled cavity between the external ear canal and the inner ear.[26] The ossicular chain and the facial nerve cross in the middle ear space and are often affected in trauma.[26] Middle ear injury occurs in up to one-third of patients, with severe head trauma, typically through direct blunt trauma to the external auditory canal or penetrating trauma.[39]

Evaluation

Patients present with ear pain, hearing loss, otorrhea (clear or bloody ear canal drainage), and tinnitus.[40] More significant injuries can have symptoms of vestibular injury including vertigo, nausea, vomiting, imbalance, or facial weakness suggesting nerve dysfunction.[40]

On a physical exam clinicians may appreciate hemotympanum, amber or clear middle ear effusion, otorrhea, hearing deficit, nystagmus, ataxia, or retroauricular hematoma.[40] The facial nerve can be tested by observing the response to commands for closing the eyes, elevating the brow and smiling/frowning.[26]

Imaging and prompt evaluation by an otolaryngologist are indicated to further assess serious middle ear trauma. Temporal Bone CT without contrast is the ideal study.[41] A noncontrast head CT is inadequate because it contains cuts that are too broad.[41]

CLINICS CARE POINTS

- Ensuring tissue coverage of exposed cartilage is key during auricular laceration repair to avoid disfiguring complications.
- The cornerstones of auricular hematoma management are prompt drainage and prevention of reaccumulation,
- Most cases of tympanic membrane rupture are suitable for outpatient follow-up with thorough discharge instructions and outpatient otolaryngology follow-up as appropriate.
- In patients with concern for serious middle ear injury prompt otolaryngology evaluation and a Temporal bone CT without contrast is indicated.

NASAL TRAUMA
Introduction

Nasal soft tissue injuries and fractures are common with facial trauma. This section will review the emergency management of nasal fractures, septal hematomas, and epistaxis.

Nasal Fractures

Fractures of the thin bones of the nasal bridge are the most common types of facial fracture.[42] They may be associated with other injuries, including orbital or midface fractures, and thus a careful examination of the midface is necessary[43]

Evaluation

Imaging is often unnecessary if tenderness and swelling are isolated to the bony bridge of the nose, breathing is unaffected, no deviation of septum, and no septal hematoma is present.[43] Imaging results in these cases will not alter initial treatment.

Plain films may be obtained if any of these criteria are not met and isolated nasal injury is suspected.[43] A Maxillofacial CT remains the preferred means of imaging in facial trauma and should be obtained if any concern for more extensive injury.[37]

Management

Displaced, but otherwise uncomplicated nasal fractures evaluated within six hours of injury are reduced immediately.[44] Septal hematomas should be treated promptly, discussed in detail later in discussion. Otherwise, patients are discharged home with symptomatic care and outpatient otorhinolaryngology follow-up as needed.[44]

Nasal septal hematomas

The accumulation of blood between the septum and overlying tissue can cause irreversible septal necrosis within 72–96 hours.[45] Destruction of the septal cartilage can lead to a "saddle nose" deformity.[5] Hematomas can also become infected creating a nasal septal abscess, with risk of extension into the face and brain[45] A hematoma is described as bluish in color and should be fluctuant, unlike a deviated septum, which may appear bluish, but will be firm (**Fig. 6**).[46]

Management

The mainstay of treatment is drainage. The hematoma should be incised 5 to 10 mm and drained.[46] After completion nare should be anteriorly packed, typically with an inflatable nasal tampon.[46] Pt are discharged home with oral antibiotics to cover Staph Aureus, including MRSA.[45] Packing should be removed in 3 days and the patient should be provided otorhinolaryngology follow-up.[45]

Epistaxis

Historically a dreaded chief complaint secondary to its potentially time-consuming and difficult management. Epistaxis is a common problem, occurring in 60% of the general population[47] Most are uncomplicated and self-limited. 90% of nosebleeds are anterior coming from the vascular watershed of the nasal septum known as Kies-selbach's Plexus.[48] Posterior bleeds most commonly come from the posterolateral branches of the sphenopalatine artery and can result in significant hemorrhage.[48]

Evaluation

The clinician should be aware of conditions that predispose to more severe bleeding including a patient history of tumors, coagulation disorders, anticoagulation medications, intranasal glucocorticoids, cirrhosis, HIV or intranasal cocaine use.[49]

   Labs are typically not indicated as routine tests but should be ordered in anticoagulated patients.[50] If there is clinical concern for massive or prolonged hemorrhage labs including coags, type and screen, and 2 large Bore IVs are indicated.[50]

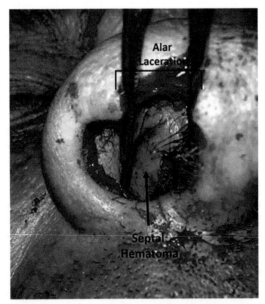

Fig. 6. Nasal septal hematoma prior to drainage. Black arrow indicates the nasal septal hematoma. (*From* [Puricelli MD, Zitsch RP. Septal Hematoma Following Nasal Trauma. *The Journal of Emergency Medicine*. 2016; *50*(1): 121-122.] with permission.)

Management

Initial tamponade

Ask the patient to blow their nose to remove blood and clots. Clinicians then spray nares with oxymetazoline (Afrin). Instruct the patient to pinch alae tightly against septum and hold continuously for 10 minutes. One retrospective study found Afrin stopped bleeding in 65% of patients presenting to the emergency department.[51] If bleeding stops observe the patient for 30 minutes for recurrent bleeding. If there is no evidence of rebleeding, studies have suggested no need for further intervention.[51]

Cautery

If initial tamponade is unsuccessful and an anterior source of bleeding is visualized, cautery is the next step.[52] Chemical cautery is typically achieved with silver nitrate sticks after topical anesthetic with cotton swabs soaked in an anesthetic and vaso-constrictive agent.[52] Once anesthetized the applicator tip is applied to a small area, starting proximally. Avoid cauterizing large areas.[52] Cautery is applied for a few seconds until a white precipitate forms.[52]

Tranexamic acid

Tranexamic acid (TXA) is a synthetic derivative of the amino acid lysine that exerts its antifibrinolytic effect through the reversible blockade of lysine binding sites on plasminogen molecules.[53] Topical application of TXA to the bleeding surface has the potential to inhibit local fibrinolysis at the site of bleeding, reducing bleeding with minimal systemic effects.[53]

Topical TXA has been a popular addition to the emergency room treatment of epistaxis, but the evidence regarding its use is limited. A multicenter trial randomly assigned subjects to receive 10 to 20 minutes of treatment with either cotton soaked in 400 mg of TXA or Saline after both received initial management with compression or ice.[54] No difference among groups was found in bleeding cessation or in the need for packing over the next seven days.[54]

Nasal packing

If cautery is unsuccessful, nasal packing to tamponade local bleeding is the next step.[52] Several packing options are available and will vary based on your institution. Common products include nasal tampons, gauze packing, and nasal balloon catheters such as the Rapid Rhino.

If there is persistent bleeding after packing the bleeding naris, the contralateral naris may be packed, thereby providing a counterforce to promote tamponade.[52] Nasal packing in anterior bleeding has about a 90–95% success rate.[55] If bilateral packing fails, the odds of a posterior source increase greatly.[52]

If there is persistent bleeding after bilateral anterior packing, Emergent ENT consultation and posterior packing are indicated. Posterior packing can be achieved with specific posterior balloon catheters, but may not be readily available. As an readily available alternative a 10 to 14 French Foley catheter may be used.[56]

Patients with anterior packing are often discharged home with otorhinolaryngology follow-up in 24–48 hours. Despite the lack of proven efficacy many specialists recommend antibiotic prophylaxis for toxic shock syndrome.[57] Patients have commonly prescribed Augmentin, a first-generation cephalosporin, or topical Mupirocin for the duration of the packing.[57]

Many with a suspected posterior source and packing require hospitalization in a bed with cardiac monitoring.[52] Hospitalization allows for the close observation of rebleeding or dysrhythmias and assessment of the need for further intervention with surgery or angiographic embolization.[52]

CLINICS CARE POINTS

- Uncomplicated nasal fractures don't require imaging and can be discharged home with symptomatic care and ENT follow-up as necessary
- Septal hematomas if not drained can lead to irreversible septal necrosis and deformity
- Epistaxis management typically starts with an initial tamponade attempt with proper patient positioning and Afrin followed by cautery or packing if unsuccessful.

ESOPHAGEAL TRAUMA
Introduction

Esophageal traumatic injuries are rare and are often masked by other associated injuries, with most large trauma centers only treating a few cases a year.[58] It occurs more frequently with penetrating trauma, most commonly gunshot wounds.[59] Although traumatic esophageal perforations are rare they can be life-threatening. Therefore, emergency providers must be knowledgeable in their diagnosis and management.

Evaluation

The clinical signs and symptoms include dysphagia, neck pain, neck swelling, retrosternal fullness, hematemesis, odynophagia and subcutaneous emphysema.[60] However, these are not reliably present; therefore, it is critical for clinicians to maintain a high degree of suspicion based on the mechanism and the injuries' proximity to the esophagus.[60]

A CT of the neck is commonly obtained, however, the overall sensitivity for esophageal injury is low.[61] Given the limitations of CT, esophagoscopy and esophagography, a series of x-ray pictures of the esophagus taken after the patient drinks barium, are used to directly visualize esophageal injury and perforation.[62]

In patients who are clinically stable, flexible esophagoscopy is used first to establish the diagnosis of esophageal perforation.[62] If the endoscopy is not possible or the results are equivocal, then esophagography can be performed. In patients who are clinically unstable or intubated flexible esophagoscopy should be performed in the ICU or operating room.[62]

Management

A timely diagnosis is the key to management. Initial management includes securing the airway, given the association of airway injury, endoscopic assessment of the airway is often necessary.[3] Broad spectrum intravenous antibiotics should be administered covering aerobes and anaerobes.[3] When esophageal injury is diagnosed the definitive management will be determined by the patients clinical stability[63] Hemodynamically unstable patients will require emergent surgical exploration and repair.[63] Clinical stable patients may be managed nonoperatively.[63]

CLINICS CARE POINTS

- The clinical signs, symptoms, and CT imaging findings of esophageal injuries are not reliably present.

- Clinicians must have a high degree of suspicion of injury based on the mechanism and injury's proximity to the esophagus.

DISCLOSURE

The authors have nothing to disclose.

REFERENCES

1. Négrel AD, Thylefors B. The global impact of eye injuries. Ophthalmic Epidemiol 1998;5(3):143–69.
2. Ehlers JP, Shah CP. Trauma. Wills Eye Man 2008;5:12.
3. Romaniuk VM. Ocular trauma and other catastrophes. Emerg Med Clin North Am 2013;31(2):399–411.
4. Bagheri N, Wajda BN. Traumatic retrobulbar hemorrhage. Wills Eye Man 2017; 7:35.
5. Lima V, Burt B, Leibovitch I, et al. Orbital compartment syndrome: the ophthalmic surgical emergency. Ophthalmol 2009;54(4):441–9.
6. Sun M, Chan W, Selva D. Traumatic orbital compartment syndrome: Importance of the lateral canthotomy and cantholysis. Emerg Med Australasia 2014;26(3): 274–8.
7. Larner AJ. A dictionary of neurological signs. Switzerland: Springer; 2006. p. 48.
8. Thompson HS, Corbett JJ, Cox TA. How to measure the Relative Afferent Pupillary Defect. Druv Ophthalmol 1981;26:39–42.
9. Hayreh SS, Kolder WE, Weingeist TA. Central retinal artery occlusion and retinal tolerance time. Ophthalmology 1980;87:75–8.
10. Vassallo S, Hartstein M, Howard D, et al. Traumatic retrobulbar hemorrhage: emergent decompression by lateral canthotomy and cantholysis. J Emerg Med 2002;22(3):251–6.
11. Kuhn F, Morris R, Mester V, et al. Terminology of mechanical injuries: the birmingham eye trauma terminology. Ocul Traumatol 2008;5:3–12.
12. Colby K. Management of open globe injuries. Int Ophthalmol Clin 1999;39(1):59.
13. Crowell E, Koduri V, Supsupin E, et al. Accuracy of computed tomography imaging criteria in the diagnosis of adult open globe injuries by neuroradiology and ophthalmology. Acad Emerg Med 2017;24(9):1072–9.
14. Miller S, Fliotsos M, Justin G, et al. Global current practice patterns for the management of open globe injuries. Am J Ophthalmol 2022;(234):259–73.
15. Kresloff MS, Castellarin AA, Zarbin MA. Endophthalmitis. Surv Ophthalmol 1998; 43(3):193–224.
16. Huang JM, Pansick AD, Blomquist PH. Use of intravenous vancomycin and cefepime in preventing endophthalmitis after open globe injury. J Ocul Pharmacol 2016;7:437–41.
17. René C. Update on orbital anatomy. Eye 2006;20:1119–29.
18. Fujino T, Sugimoto C, Tajima S, et al. Mechanism of orbital blowout fracture: II. Analysis by high speed camera in two dimensional eye model. Keio J Med 1974;23:115–24.
19. Kersten RC. Blowout fracture of the orbital floor with entrapment caused by isolated trauma to the orbital rim. Am J Ophthalmol 1987;103:215–20.
20. Gart Michael, Gosain Arun. Evidence-based medicine: orbital floor fractures. Plast Reconstr Surg 2014;134(6):1345–55.

21. Cruz AA, Eichenberger GC. Epidemiology and management of orbital fractures. Curr Opin Ophthalmol 2004;15(5):416.
22. Brandt MT, Haug RH. Traumatic hyphema: a comprehensive review. J Oral Maxillofac Surg 2001;59:1492.
23. Katia C, Genadry, Shrock C, et al. Traumatic Hyphema. J Emerg Med 2021;61(6):740–1.
24. Sankar PS, Chen TC, Grosskreutz CL, et al. Traumatic hyphema. Int Ophthalmol Clin 2002;42(3):57.
25. Walton W, Von Hagen S, Grigorian R, et al. Surv. Management of traumatic hyphema. Surv Ophthalmol 2002;47(4):297.
26. Parrviz J, Peter AD, Azar N. Orbit. In: Surgical anatomy of head and neck. Harvard University Press; 2001. p. 150.
27. Brown DJ, Jaffe JE, Henson JK. Advanced laceration management. Emerg Med Clin North Am 2007;25:83.
28. Lavasani L, Leventhal D, Constantinides M, et al. Management of acute soft tissue injury to the auricle. Facial Plast Surg 2010;26(6):445–50.
29. Sabatino F, Moskovitz JB. Facial wound management. Emerg Med Clin North Am 2013;31(2):529–38.
30. Greywoode JD, Pribitkin EA, Krein H. Management of auricular hematoma and the cauliflower ear. Facial Plast Surg 2010;26(6):451.
31. Dalal P, Purkey M, Price C, et al. Risk factors for auricular hematoma and recurrence after drainage. Laryngoscope 2020;130(3):628–31.
32. Jones SE, Mahendran SJ. Interventions for acute auricular haematoma. Cochrane Database Syst Rev 2004;1465–75.
33. Riviello RJ, Brown NA. Otolaryngologic procedures. Clin Procedures Emerg Med 2010;5:1178.
34. Giles WC, Iverson KC, King JD, et al. Incision and drainage followed by mattress suture repair of auricular hematoma. Laryngoscope 2007;117(12):2097.
35. Brickman K, Adams DZ, Akpunonu P, et al. Acute management of auricular hematoma: a novel approach and retrospective review. Clin J Sport Med 2013;23(4):321.
36. Sagiv D, Migirov L, Glikson E. Traumatic perforation of the tympanic membrane: a review of 80 cases. J Emerg Med 2018;54:186–90.
37. Henry M, Hern GH. Traumatic injuries of the ear, nose and throat. Emerg Med Clin North Am 2018;37(1):131–6.
38. Orji FT, Agu CC. Determinants of spontaneous healing in traumatic perforations of the tympanic membrane. Clin Otolaryngol 2008;33(5):420.
39. Ort S, Beus K, Isaacson J. Pediatric temporal bone fractures in a rural population. Otolaryngol Head Neck Surg 2004;131(4):433.
40. Lasak J, Ess M, Kryzer T, et al. Penetrating middle ear trauma through the external auditory canal. Otolaryngology-head Neck Surg 2004;131(2):92.
41. Johnson F, Semaan MT, Megerian CA. Temporal bone fracture: evaluation and management in the modern era. Otolaryngol Clin North Am 2008;41(3):597.
42. Rhee SC, Kim YK, Cha JH. Septal fracture in simple nasal bone fracture. Plast Reconstr Surg 2004;113:45–52.
43. Basheeth N, Donnelly M, David S, et al. Acute nasal fracture management: a prospective study and literature review. Laryngoscope 2015;125(12):2677–84.
44. Mondin V, Rinaldo A, Ferlito A. Management of nasal bone fractures. J Otolaryngol 2005;26(3):181.
45. Sanyaolu L, Farmer S, Cuddihy P. Nasal septal haematoma. BMJ : Br Med J 2014;349.

46. Puricelli MD, Zitsch RP. Septal hematoma following nasal trauma. J Emerg Med 2016;50(1):121–2.
47. Kucik CJ, Clenney T. Management of epistaxis. Am Fam Physician 2005; 71(2):305.
48. Schlosser RJ. Clinical practice. Epistaxis. N Engl J Med 2009;360(8):784.
49. Abrich V, Brozek A, Boyle TR, et al. Risk factors for recurrent spontaneous epistaxis. Mayo Clin Proc 2014;89(12):1636–43.
50. Thaha MA, Nilssen EL, Holland S, et al. Routine coagulation screening in the management of emergency admission for epistaxis–is it necessary? J Laryngol Otol 2000;114(1):38.
51. Krempl GA, Noorily AD. Use of oxymetazoline in the management of epistaxis. Ann Otol Rhinol Laryngol 1995;104(9 Pt 1):704.
52. Mudunuri RK, Murthy MA. The treatment of spontaneous epistaxis: conservative vs cautery. J Clin Diagn Res 2012;6(9):1523.
53. Dunn CJ, Goa KL. Tranexamic acid: a review of its use in surgery and other indications. Drugs 1999;57(6):1005.
54. Reuben A, Appelboam A, Stevens KN, et al. The use of tranexamic acid to reduce the need for nasal packing in epistaxis (NoPAC): randomized controlled trial. Ann Emerg Med 2021;77(6):631.
55. Corbridge RJ, Djazaeri B, Hellier WP, et al. A prospective randomized controlled trial comparing the use of merocel nasal tampons and BIPP in the control of acute epistaxis. Clin Otolaryngol Allied Sci 1995;20(4):305.
56. McFerran DJ, Edmonds SE. The use of balloon catheters in the treatment of epistaxis. J Laryngol Otol 1993;107(3):197.
57. Rejas UE, Trinidad RG, Alvarez DJ, et al. Utility of the surgical treatment for severe epistaxis by endoscopic approach of sphenopalatine and ethmoidal arteries. Acta Otorrinolaringol Esp 2006;57(5):228.
58. Bryant AS, Cerfolio RJ. Esophageal trauma. Thorac Surg Clin 2007;17:63–72.
59. Xu AA, Breeze JL, Paulus JK, et al. Epidemiology of traumatic esophageal injury: an analysis of the national trauma data bank. Am Surg 2019;85(4):342.
60. Biff WL, Morre EE, Feliciano DV, et al. Western Trauma Association critical decisions in trauma: diagnosis and management of esophageal injuries. J Trauma Acute Care Surg 2015;79(6):1089–95.
61. Kazi M, Junaid M, Khan MJ, et al. Masoom Utility of clinical examination and CT scan in assessment of penetrating neck trauma. J Coll Physicians Surg Pak 2013; 23(4):308.
62. Srinivasan R, Haywood T, Horwitz B, et al. Role of flexible endoscopy in the evaluation of possible esophageal trauma after penetrating injuries. J Gastroenterol 2000;95(7):1725.
63. Petrone P, Kassimi K, Jiménez-Gómez M, et al. Management of esophageal injuries secondary to trauma. Inj 2017;48(8):1735–42.

High Stakes Pediatrics: Resuscitation and the MISFITS

Adam Broughton, MSc^PA, PA-C*

KEYWORDS

- Pediatric - Resuscitation - Critical - Sepsis - Seizure

KEY POINTS

- Clinicians can follow a sequential approach to the resuscitation of unstable or critically ill pediatric patients.
- Causes of critical illness in the pediatric population differ from the adult population.
- The use of the mnemonic MISFITS can remind clinicians of the unique causes of illness in neonates and infants.
- Treatment protocols for sepsis and seizure can aid in clinical care.

INTRODUCTION

Every presentation of a pediatric patient is high stakes considering the preciousness of life and the expected long life of the child. The following chapter focuses on initial treatments including the resuscitation of the undifferentiated critically ill pediatric patient followed by brief discussions of disease states in the pediatric population that are unique or differ slightly from adult emergency medicine (EM).

GENERAL APPROACH TO THE CRITICALLY ILL PEDIATRIC PATIENT

Background: To improve outcomes and begin resuscitation early, it is essential that the EM clinicians recognize the features of a critically ill neonate, infant, or child which may differ slightly from adolescents and adults including limited communication from the patient and potentially an incomplete history of events. Clinicians must quickly and accurately interpret visual clues, vital signs (VS), and physical examination findings to start early, aggressive resuscitation in undifferentiated shock without a complete history and before confirmatory testing and imaging.

Northeastern University, Department of Medical Sciences | Physician Assistant Program202 Robinson Hall, 360 Huntington Avenue, Boston, MA 02115, USA
* 28 Juniper Street, Wenham, MA 01984.
E-mail address: a.broughton@northeastern.edu

Physician Assist Clin 8 (2023) 95–108
https://doi.org/10.1016/j.cpha.2022.08.012
2405-7991/23/© 2022 Elsevier Inc. All rights reserved.

Pearls and Pitfalls: The first step in recognizing a potentially critically ill child is a careful examination of the vital signs. Pediatric vital signs vary by age as illustrated in **Table 1**. Even vital signs, however, can be misleading with most pediatric patients having robust cardiovascular reserves allowing them to maintain blood pressure (BP) within normal range while in early shock states, known as compensated shock. Unrecognized and untreated, this will lead to the "crashing patient" with sudden and precipitous drops in BP and cardiovascular collapse. This is known as decompensated shock defined by a low mean arterial pressure (MAP) resulting in global hypoperfusion often first manifested in an alteration in mental status. Goals for MAP will be discussed later and are listed in **Table 2**.

A declining mental status can also be difficult to interpret in patients with limited communication requiring careful history taking and physical examinations. Frequent re-evaluation looking for poor perfusion including skin changes and poor capillary refill as well as monitoring of vital signs, especially the heart and respiratory rate are crucial in the early identification of the critically ill pediatric patient.

The pediatric assessment triangle (PAT)[1] depicted in **Figure 1** is a rapid observational tool using visual clues to predict the etiology and severity of the undifferentiated sick child. It has been taught in the pediatric resuscitation curriculum and assessed in a prospective observational study[2] showing reliable identification of high-acuity patients and their category of illness. The PAT requires no equipment, only evaluation of the child's appearance, work of breathing, and circulation to the skin looking for the following features (**Fig. 1**):

1. *Appearance* – tone, interaction, consolable, look/gaze, speech cry (abbreviated TICLS)
2. Work of Breathing – abnormal sounds, positioning, retractions, nasal flaring, apnea/gasping
3. *Circulation* to skin – pallor, mottling, cyanosis

Using these 3 categories as representations of brain perfusion, respiratory status, and cardiovascular performance, a clinician can accurately predict the etiology of the undifferentiated sick infant. Most times, if all 3 are normal the patient is stable, while abnormal findings in 1, 2, all 3 categories can point toward a cause. Pure respiratory distress will have normal skin and brain perfusion, while respiratory failure will first result in altered mental status (AMS). Similarly, early cardiovascular impairments will lead to skin changes such as mottling, pallor, and poor capillary refill, followed by

Table 1 Normal pediatric vital signs				
Age	HR	SBP	DBP	RR
Premature	110–170	55–75/	/35–45	40–70
0–3 mo	110–160	65–85/	/45–55	35–55
3–6 mo	110–160	70–90/	/50–65	30–45
6–12 mo	90–160	80–100/	/55–65	22–38
1–3 y	80–150	90–105/	/55–70	22–30
3–6 y	70–120	95–110/	/60–75	20–24
6–12 y	60–110	100–120/	/60–75	16–22
>12 y	60–100	110–135/	/65–85	12–20

HR, heart rate, SBP, systolic blood pressure, RR, respiratory rate.

Table 2
Goal systolic blood pressure (SBP) and mean arterial pressure (MAP) for age

Age	Goal SBP > 5th Percentile for Age	Goal SBP > 50th Percentile for Age	Goal MAP at 50th Percentile
Newborn	>60	90	55 mm Hg
1–12 mo	>70	90	55 mm Hg
2 year old	>74	94	58 mm Hg
4 year old	>78	98	61 mm Hg
7 year old	>84	104	65 mm Hg
10 year old	>90	110	70 mm Hg

AMS in shock. A change in "Appearance" without any indication of respiratory or circulatory compromise points toward a metabolic cause such as hypoglycemia or a pure central nervous system (CNS) etiology.

Easy access to printed or digital reminders of pediatric VS and the PAT can be found online and make for great reminders, rather than relying on memory alone. Broselow tape is also a handy estimate of pediatric drug dosing that is often found in emergency departments with corresponding color-coded drawers for common medications.

PEDIATRIC RESUSCITATION

Introduction: Regardless of the cause of cardiopulmonary collapse, the steps in early resuscitation of the neonate, infant, and child are similar in each age group and aimed at restoring airway patency, normal breathing, and adequate circulation. Clinicians should be trained in and follow the protocols of Pediatric Advanced Life Support (PALS) with key elements highlighted here. This is not a substitute for certification in PALS and should be viewed as a summary.

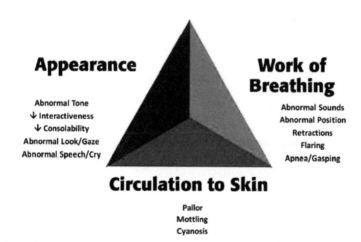

Fig. 1. The Pediatric Assessment Triangle and its components from Horeczko T, Enriquez B, McGrath NE, Gausche-Hill M, Lewis RJ. The pediatric assessment triangle: Accuracy of its application by nurses in the triage of children. Journal of emergency nursing. 2013;39(2):182-189; with permission (see **Fig. 1** in original).

Always consider sepsis as a cause of cardiovascular collapse, especially in the neonate under 30 days with a low threshold to give empiric broad-spectrum antibiotics early. Genetic abnormalities often show abnormal physiology in the first month of life and can result in hypoperfusion and shock states. Hypoglycemia is common in sepsis and in-born errors of metabolism.

INITIAL IMPRESSION

1. Using the Pediatric Assessment Triangle,[1] a provider can visually assess the child's appearance, circulation, and work of breathing to formulate a general idea of the cause of illness with visual clues of respiratory causes, CNS or metabolic etiology, cardiovascular collapse (shock), or complete cardiopulmonary failure (arrest).
2. Recognizing the critically ill neonate
   a. Poor perfusion – mottled/gray, delayed cap refill, tachycardic
   b Respiratory distress – grunting is auto-peep (may need positive pressure), tachypnea
   c Altered mental status (AMS) – lethargic, not responding to noxious stimuli
   d Poor tone – floppy baby

Vital signs: Vital signs vary dramatically by age with a quick reference later in discussion in **Table 1**.
Normal Vital Signs:

THE A, B, C, D², E² METHOD

Primary Assessment: The primary assessment includes the evaluation and management of the airway, breathing, circulation, (A, B, C) as well as a quick neurologic evaluation (disability = D) and exposure (E) of the skin to look for rashes or other clues. After exposure, including the diaper area and back, clinicians should ensure no further heat loss, especially in neonates as well as prevent hyperthermia. Because hypoglycemia can be a cause or a result of critical illnesses, early monitoring, and correction with dextrose (D) is essential, as are extra tests (E) depending on the presentation.

Because infants have low glucose reserves and may have unrecognized metabolic derangement, the early assessment and correction of hypoglycemia are encouraged. This can be expressed as an additional "D" for dextrose in the sequence of evaluation as well as an extra "E" for extra testing that needs to be addressed simultaneously, such as vascular access, abdominal examination, and focused assessment with sonography in trauma (FAST), obtaining urine and blood for cultures and laboratories, and so forth. This can easily be remembered as A, B, C, D², and E².

AIRWAY

- Assess for patency: start with maneuvers to open the airway (jaw-thrust, head-tilt, shoulder elevation for large occiput) being cautious not to excessively move the cervical spine if suspicious of trauma
- Remove obstructions or potential obstructions manually or with suction (food, foreign body). Upper airway obstructions tend to cause stridor and usually can be removed with McGill forceps if visualized. If there is stridor without visible obstruction, be cautious of epiglottis, larynx, or trachea foreign body or inflammation.
- Administer medications such as racemic epinephrine for croup with stridor. Consider epiglottitis or other dangerous causes of upper airway obstruction that may need controlled intubation.
- Do not delay the administration of intramuscular (IM) epinephrine for anaphylaxis.

BREATHING

- Assess rate and effort of breathing visually and auscultate for wheezing or rales that might be a clue to a diagnosis.
- Pulse oximetry assessment and oxygen intervention as needed. Provide 100% oxygen by nasal cannula if oxygen saturation is less than 94% or according to clinician judgment.
- Proceed to bag valve mask or positive pressure ventilation for continued hypoxia or poor ventilatory effort.
- If in respiratory failure, or concern for impending respiratory arrest, proceed to intubation as indicated. Be cautious in children with rapid respiratory rate due to metabolic acidosis because artificial ventilators may not be able to replicate the rate needed to compensate for acidosis.
- Initiate treatment of any conditions found to compromise respiration or ventilation such as albuterol and epinephrine for asthma.
- Monitor ventilation with end-tidal carbon dioxide if intubated or for the close assessment of potential ventilatory failure on supplemental oxygen that may have a rise in $CO2$ before a decline in oxygen.

CIRCULATION

- Assess perfusion through skin color, temperature, capillary refill, and strength of peripheral pulses.
- Auscultate heart sounds for clues to etiology.
- Measure blood pressure (BP) frequently.
- Early recognition of shock in pediatric patients is key because a drop in BP is usually a late finding with tachycardia and poor capillary refill seen early. Sepsis or anemia may have very high cardiac output yet produce shock. Low cardiac output will often be compensated early with increased heart rate, venous tone, arterial resistance, and inotropy that can result in a systolic BP (SBP) in the normal range.
- Decompensated shock is defined in PALS as the following, although clinicians should rely on experience and gestalt to start treatment early.
  - Goal systolic blood pressure (SBP) are calculated for <5th percentile = 70 mm Hg + (child's age in years x 2) SBP considered normal at 50th percentile = 90 mm Hg + (age in years x2).
  - It is recommended to maintain MAP between 5th and 50th percentile for age recommended by Surviving Sepsis Campaign[3] with insufficient evidence for a narrower recommendation. Aiming for a mean arterial pressure (MAP) at the 50th percentile may be preferable[4] (calculated as 55 + 1.5 x age in years). These are listed for quick reference in **Table 2**.
- Begin volume expansion as needed
  - Initial fluid bolus IV 10 to 20 mL/kg isotonic fluid
  - Transfuse PRBC 10 mL/kg if indicated
  - Follow massive transfusion protocol for trauma with hemorrhage.

DISABILITY

A rapid neurologic evaluation should include pupillary response to light and level of consciousness. The AVPU scale seen in **Table 3** assesses if the child is spontaneously alert, responsive to voice or pain only, or completely unresponsive is a rapid test for level of consciousness.

Table 3	
AVPU scale for level of consciousness	
A	**Awake**
V	Responds to verbal stimuli
P	Responds to painful stimuli
U	Unresponsive

The use of the Glasgow Coma Scale (GCS) in pediatric trauma patients ≤ 3 years old has not been shown to be very reliable[5] with routine intubation of trauma patients with a GCS of ≤ 8 possibly harmful.[6] Other more complex scoring systems such as the revised trauma score[7] (correlates strongly with patient survival and whether the patient should be transferred to a trauma center) or the pediatric age-adjusted shock index[8] can be used to identify severely injured children but are more cumbersome and offer less immediate guidance. These can be calculated in secondary or tertiary surveys.

DEXTROSE

Obtain rapid bedside glucose test and treatment with dextrose. The "Rule of 50" below is recommended by PALS[9] when treating for hypoglycemia to give 50 g of dextrose. Adults are typically given "1 amp" or 50 mL of D50, while infants and children should be given less concentrated solutions to avoid sclerosing the veins. A quick reference is found in **Table 4**.

If D10 W and D25 W are not available, dilution of D50 can easily be made[10] by using 10 mL of D50 with 40 mL of sterile water to create D10 W and 25 mL of D50 with 25 mL of sterile water to create D25 W, both a total volume of 50 mL.

EXPOSURE

All skin areas must be examined for any evidence of bruising, trauma, rashes, or other skin findings. Temperatures obtained with rectal temperatures are most accurate[11] and a reflection of core temperature under 5 years old.[12,13] This is also extremely important in the evaluation of nonaccidental trauma (NAT) discussed later.

EXTRA TESTING

A focused physical examination will include other areas not addressed in the airway, breathing, circulation primary assessment depending on the presentation and differential diagnosis considered. More extensive guidance will be given in the following section on common causes of critically ill pediatric presentations.

SECONDARY AND TERTIARY ASSESSMENT

This includes a focused history with caregivers and patient if possible. Key historical questions pertinent to the pediatric population are included here in **Table 5**.

Table 4			
Dextrose dosing in pediatric hypoglycemia			
Patient	**Dextrose Concentration**	**Dose**	**Concentration x Dose = 50**
Newborn/infant	D10 W	5 mL/kg	50
Child	D25 W	2 mL/kg	50
Adolescent	D50 W	1 mL/kg	50

Table 5
Helpful historical questions

Question	May Identify
Familial genetic/inherited diseases?	Congenital heart disease, cystic fibrosis, metabolic disorder
Prenatal care?	Genetic disorder (cystic fibrosis, muscular dystrophy, hemophilia A, kidney disease, sickle cell, Tay-Sachs, thalassemia), heart defect on ultrasound screening
Birth outside of hospital?	Lack of screening tests or vitamin K administration at birth
Preterm birth?	Risk factor for pulmonary diseases, serious bacterial infection, necrotizing enterocolitis, jaundice, anemia
Vaccinations since birth?	Risk for influenza, hepatitis B, hemophilus influenza, measles, pneumococcal disease, rotavirus, diphtheria, pertussis, rubella, varicella
Formula fed and how is formula mixed?	Hypotonic hydration, hypoglycemia
Sweating or crying when feeding?	Congenital heart disease
Hungry after feeding and vomiting?	Pyloric stenosis

By this time, a clinician may have a suspicion of etiology, nature, treatment of illness/injury and will order ancillary studies according to clinical suspicion. For the undifferentiated crashing pediatric patient or neonate, consider THE MISFITS[14] which is listed in **Table 6** with a brief description of treatment guidelines.

Table 6
Differential diagnosis of the undifferentiated neonate in distress

Trauma	A Wide Range of Presentation Should Be Treated according to ATLS Guidelines with Head Trauma a Leading Cause of Death
Hypovolemia and Heart disease	Volume expansion and Cardiovascular and arrhythmia management according to PALS guidelines
Endocrine	Consider congenital adrenal hypoplasia in fluid refractory shock, correct electrolyte and glucose abnormalities as needed
Metabolic	Check and correct glucose early, manage electrolyte and acid/base derangement
Inborn errors of metabolism	Rare, most diagnosed at birth, hypoglycemia is common, fluid resuscitation may be needed
Sepsis	Leading cause of neonatal mortality that requires rapid resuscitation and treatment
Intestinal catastrophes	Sometimes surgical emergencies that are unique to the pediatric population
Toxins	Consult Poison Control early, obtain ECG, glucose, and electrolytes early, extremely wide range of management
Seizures	Often simple self-resolving febrile seizure. Status epilepticus requires prompt management.

From the preceding list, several categories have highly specified treatments for the many different congenital abnormalities and pathologic states. Because sepsis is the leading cause of childhood death,[15] it will be discussed in detail later in discussion, along with the actively seizing pediatric patient.

SEPSIS

Pediatric Sepsis Protocol: The development of a pediatric sepsis protocol has been shown to improve outcomes even in hospitals with limited resources;[16] however, single screening tools and universal resuscitation bundles, especially in pediatric sepsis, remain controversial with weak evidence to support a single approach.[17] Despite this, the following are key points from the Surviving Sepsis Campaign[18] and Society of Critical Care Medicine.[19]

A 2-step process of first-contact triage nurse or provider screening with a system alert for a clinician evaluation.[17] The use of qSOFA is not recommended[18] with authors recommending the combination of triage evaluation, pediatric SIRS[20] and/or PEWS[21] score, in addition to risk factor screening.[17]

1) Initial laboratories and work-up may be dependent on the patient's age with most children who meet the definition of sepsis receiving the full work-up if no obvious source.
2) Obtain blood cultures before antibiotics unless it will delay antimicrobial therapy.
3) Empiric broad-spectrum antibiotics to cover all likely pathogens recommended within 60 minutes
   a) Previously healthy, immunocompetent children: Ceftriaxone (or Cefotaxime if under 1 month) AND Vancomycin.
   b) Immunocompromised or hospitalized patients should have antipseudomonal coverage (third or higher-generation cephalosporin ie, cefepime) AND a broad-spectrum carbapenem (meropenem, imipenem/cilastatin) OR extended range penicillin/beta-lactamase inhibitor (piperacillin/tazobactam)
   c) Neonates: consider ampicillin for listeria and acyclovir for HSV
4) Respiratory support:
   a) Treat hypoxia without respiratory distress with oxygen by face mask or high-flow nasal cannula
   b) Nasal CPAP can be considered in respiratory distress with hypoxia.
   c) For respiratory failure despite initial oxygenation or respiratory impending failure, intubate. RSI can cause significant hypotension so fluid resuscitation prior when able is best.
   d) Noninvasive ventilation can be considered in patients responding to therapy.
5) Airway management
   a) Trial of noninvasive ventilation is reasonable before RSI.
   b) Optimize RSI with adequate fluid resuscitation prior.
   c) Sedation – ketamine or fentanyl, avoid etomidate
   d) Succinylcholine or rocuronium
6) Fluid resuscitation should start within 30 minutes ideally.
   a) A bolus of 20 mL/kg IV crystalloid is the minimum starting dose.
   b) Start with 40 mL/kg especially for age over 2 years as this has been shown to decrease mortality.[22]
   c) Adult studies[23,24] favor balanced crystalloids (lactated ringers, Plasma-Lyte) over normal saline which can produce a metabolic acidosis in large volumes with clinical trials in pediatrics ongoing.[25]
7) Blood transfusion if hemoglobin of less than 7 g/dL. No clear guidelines above 7.

8) Maintain MAP between 5th and 50th percentile for age recommended by Surviving Sepsis Campaign[3] with insufficient evidence for a narrower recommendation. Aiming for a mean arterial pressure (MAP) at the 50th percentile may be preferable[4] (calculated as 55 + 1.5 x age in years). This goal at the 50th percentile is calculated later in discussion in **Table 7**.

9) Perfusion goals should include capillary refill of less than 2 seconds, normal pulses, warm extremities, urine output >1 mL/kg/h, normal glucose and ionized calcium, and normal mental status.

10) Central or peripheral inotropes should be started within 60 minutes, ideally as soon as refractory shock is recognized with the ability to titrate medications down if needed.

11) Inotropic support (pressors) include:
   a) Peripheral epinephrine at 0.05–0.3 μg/kg/min initially and can be given centrally if needed for "cold shock" with mottled, cool, vasoconstricted extremities
   b) Norepinephrine starting at 0.05 μg/kg can be used if "warm shock" seen in a vasodilated patient.
   c) Central dopamine titrated to a max of 10 μg/kg/min if unable to use epinephrine or norepinephrine.

12) Add IV hydrocortisone 2 mg/kg initially for fluid and vasopressor resistant hypotension[26] or known adrenal insufficiency which can be 2–3 mg/kg starting up to a maximum of 100 mg.

13) Monitor and support blood glucose greater than 50 and less than 180, and follow serial lactate and anion gap measures at least every hour. Continuous pulse oximetry, ECG and telemetry monitoring, core temperature, and urine output are all strongly recommended.

PEDIATRIC SEIZURE

Treatment: Management of acutely seizing child in the ED consists of the following:

1. Support brain oxygenation and cardiorespiratory function according to PALS guidelines including supplemental oxygen and airway management with positioning and intervention with RSI if needed for severe hypoxia or status epilepticus.[27]
2. Terminate seizure activity usually with benzodiazepine (lorazepam or diazepam) and a loading dose of phenytoin.[27]
3. Correct potential nonepileptic cause: hypoglycemia, infection, electrolyte imbalance, fever, or other causes.
4. Prevent and treat status epilepticus usually with barbiturate coma using thiopental.[27]

Table 7
Quick reference for goal MAP at 50th percentile of child of average height

Age	Calculation	Goal MAP
Newborn	55 + 1.5 x age in years	55 mm Hg
2 year old	55 + 1.5 x age in years	58 mm Hg
4 year old	55 + 1.5 x age in years	61 mm Hg
7 year old	55 + 1.5 x age in years	65 mm Hg
10 year old	55 + 1.5 x age in years	70 mm Hg

Table 8
Antiseizure medications

Medication	Route	Dose	Max
Lorazepam	IV	0.1 mg/kg	4 mg
Diazepam	IV/IO	0.15–0.2 mg/kg	10 mg
	Rectal	0.2–0.5 mg/kg	20 mg
	Buccal	0.5 mg/kg	10 mg
Midazolam	IM	0.2 mg/kg	10 mg
	Intranasal	0.2 mg/kg	10 mg
Valproic acid	IV/IO	20 mg/kg	3000 mg
Fosphenytoin	IV	20 PE*/kg	1500 PE[a]
Phenobarbital	IV	15–20 mg/kg	20 mg/kg
Levetiracetam	IV	30–60 mg/kg	4500 mg

[a] PE = phenytoin equivalents.

Treatment with antiepileptic drugs (AED) after a first seizure has not been shown to improve prognosis.[28] Treatment with AED after the first seizure may be considered in circumstances whereby the benefits of reducing the risk of a second seizure outweigh the risks of pharmacologic and psychosocial side effects which must be understood by the prescriber. There is a paucity of evidence to suggest the use of IV lorazepam over diazepam and if no IV access is available, buccal midazolam or rectal diazepam are acceptable.

STATUS EPILEPTICUS

Clinical practice: For seizures that persist despite treatment with benzodiazepine, and phenytoin and/or phenobarbitone, consider status epilepticus and treatment with thiopental (barbiturate coma) or continuous benzodiazepine drip. ED providers may be more comfortable with benzodiazepines such as diazepam at a starting dose of 0.01 mg/kg/min or midazolam infusion starting with 2 μg/kg/min up to 12 μg/kg/min.[28] Intravenous Valproate 30 mg/kg diluted 1:1 in normal saline over 2 to 5 min is an alternative to benzodiazepine drip. If still unsuccessful, Levetiracetam 40 mg/kg at 5 mg/kg/min can be infused after valproate before initiating thiopental coma.[27] Ketamine, lidocaine, and propofol are all alternative options with ketamine probably the most comfortable option for ED providers.

To simplify the approach, authors have suggested a sequential approach to the pediatric patient in status epilepticus like other "code" situations with algorithms like ACLS.[29] By drawing on other literature and evidence, a "seizure code" could simplify the approach with regard to variations in presentation and medication dosing. A summary of this plan adopted from the Neurocritical Care Society and American Epilepsy Society by Stredny and colleagues[29] is included here for quick reference.

1) Initial medication – IV lorazepam or diazepam. If IV access not available, rectal diazepam or intranasal or buccal midazolam.
2) Repeat benzodiazepine if seizure persists at 5 minutes.
3) At 10 minutes consider status epilepticus and add a second agent. Medications options include fosphenytoin, valproic acid, levetiracetam, or phenobarbital.
4) Consult pediatric neurology.
5) At 15 minutes, continuous seizure may be treated with a repeat dose of the second agent chosen, switch to a different agent above, or start continuous infusion. **Table 8** shows the initial and maximum dosing of common seizure medications by the route.

SUMMARY

The crashing pediatric patient, including neonates, requires immediate action to correct pathologic states leading to airway, breathing, and cardiovascular compromise. The most common cause of mortality in infants and children remains sepsis which should be promptly considered and treated. Pediatric seizures present in a much different fashion but can be equally anxiety provoking. A systemic approach to both can aid providers in performing excellent pediatric resuscitation.

CLINICS CARE POINTS

- Care of the critically ill pediatric patient can be anxiety provoking, and clinicians can benefit from a simplified approach focusing on the core principles of resuscitation.
  - Pitfall: Avoid becoming preoccupied with recognition and treatments for rare pediatric illnesses while forgetting to address the basics of emergency medicine
- The first step is the recognition of compensated and decompensated shock states requiring early intervention.
  - Pitfall: Do not rely on BP and MAP alone to recognize shock as children usually have robust cardiovascular reserves that maintain BP until a precipitous crash.
- The Pediatric Assessment Triangle is a validated, rapid observational tool to quickly delineate a potential cause of undifferentiated shock.
  - Pitfall: Trying to memorize normal vital signs can be difficult and delay rapid evaluation and intervention.
- The A, B, C, D2, and E2 sequence in neonatal and pediatric resuscitation is a memory aid for airway, breathing, circulation, disability, dextrose, exposure, and extra tests.
  - Pitfall: Neonates can exhaust glucose reserves and lose body heat rapidly, thus correcting hypoglycemia and preventing hypothermia should be part of resuscitation.
- For the undifferentiated crashing pediatric patient or neonate, consider THE MISFITS: Trauma, Hypovolemia and Heart disease, Endocrine diseases, Metabolic derangements, Inborn errors of metabolism, Sepsis, Intestinal catastrophes, Toxin exposure, and Seizures. Of these, sepsis is the leading cause of pediatric death.
  - Pitfall: Do not delay early broad-spectrum antibiotics and lab tests and cultures necessary for the diagnosis and treatment of sepsis while waiting for confirmatory testing.
- Perfusion goals in septic shock include a MAP between the 5th and 50th percentile, capillary refill of less than 2 seconds, normal pulses, warm extremities, urine output >1 mL/kg/h, normal glucose and ionized calcium, and normal mental status.
  - Pitfall: Do not delay early, aggressive IV fluid resuscitation starting at 20 mL/kg with 40 mL/kg recommended over the age of 2.
- Inotropic support in septic shock should be started within 60 minutes or whenever a refractory shock is recognized.
  - Pitfall: Adrenal insufficiency can be a missed cause of fluid and vasopressor-resistant hypotension.
- A sequential approach to actively seizing pediatric patient, much like other algorithms such as ACLS, can result in better outcomes.
  - Pitfall: Do not delay the administration of benzodiazepines in seizing children with buccal midazolam and rectal diazepam available.

DISCLOSURE

The authors have nothing to disclose.

REFERENCES

1. Dieckmann RA, Brownstein D, Gausche-Hill M. The pediatric assessment triangle: A novel approach for the rapid evaluation of children. Pediatr Emerg Care 2010;26(4). https://doi.org/10.1097/PEC.0b013e3181d6db37. Available at: https://pubmed-ncbi-nlm-nih-gov.ezproxy.neu.edu/20386420/. Accessed February 17, 2022.

2. Horeczko T, Enriquez B, McGrath NE, et al. The pediatric assessment triangle: Accuracy of its application by nurses in the triage of children. J Emerg Nurs 2013;39(2):182–9.

3. SCCM | pediatric patients. Society of Critical Care Medicine (SCCM) Web site. Available at: https://sccm.org/SurvivingSepsisCampaign/Guidelines/Pediatric-Patients. Accessed February 26, 2022.

4. Haque IU, Zaritsky AL. Analysis of the evidence for the lower limit of systolic and mean arterial pressure in children. Pediatr Crit Care Med 2007;8(2):138–44. https://doi.org/10.1097/01.PCC.0000257039.32593.DC. Accessed March 26, 2022.

5. DiBrito SR, Cerullo M, Goldstein SD, et al. Reliability of glasgow coma score in pediatric trauma patients. J Pediatr Surg 2018;53(9):1789–94. https://doi.org/10.1016/j.jpedsurg.2017.12.027. Available at: https://www.sciencedirect.com/science/article/pii/S0022346818300101. Accessed Apr 11, 2022.

6. Jakob DA, Lewis M, Benjamin ER, et al. Isolated traumatic brain injury: Routine intubation for glasgow coma scale 7 or 8 may be harmful. J Trauma Acute Care Surg 2021;90(5):874–9. https://doi.org/10.1097/TA.0000000000003123. Available at: https://journals.lww.com/jtrauma/Abstract/2021/05000/Isolated_traumatic_brain_injury__Routine.13.aspx. Accessed April 11, 2022.

7. Eichelberger MR, Gotschall CS, Sacco WJ, et al. A comparison of the trauma score, the revised trauma score, and the pediatric trauma score. Ann Emerg Med 1989;18(10):1053–8. https://doi.org/10.1016/S0196-0644(89)80930-8. Available at: https://www.sciencedirect.com/science/article/pii/S0196064489809308. Accessed April 11, 2022.

8. Reppucci ML, Phillips R, Meier M, et al. Pediatric age-adjusted shock index as a tool for predicting outcomes in children with or without traumatic brain injury. J Trauma Acute Care Surg 2021;91(5):856–60. https://doi.org/10.1097/TA.0000000000003208. Available at: https://journals.lww.com/jtrauma/Abstract/2021/11000/Pediatric_age_adjusted_shock_index_as_a_tool_for.13.aspx. Accessed April 11, 2022.

9. Kleinman ME, Chameides L, Schexnayder SM, et al. Part 14: Pediatric advanced life support. Circulation 2010;122(18_suppl_3):S876–908. https://doi.org/10.1161/CIRCULATIONAHA.110.971101. Available at: https://www.ahajournals.org/doi/full/10.1161/CIRCULATIONAHA.110.971101. Accessed February 17, 2022.

10. Young TP, Borkowski CS, Main RN, et al. Dextrose dilution for pediatric hypoglycemia. Am J Emerg Med 2019;37(10):1971–3. https://doi.org/10.1016/j.ajem.2019.03.054. Available at: https://www.sciencedirect.com/science/article/pii/S0735675719302207. Accessed April 11, 2022.

11. Siberry GK, Diener-West M, Schappell E, et al. Comparison of temple temperatures with rectal temperatures in children under two years of age. Clin Pediatr (Phila) 2002;41(6):405–14. https://doi.org/10.1177/000992280204100605. Available at: https://pubmed.ncbi.nlm.nih.gov/12166792/. Accessed February 15, 2022.

12. Reynolds M, Bonham L, Gueck M, et al. Are temporal artery temperatures accurate enough to replace rectal temperature measurement in pediatric ED patients? J Emerg Nurs 2014;40(1):46–50. https://doi.org/10.1016/j.jen.2012.07.007. Available at: https://pubmed.ncbi.nlm.nih.gov/23142099/. Accessed February 15, 2022.

13. Mogensen CB, Wittenhoff L, Fruerhøj G, et al. Forehead or ear temperature measurement cannot replace rectal measurements, except for screening purposes. BMC Pediatr 2018;18(1):15. https://doi.org/10.1186/s12887-018-0994-1. https://www.ncbi.nlm.nih.gov/pubmed/29373961.

14. S Am, LI N. The critically ill infant with congenital heart disease. Emerg Med Clin North Am 2015;33(3). https://doi.org/10.1016/j.emc.2015.04.002. Available at: https://www-clinicalkey-com.ezproxy.neu.edu/#!/content/playContent/1-s2.0-S0733862715000267?returnurl=null&referrer=null. Accessed February 28, 2022.

15. Harley A, Schlapbach LJ, Johnston ANB, et al. Challenges in the recognition and management of paediatric sepsis — the journey. Australas Emerg Care 2022; 25(1):23–9.

16. Medeiros DNM, Mafra AC, Nunes C, Carcillo JA, et al. A pediatric sepsis protocol reduced mortality and dysfunctions in a brazilian public hospital. Front Pediatr 2021;0. https://doi.org/10.3389/fped.2021.757721. Available at: https://www.frontiersin.org/articles/10.3389/fped.2021.757721/full. Accessed February 26, 2022.

17. Cruz, Lane, Balamuth, et al. Updates on pediatric sepsis. J Am Coll Emerg Physicians Open 2020;1(5):981.

18. Evans L, Rhodes A, Alhazzani W, et al. Surviving sepsis campaign: International guidelines for management of sepsis and septic shock 2021. Crit Care Med 2021;49(11):e1063. https://doi.org/10.1097/CCM.0000000000005337. Available at: https://journals.lww.com/ccmjournal/Fulltext/2021/11000/Surviving_Sepsis_Campaign__International.21.aspx. Accessed February 27, 2022.

19. Davis AL, Carcillo JA, Aneja RK, et al. American college of critical care medicine clinical practice parameters for hemodynamic support of pediatric and neonatal septic shock. Crit Care Med 2017;45(6):1061–93. https://doi.org/10.1097/CCM.0000000000002425. Available at: https://www.ncbi.nlm.nih.gov/pubmed/28509730.

20. Goldstein B. Pediatric SIRS, sepsis, and septic shock criteria. MDCalc Web site. Available at: https://www.mdcalc.com/pediatric-sirs-sepsis-septic-shock-criteria. Accessed February 27, 2022.

21. Monaghan A. Pediatric early warning score (PEWS). MDCalc Web site. Available at: https://www.mdcalc.com/pediatric-early-warning-score-pews. Accessed February 27, 2022.

22. Oliveira CF, Nogueira de Sá, Flávio R, et al. Time- and fluid-sensitive resuscitation for hemodynamic support of children in septic shock: Barriers to the implementation of the american college of critical care medicine/pediatric advanced life support guidelines in a pediatric intensive care unit in a developing world. Pediatr Emerg Care 2008;24(12):810–5. https://doi.org/10.1097/PEC.0b013e31818e9f3a. Available at: https://pubmed.ncbi.nlm.nih.gov/19050666/. Accessed February 27, 2022.

23. Rochwerg B, Alhazzani W, Gibson A, et al. Fluid type and the use of renal replacement therapy in sepsis: A systematic review and network meta-analysis. Intensive Care Med 2015;41(9):1561–71. https://doi.org/10.1007/s00134-015-3794-1. Accessed February 27, 2022.

24. Annane D, Siami S, Jaber S, et al. Effects of fluid resuscitation with colloids vs crystalloids on mortality in critically ill patients presenting with hypovolemic shock: The CRISTAL randomized trial. JAMA 2013;310(17):1809–17. Accessed February 26, 2022.
25. Weiss SL, Balamuth F, Long E, et al. PRagMatic pediatric trial of balanced vs nOrmaL saline FlUid in sepsis: Study protocol for the PRoMPT BOLUS randomized interventional trial. Trials 2021;22(1):776. Accessed February 26, 2022.
26. Noori S, Friedlich P, Wong P, et al. Hemodynamic changes after low-dosage hydrocortisone administration in vasopressor-treated preterm and term neonates. Pediatrics 2006;118(4):1456–66. Accessed February 27, 2022.
27. Sasidaran K, Singhi S, Singhi P. Management of acute seizure and status epilepticus in pediatric emergency. Indian J Pediatr 2011;79(4):510–7. Available at: https://link.springer.com/article/10.1007/s12098-011-0604-9.
28. Hirtz D, Berg A, Bettis D, et al. Practice parameter: Treatment of the child with a first unprovoked seizure. Approved by Qual Stand Subcommittee 2003;60(2).
29. Stredny CM, Abend NS, Loddenkemper T. Towards acute pediatric status epilepticus intervention teams: Do we need "Seizure codes". Seizure (London, England) 2018;58:133–40.

Obstetric Emergency Update

Severe Acute Respiratory Syndrome COVID-19 and Hypertension

Lori J. Stack, MD[a], Allisyn Brady, PA-C[b],*

KEYWORDS

- COVID-19 • Pregnancy • Assessment • Management • Preeclampsia
- Gestational hypertension • Severe hypertension of pregnancy • Eclampsia

KEY POINTS

- Pregnant women are at higher risk of COVID-19 infection, severe disease, morbidity, and mortality than their nonpregnant counterparts; fetal risks include preterm delivery, cesarean delivery, and stillbirth.
- A high index of suspicion is essential because symptoms of COVID-19 can be mistaken for or may mimic physiologic conditions and complications of pregnancy.
- Assessment and management of COVID-19-positive pregnancies should follow the ACOG and Society for Maternal-Fetal Medicine guidelines.
- Hypertension in the pregnant or postpartum patient should be immediately recognized and addressed because Hypertension (systolic >140 mm Hg and/or diastolic >90 mm Hg) in the pregnant or postpartum patient it is a leading contributor to both maternal and perinatal morbidity and mortality.
- Hypertension in pregnancy and the postpartum period (up to 12 months after delivery) can be habringers of cardiovascular disease, stroke, renal failure, and eclamptic seizures.
- Although the postpartum period is typically considered to be from birth to up to 6 weeks afterward, hypertension and cardiovascular complications may arise as late as 12 months after delivery.

SEVERE ACUTE RESPIRATORY SYNDROME CORONAVIRUS 2 AND PREGNANCY
Introduction

Much of the study of severe acute respiratory syndrome coronavirus 2 (SARS-COV-2) remains in its infancy, especially regarding pregnancy. Although the absolute risk of

[a] Center for Fetal Diagnosis and Treatment, Children's Hospital of Philadelphia, 3401 Civic Center Boulevard, Philadelphia, PA 19104, USA; [b] Cambridge Health Alliance, Department of Obstetrics and Gynecology, 1493 Cambridge Street, Cambridge, MA 02139, USA
* Corresponding author. Department of Obstetrics and Gynecology, Cambridge Health Alliance, 8 Camelia Avenue, Cambridge, MA 02139.
E-mail address: albrady@challiance.org

Physician Assist Clin 8 (2023) 109–122
https://doi.org/10.1016/j.cpha.2022.08.010
2405-7991/23/© 2022 Elsevier Inc. All rights reserved.

physicianassistant.theclinics.com

severe morbidity and mortality remains low, data from the Centers for Disease Control and Prevention indicate that the risk for both intensive care unit (ICU) admission and invasive ventilation in pregnant symptomatic women is increased 3-fold compared with nonpregnant symptomatic women,[1] whereas the risk of extracorporeal membrane oxygenation is increased 2.4-fold and the risk of death from coronavirus disease 2019 (COVID-19) is increased by 70%. Women with comorbidities, those older than 35 years, and Latina and black women are all at increased risk for adverse maternal outcomes.[2] Severe-critical disease in pregnancy is associated with worse outcomes, and the Delta variant brought additive risk for severe-critical disease and death.[2,3]

The care of all COVID-19-positive pregnant patients requires a high index of suspicion and meticulous follow-up planning. Management of severe-critical patients requires complex care by a team including obstetrics, maternal-fetal medicine, neonatology, critical care, infectious disease, and obstetric anesthesiology.[3]

Immunology and Physiology of Pregnancy

Immunologic changes that occur routinely in pregnancy may lead to worse outcomes in COVID-19-positive women. Researchers at Johns Hopkins University noted a reduced antiviral antibody response in COVID-19-positive pregnancies.[4] In addition, the immune response in pregnancy naturally heightens cellular/innate immunity, which functions to prevent the fetus from being seen as "foreign." However, the compensatory or relative decrease in adaptive/humoral immunity leaves the mother more susceptible to infection. These changes may predispose pregnant women to increased severity with COVID-19 infection.[5]

Many of the normal physiologic changes of pregnancy leave expectant mothers with limited reserve as well as symptoms resembling those of COVID-19. Again, it is essential to consider many of these symptoms as ramifications of COVID-19 until proven otherwise. That is to say, the symptoms should not be considered as those of normal pregnancy without seeing and evaluating the patient. **Table 1** delineates important physiologic changes of pregnancy that place expectant mothers at increased risk when infected with COVID-19.[6]

COVID-19-Related Complications in Pregnancy

COVID-19 brought significant additional risk of specific pregnancy complications including venous thromboembolism, hypertensive disorders of pregnancy, cesarean delivery, preterm birth, and stillbirth.

Venous thromboembolism includes cerebral venous sinus thrombosis, arterial thrombosis, cerebral vascular accident, pulmonary embolism, and deep vein thrombosis. A study by the National Institute of Child Health and Human Development Maternal Fetal Medicine Units Network reported thromboembolism rates in severe-critical, mild-moderate, and asymptomatic pregnant women with COVID-19 as 6%, 0.2%, and 0%, respectively.[7]

Hypertensive disorders, including hemolysis, elevated liver enzymes, low platelets (HELLP) syndrome, eclampsia, preeclampsia with or without severe features, gestational hypertension, and chronic hypertension with superimposed preeclampsia, were present in 40.4% of pregnancies with severe-critical disease versus 18.8% of pregnancies with asymptomatic COVID-19 positivity.[6] Although an elevated incidence in severe-critical disease may be anticipated, it is crucial to note that the risk of hypertensive disease is significantly elevated in asymptomatic, COVID-19-positive pregnancies. Many of the laboratory abnormalities seen with COVID-19 will be the same as those seen with hypertensive complications of pregnancy. It is essential to determine the cause of these laboratory abnormalities because treatment will differ

Table 1
Physiologic changes of pregnancy that place expectant mothers at increased risk during coronavirus disease infection

	Cardiovascular	Effect
Increased	Plasma volume by 40–50%, but erythrocyte volume by only 20%	Dilutional anemia results in decreased oxygen-carrying capacity
	Heart rate by 15–20 bpm	Increased CPR circulation demands
	Clotting factors susceptible to thromboembolism	Increased CPR circulation demands
	Dextrorotation of the heart	Increased ECG left axis deviation
	Estrogen effect on myocardial receptors	Supraventricular arrhythmias
Decreased	Supine blood pressure and venous return with aortocaval compression	Decreases cardiac output by 30%
		Susceptible to cardiovascular insult
	Arterial blood pressure by 10–15 mm Hg	Sequesters blood during CPR
		Susceptible to third spacing
	Systemic vascular resistance	Susceptible to pulmonary edema
	COP	
	PCWP	

	Respiratory	Effect
Increased	Respiratory rate (progesterone mediated)	Decreased buffering capacity
		Rapid decrease of Pao_2 in hypoxia
	Oxygen consumption by 20%	Decreased buffering capacity
	Tidal volume (progesterone mediated)	Compensated respiratory alkalosis
		Failed intubation
	Minute ventilation	Failed intubation
	Laryngeal angle	Difficult nasal intubation
	Pharyngeal edema	
	Nasal edema	
Decreased	Functional residual capacity by 25%	Decreases ventilatory capacity
	Arterial Pco_2	Decreases buffering capacity
	Serum bicarbonate	Compensated respiratory alkalosis

	Gastrointestinal	Effect
Increased	Intestinal compartmentalization	Susceptible to penetrating injury
Decreased	Peristalsis, gastric motility	Aspiration of gastric contents
	Gastroesophageal sphincter tone	Aspiration of gastric contents

	Uteroplacental	Effect
Increased	Uteroplacental blood flow by 30% of cardiac output	Sequesters blood in CPR
		Decreases cardiac output by 30%
	Aortocaval compression	Aspiration of gastric contents
	Elevation of diaphragm by 4–7 cm	
Decreased	Autoregulation of blood pressure	Uterine perfusion decreases with drop in maternal blood pressure

Abbreviations: COP, colloid oncotic pressure; CPR, cardiopulmonary resuscitation; ECG, electrocardiography; PCWP, pulmonary capillary wedge pressure.

depending on the underlying etiology. The diagnosis and management of hypertension in pregnancy are robust topics deserving significant attention; therefore the subject is discussed in detail later in this article.

Cesarean birth occurred in 59.6% of severe-critical disease pregnancies compared with 11.9% of asymptomatic patients.[7] Preterm delivery has been documented in 16.4% to 41.8% of pregnancies with severe-critical disease, depending on the reporting entity.[2,7] Some of the early data may have been skewed by iatrogenic causes versus spontaneous preterm labor. More than 1.25 million women have delivered since the onset of COVID-19 in the United States. A recent retrospective study revealed an increased risk of severe maternal morbidity and mortality from obstetric causes (i.e. ICU admission and blood transfusion of 4 or more liters) in Covid positive pregnancies.[8] Data collected between March 2020 and September 2021 show that the adjusted relative risk of stillbirth was 0.59 before COVID-19, whereas that risk increased to 1.47 in the period before the arrival of the Delta variant. Within the Delta-predominant period, relative risk further increased to 4.4 or 2.07% of COVID-19-positive pregnancies.[9]

Triage

American College of Obstetricians and Gynecologists/Society for Maternal-Fetal Medicine Outpatient Assessment and Management for Pregnant Women with Suspected or Confirmed COVID-19 provides the current guidelines for triage. This flowsheet should be followed for guidance with assessment, triage, intensified outpatient monitoring, transfer to obstetric unit or ICU, or transfer to outside facility (**Fig. 1**).

Patient Evaluation

The patient should be assessed in an isolation room, and the patient should wear a mask. Health care workers should maintain droplet and contact precautions using gowns, gloves, masks, face shields, and goggles. N-95 masks have been reserved for cesarean delivery, second stage of labor, operating room (O.R) management of postpartum hemorrhage, and intubation.[3]

Clinical risks and exposure history should be assessed. Pregnancy alone is a risk factor for poor outcomes. Importantly, outcomes worsen in those with hypertensive

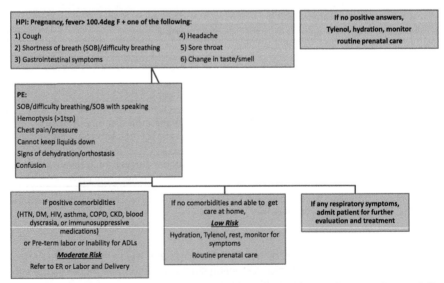

Fig. 1. HPI-history of present illness, SOB-shortness of breath, HTN-hypertension, DM-diabetes, COPD-chronic obstructive pulmonary disease, ADL-activities of daily living. *Adapted from* ACOG, Outpatient Assessment and Management for Pregnant Women With Suspected or Confirmed Novel Coronavirus (COVID-19).

disorders (preexisting or pregnancy-induced), chronic cardiopulmonary disease, diabetes (preexisting or gestational), obesity, renal disease, advanced maternal age, cancer, sickle cell disease, body mass index greater than 35 kg/m^2; immunocompromised state, and tobacco use.[10]

Physical Examination

Upon presentation, vital signs should be promptly obtained, including pulse oximetry reading. The normal oxygen saturation as measured by pulse oximetry (Spo$_2$) in a healthy pregnant woman is greater than or equal to 94% on room air. Also, the degree of hypoxia is often worse than what the clinical symptoms may suggest.[11] Fetal heart monitoring should be initiated if estimated gestational age is greater than or equal to 24 weeks. Supine positioning should be avoided to allow adequate blood flow to the fetus, especially after 24 weeks' gestation. A routine physical examination should be performed with detailed attention to lungs and heart. Laboratory parameters should be obtained including the following:

- Expedited COVID-19 polymerase chain reaction (PCR) test upon arrival (be aware that PCR can be false-negative; therefore, treat any symptomatic pregnant patient as if they are PCR positive)
- Complete blood cell count to evaluate for thrombocytopenia/hemolysis
- Comprehensive medical panel for abnormal liver function tests
- Arterial blood gases in patients with low SpO$_2$ (normal pregnancy values differ from those of nonpregnant patients. Normal first-trimester values: pH, 7.42–7.46; Pao$_2$, 105–106; Paco$_2$, 28–29; serum HCO$_3$, 18. Normal third-trimester values: pH, 7.43; Pao$_2$, 101–106; Paco$_2$, 26–30; serum HCO$_3$ 17.[6]
- Urine protein or protein/creatinine ratio in patients with suspicion for gestational hypertension/preeclampsia
- Prothrombin time/partial thromboplastin time/international normalized ratio
- Ferritin levels in the presence of concern for cytokine storm[10]

D-dimer is naturally elevated in pregnancy and is thus not useful. Chest radiograph, if indicated, should be performed with an abdominal shield.

An obstetrician should be notified immediately of any PCR-positive patient or patient under investigation and any abnormality in vital signs, physical examination, or radiologic or laboratory studies.

Disease Severity and Disposition

Table 2 outlines disease severity, symptoms, findings, and appropriate disposition for COVID-19-positive pregnant women.

Management

Therapeutic options
In general, the National Institutes of Health COVID-19 treatment guideline therapies that would be given otherwise should not be withheld in the treatment of COVID-19-positive pregnant/lactating women. Still, it is prudent to consult an obstetrician before initiating medical therapy.

- Antenatal steroids for the sole purpose of fetal lung maturity: Use with caution and only before 34 weeks' gestation.[5]
- Anticoagulants in ICU setting. Consider in all hospitalized COVID-19-positive patients.[5]

Table 2
Severity scale for COVID-19 in pregnancy[9]

Severity at Presentation	Findings/Symptoms	Disposition
Asymptomatic	• Positive PCR test • No symptoms	• Home with precautions and daily self-monitoring, consider home pulse oximeter and/or BP cuff, prompt and regular follow-up with OB. • Be seen if increased SOB; tachypnea; unremitting temperature > 39°C; SpO_2 < 95%: nontolerance of medications or fluids; confusion/lethargy; pleuritic chest pain; cyanotic lips/fingertips; preterm contractions, vaginal bleeding or decreased fetal movement[9,10]
Mild disease	• Positive test • Flulike symptoms without dyspnea, shortness of breath, or abnormal chest imaging findings	• Home with precautions. • IV fluids if indicated • Consider home pulse oximeter and/or BP cuff • Admit if unable to tolerate p.o. • Prompt follow-up with OB
Moderate disease	• $SpO_2 \geq 95\%$ on room air • Evidence of lower respiratory tract disease with dyspnea, pneumonia on imaging, abnormal blood gases, or refractory temperature $\geq 39°C$	• Admit for maternal/fetal assessment and treatment on obstetric unit • Consider antibiotics for pneumonia, avoid quinolones if possible • Consider anticoagulation to prevent venous thromboembolism • Consider delivery for standard fetal indications
Severe disease	• $SpO_2 \leq 94\%$ on room air • Respiratory rate >30 bpm • Po_2/Fio_2 < 300 mm Hg[10] • >50% lung involvement on imaging	• Admit to ICU with consults • Include management listed under moderate disease
Critical disease	• Multiorgan failure or dysfunction • Shock	• Admit to ICU with multispecialty care team • Include management under moderate disease • Need for ventilation or high-flow nasal canula[9]

Abbreviations: BP, blood pressure; bpm, beats per minute; Fio_2, fraction of inspired oxygen; IV, intravenous; OB, obstetrician; p.o., per mouth; SOB, shortness of breath.

Adapted from Society For Maternal Fetal Medicine Management Considerations for Pregnant Patients With COVID-19 Developed with Guidance from Torre Halscott, MD, MS, Jason Vaught, MD, and Emily Miller, MD, MPH. 6-16-2020 (this is an update of the draft originally posted on 4-30-20).

• Antibiotics for the treatment of pneumonia are acceptable. Try to avoid quinolones.
• Acetaminophen: Consider as the first-line analgesia in milder cases.

- Nonsteroidal anti-inflammatory drugs: Consider over opioids for additional analgesia with obstetric consult. Opioids may pose higher clinical risk.[3]
- Avoid nitrous oxide in suspected or confirmed patients with COVID-19.
- Oxygen: Consider in the presence of maternal hypoxia. Consider for fetal indications.
- Magnesium sulfate: For seizure prophylaxis only in preeclampsia with severe features. Consider risk of eclampsia versus risk of respiratory depression.[3] Seizure prophylaxis dose is 4-6g load over 20-30 minutes followed by 2 g/h.
- Monoclonal antibodies: Accepted treatment of infected as well as inadequately vaccinated exposures
- Remdesivir: Accepted[2]
- Dexamethasone: If indicated, use fetal lung maturity dosing for the first 2 days of use if less than 34 weeks' gestation.[5]
- Baricitinib: If patient meets clinical US Food and Drug Administration (FDA) qualifications[2]
- Tocilizumab: If patient meets clinical FDA qualifications.[2]
- Paxlovid: If patient meets clinical FDA qualifications.[12]

Obstetric Management

Obstetric care/intervention for COVID-19-positive patients without severe-critical disease is similar to that for non-COVID-19 pregnancies. In less severe disease, induction of labor and cesarean delivery are reserved for normal obstetric indications. The risks of preterm delivery versus the risk of prolonged fetal hypoxemia should be considered in cases of prolonged maternal hypoxemia.[3]

Postpartum Management

Decision regarding keeping the infant with or separated from a COVID positive or COVID suspected mother should be made on a case by case basis by the mother and the care team.[8] The mother should be monitored/advised of potential COVID-19 complications up to 6 weeks postpartum.

HYPERTENSION IN PREGNANCY AND POSTPARTUM
Introduction

Hypertension in the pregnant or postpartum patient should be immediately recognized and addressed because it is a leading contributor to both maternal and perinatal morbidity and mortality.[13]

In pregnancy and the postpartum period, the diagnosis of hypertension is defined as systolic blood pressure equal to or greater than 140 mm Hg and/or a diastolic pressure equal to or greater than 90 mm Hg in at least two readings more than 4 hours apart.[13] Although most diagnoses of postpartum hypertension disorders are made within weeks of delivery, signs and symptoms can present as late as one year after birth.[14] For nonobstetric providers in the urgent care and emergency setting, it is crucial for enhanced awareness of hypertension in pregnancy and the potential for late presentation in the postpartum setting.

There are several classifications of hypertension in pregnancy (**Table 3**).[15] Each one of these classifications have their own indications for timing of delivery and also postpartum follow-up. Any patient with a diagnosis of hypertension in pregnancy, despite the classification, could develop preeclampsia and has the potential to develop severe range blood pressures. For the pregnant or postpartum patient, severe range blood pressures are defined as systolic blood pressure greater than or equal to 160 mm

Table 3
Classification of hypertensive disorders in pregnancy

Disorder	Characteristics
Chronic hypertension	Systolic blood pressure of 140 mm Hg or greater, diastolic blood pressure of 90 mm Hg or greater, or both known to predate consumption or detected before 20 wk of gestation
Gestational hypertension	New-onset hypertension that develops after 20 wk of gestation; in the absence of proteinuria[a]
Preeclampsia-eclampsia	Development of hypertension presenting after 20 wk of gestation with proteinuria[a]; in the absence of proteinuria, preeclampsia can manifest as new-onset hypertension with any of the following features: thrombocytopenia, renal insufficiency, impaired liver function, pulmonary edema, or cerebral or visual symptoms; eclampsia is the presence of new-onset grand mal seizures in a pregnant woman with preeclampsia
Chronic hypertension with superimposed preeclampsia	The onset of features diagnostic of preeclampsia in a woman with chronic hypertension beyond 20 wk of gestation

[a] Proteinuria is defined as 300 mg or more of protein in 24-h urine collection or the ratio of measured protein level to creatinine level in a single voided urine collection that equals or exceeds 3 (each measured as mg/dL), termed the protein-to-creatinine ratio.
Reprinted with permission from Schmitz PG, Nguyen T. Hypertension. Clin Update Womens Health Care 2016;XV(1):1–114. Available at: https://www.acog.org/clinical/journals-and-publications/clinical-updates.

Hg and/or diastolic blood pressure greater than or equal to 110 mm Hg and should be immediately identified to determine which treatment is warranted. This severe hypertension for pregnant and postpartum patients will give them the diagnosis of preeclampsia with severe features.[13] Consideration should be given to any severe range blood pressure because it could be a sign of preeclampsia and impending eclampsia and should be treated to prevent congestive heart failure, myocardial ischemia, renal injury or failure, and ischemic or hemorrhagic stroke.[13] The parameters of severe hypertension are much lower in pregnant and postpartum patients than the general population.

DISCUSSION
Gestational Hypertension

Gestational hypertension is defined as elevation in blood pressure after 20 weeks gestation, two elevations more than 4 hours apart, in a patient with no previous history of hypertension.[13] These patients do not have laboratory abnormalities or proteinuria; however, they are monitored closely and could develop preeclampsia. In fact, patients with gestational hypertension are managed similarly to patients with preeclampsia and may not be distinguishable. Patients with gestational hypertension should have a way of monitoring their blood pressure and be aware of any signs or symptoms of preeclampsia, because any patient with gestational hypertension could move on to develop preeclampsia and/or severe hypertension.

Chronic Hypertension

Patients who have been identified as having hypertension before 20 weeks' gestation are thought to have a history of chronic hypertension. Chronic hypertension can just

---

Box 1
Diagnostic criteria for preeclampsia

Blood pressure:
- Systolic blood pressure of 140 mm Hg or more or diastolic blood pressure of 90 mm Hg or more on two occasions at least 4 hours apart after 20 weeks' gestation in a woman with a previously normal blood pressure
- Systolic blood pressure of 160 mm Hg or more or diastolic blood pressure of 110 mm Hg or more. (Severe hypertension can be confirmed within a short interval (minutes) to facilitate timely antihypertensive therapy.)
and

Proteinuria
- 300 mg or more per 24-hour urine collection (or this amount extrapolated from a timed collection) or
- Protein/creatinine ratio of 0.3 mg/dL or more or
- Dipstick reading of 2+ (used only if other quantitative methods not available)

Or in the absence of proteinuria new-onset hypertension with the new onset of any of the following:
- Thrombocytopenia: Platelet count less than $100,000 \times 10^9$/L
- Renal insufficiency: Serum creatinine concentrations greater than 1.1 mg/dL or a doubling of the serum creatinine concentration in the absence of other renal disease
- Impaired liver function: Elevated blood concentrations of liver transaminases to twice normal concentration
- Pulmonary edema
- New-onset headache unresponsive to medication and not accounted for by alternative diagnoses or visual symptoms

Adapted from ACOG practice bulletin Number 222: Gestational hypertension and preeclampsia, June 2020.

---

be a history of hypertension before pregnancy, or if someone has not been diagnosed with a hypertensive disorder before pregnancy but present early in their pregnancy before 20 weeks' gestation with hypertension.[16] Patients with chronic hypertension can develop superimposed preeclampsia, so they should be monitored for signs and symptoms of preeclampsia. These patients should also have baseline laboratory test results including evaluation for proteinuria to see if there are any underlying signs of end-organ damage and can also be used if these laboratory values change during their pregnancy.

Preeclampsia/Eclampsia

Preeclampsia is defined as elevated blood pressure on two occasions (more than 4 hours apart) with proteinuria, usually after 20 weeks' gestation. Patients can become preeclamptic without having proteinuria based on certain laboratory values or symptoms alone (preeclampsia with and without severe features: **Boxes 1** and **2**).[13] There are two types of preeclampsia: preeclampsia without severe features and preeclampsia with severe features. A patient having "preeclampsia without severe features" needs to be monitored closely. Should a patient develop severe range blood pressure on two readings greater than 4 hours apart, the diagnosis becomes "preeclampsia with severe features," which requires treatment with magnesium sulfate for seizure and eclampsia prophylaxis. Two documented severe range blood pressures or persistent severe range blood pressure also requires immediate treatment with antihypertensive medication (**Tables 4** and **5**).[13] A repeat blood pressure should be obtained within 15 minutes of any severe range reading to ensure proper diagnosis and treatment.

Box 2
Preeclampsia with severe features

- Systolic blood pressure of 160 mm Hg or more, or diastolic blood pressure of 110 mm Hg or more on two occasions at least 4 hours apart (unless antihypertensive therapy is initiated before this time)
- Thrombocytopenia (platelet count <100,000 $\times$ 10^9/L)
- Impaired liver function that is not accounted for by alternative diagnoses and as indicated by abnormally elevated blood concentrations of liver enzymes (to more than twice the upper limit of normal concentrations), or by severe persistent right upper quadrant or epigastric pain unresponsive to medications
- Renal insufficiency (serum creatinine concentration more than 1.1 mg/dL or a doubling of the serum creatinine concentration in the absence of other renal disease)
- Pulmonary edema
- New-onset headache unresponsive to medication and not accounted for by alternative diagnoses
- Visual disturbances

Adapted from ACOG practice bulletin Number 222: Gestational hypertension and preeclampsia, June 2020.

Preeclampsia with severe features can also be defined with certain laboratory thresholds and would require magnesium sulfate treatment (see **Box 2**).[13] Preeclampsia can happen not only during pregnancy but also in the postpartum period; this can be confusing because the cure for preeclampsia is thought to be delivery of the baby. However, someone could present with initial signs for a diagnosis of preeclampsia with or without severe features once the baby is delivered up until 6 weeks and

Table 4
Antihypertensive agents used for urgent blood pressure control in pregnancy

Drug	Dose	Comments	Onset of Action
Labetalol	10–20 mg IV, then 20–80 mg every 10–30 min to a maximum cumulative dosage of 300 mg or constant infusion 1–2 mg/min IV	Tachycardia is less common with fewer adverse effects. Avoid in women with asthma, preexisting myocardial disease, decompensated cardiac function, and heart block and bradycardia	1–2 min
Hydralazine	5 mg IV or IM, then 5–10 mg IV every 20–40 min to a maximum cumulative dosage of 20 mg or constant infusion 0.1–10 mg/min IV	Higher or frequent dosage associated with maternal hypotension, headaches, and abnormal fetal heart rate trackings; may be more common than other agents	10–20 min
Nifedipine (immediate release)	10–20 mg orally, repeat in 20 min if needed; then 10–20 mg every 2–6 h; maximum daily dose is 180 mg	May observe reflex tachycardia and headaches	5–10 min

Abbreviations: IM, intramuscularly; IV, intravenously.

Table 5 Serum magnesium concentration and toxicities			
mmol/L	mEq/L	mg/dL	Effect
2–3.5	4–7	5–9	Therapeutic range
>3.5	>7	>9	Loss of patellar reflexes
>5	>10	>12	Respiratory paralysis
>12.5	>25	>30	Cardiac arrest

Data from Duley L.Magnesium Sulphate regimens for women with eclampsia: message from the Collaborative Eclampsia Trial. Br J Obstet Gynaecol 1996;103:103-5 and Lu Jf, Nightigale CH. Magnesium sulfate in eclampsia and pre-eclampsia: pharmacokinetic principles. Clin Pharmacokinet 2000;38:305-14.

From ACOG Practice bulletin number 222: Gestational Hypertension and Preeclampsia, June 2020.

sometimes up until one year postpartum. Therefore, even in a postpartum patient, preeclampsia should be considered and treated as such.

Severe Hypertension

It is especially important to pay attention to severe range blood pressures because these thresholds are different for pregnant and postpartum patients. If a patient has blood pressures that are severe they need to be addressed immediately, sometimes within minutes. Sustained severe range blood pressure within 15 minutes warrants treatment. There are several different antihypertensives that are given to control severe range blood pressures in pregnancy (see **Table 4**).[13] There is no one antihypertensive medication that is preferred over another to control severe hypertension in pregnancy.[17] The decision can be made clinically. For example, if a patient presents and does not have intravenous (IV) access, one could consider oral nifedipine for immediate treatment. However, for all these patients IV access is indicated and should be started as soon as possible.

Dosing should be continued if the blood pressure continues to be in the severe range (see **Table 4**).[13] Any pregnant patient who has severe range blood pressure is diagnosed with severe hypertension whether it is preeclampsia (now with severe features) or severe gestational hypertension. Whenever giving an antihypertensive for a patient with severe range blood pressures, magnesium sulfate should also be given secondary to the risk of eclampsia for seizure prevention.

Preventing Eclampsia

Once a patient develops preeclampsia with severe features, magnesium sulfate should be started for seizure prophylaxis. The usual dosage of magnesium sulfate is 4-6 g IVPB loading dose followed by 2 g/h IVPB.[18] Magnesium sulfate should be given intrapartum until birth, and then continued for 24 hours postpartum. When administering magnesium sulfate, attention must be paid to clinical signs of magnesium toxicity, including loss of deep patellar reflexes and respiratory depression.[18] Magnesium needs to reach a level for therapeutic treatment, but should be discontinued if there is concern for toxicity (see **Table 2**).[13]

EVALUATION AND WORKUP FOR HYPERTENSIVE PREGNANT AND POSTPARTUM PATIENTS

Keeping all the classifications for hypertension of pregnancy in mind, one must be on alert for any blood pressure elevations in a pregnant or postpartum patient.

Signs and Symptoms

Preeclampsia can present with one or more of the following both during pregnancy and the postpartum period:

- Headache
- Visual changes, including scotomata
- Epigastric and/or right upper quadrant pain
- Edema, dependent or otherwise
- Shortness of breath
- Chest pain
- Nausea and/or vomiting
- Hyperreflexia

Laboratory Values

The following laboratory tests may be helpful in determining the diagnosis:

- Complete blood cell count: thrombocytopenia
- Renal studies: elevated creatinine
- Liver function tests: twice the upper limit of normal range
- Coagulopathy
- Proteinuria: protein/creatinine urine ratio greater than 0.30 mg/dL or 24-hour urine collection for protein greater than 300 mg.

SUMMARY

Pregnant and postpartum patients with COVID-19 and hypertension may present differently than the general populations. These patients are at high risk, in particular while pregnant because fetal outcomes need to be considered; however, they are still vulnerable and at risk postpartum up to one year after delivery. There is an interesting correlation between the fact that pregnant patients with COVID-19, whether symptomatic or asymptomatic, have a high rate of hypertensive disorders. More than 60% of pregnancy-related deaths are considered preventable[19]; significant attention should be paid to the pregnant and postpartum populations.

CLINICS CARE POINTS

- An SpO2 of less than 95% is abnormal in pregnancy and requires assessment and treatment of both the maternal and fetal dyad.
- Remember that in caring for a pregnant woman, you are caring for TWO patients, three if a twin gestation.
- Magnesium sulfate loading dose for seizure prophylaxis is 4 or 6gm IVPB, after 2gm/hour IVPB.
- Blood pressure of greater or equal to 140 systolic or greater than or equal to 90 diastolic is abnormal in a pregnant woman and requires further evaluation.
- Blood pressures of greater than or equal to 160 systolic or greater than or equal to 110 diastolic is consistent with preeclampsia with severe features and requires both antihypertensive therapy and seizure prophylaxis if persistent.
- Contrary to popular belief that the "postpartum period" is six weeks, it actually persists for 12 months, and pregnancy complications must be considered in any woman presenting within that time frame.

DISCLOSURE

L.J. Stack has no disclosures to declare. A. Brady has no disclosures to declare.

REFERENCES

1. Society for Maternal-Fetal Medicine. Provider considerations for engaging in COVID-19 vaccine counseling with pregnant and lactating patients. 2022. Available at: http://www.smfm.org; https://www.smfm.org/covidclinical. Accessed February 21, 2022.
2. Society for Maternal-Fetal Medicine. Coronavirus (COVID-19) and Pregnancy: What Maternal-Fetal Medicine Subspecialists Need to Know. 2020. Available at: http://www.smfm.org; https://www.smfm.org/covidclinical. Accessed February 21, 2022.
3. Society for Maternal-Fetal Medicine and Society for Obstetric and Anesthesia and Perinatology. Labor and Delivery COVID-19 Considerations. 2020. Available at: http://www.smfm.org; https://www.smfm.org/covidclinical. Accessed February 21, 2022.
4. Sherer ML, Lei J, Creisher PS, et al. Pregnancy alters interleukin-1 beta expression and antiviral antibody responses during severe acute respiratory syndrome coronavirus 2 infection. Am J Obstet Gynecol 2021;225(3):301.e1-14.
5. PeriFACTS OB/GYN Academy. Activity # 22001P. Available at: http://www.urmc.rochester.edu/institute-innovative-education/center-experiential-learning/perifacts.aspx. January 2022. Accessed February 21, 2022.
6. ACOG Practice Bulletin No. 211: Critical Care in Pregnancy. Obstet Gynecol 2019;133(5):e303–19.
7. Metz TD, Clifton RG, Hughes BL, et al. Disease severity and perinatal outcomes of pregnant patients with coronavirus disease 2019 (COVID-19). Obstet Gynecol 2021;137(4):571.
8. Society for Maternal-Fetal Medicine. COVID-19 and Pregnancy: What Maternal-Fetal Medicine Subspecialists Need to Know. Available at http://www.smfm.org. Accessed January 10, 2022.
9. DeSisto CL, Wallace B, Simeone RM, et al. Risk for stillbirth among women with and without COVID-19 at delivery hospitalization—United States, March 2020–September 2021. Morbidity Mortality Weekly Rep 2021;70(47):1640.
10. Society for Maternal-Fetal Medicine. Management considerations for pregnant patients with COVID-19. 2020. Available at: http://www.smfm.org; https://www.smfm.org/covidclinical 2020. Accessed February 21, 2022.
11. Society for Maternal-Fetal Medicine. Practical Guidance for Treating Pregnant Persons With COVID-19 in Resource-Limited Settings: Early Lessons From the US Epidemic. 2020. Available at: http://www.smfm.org; https://www.smfm.org/covidclinical 2020. Accessed February 21, 2022.
12. Society for Maternal-Fetal Medicine. FDA Issues EUA for the Treatment of Mild-to-Moderate COVID-19. 2021. Available at: http://www.smfm.org; https://www.smfm.org/2021press. Accessed February 21, 2022.
13. American College of Obstetrics and Gynecology: Gestational Hypertension and Preeclampsia: Practice Bulletin Number 222, June 2020. Available at: https://www.acog.org/clinical/clinical-guidance/practice-bulletin/articles/2020/06/gestational-hypertension-and-preeclampsia. Accessed February 21, 2022.
14. Pregnancy Mortality Surveillance System. In: Center for Disease Control and Prevention. Available at: https://www.cdc.gov/reproductivehealth/maternal-mortality/pregnancy-mortality-surveillance-system.htm. Accessed February 21, 2022.

15. American College of Obstetrics and Gynecology: Hypertension, Clinical updates in Women's Health Care, January 2016. Available at: https://www.acog.org/clinical/journals-and-publications/clinical-updates/2016/01/hypertension. Accessed February 21, 2022.
16. American College of Obstetrics and Gynecology: Chronic Hypertension in Pregnancy: Practice Bulletin Number 203 January 2019. Available at: https://www.acog.org/clinical/clinical-guidance/practice-bulletin/articles/2019/01/chronic-hypertension-in-pregnancy. Accessed February 21, 2022.
17. Duley L, Meher S, Jones L. Drugs for treatment of very high blood pressure during pregnancy. Cochrane Database Syst Rev 2013;(7):CD001449.
18. Euser A, Cipolla M. Magnesium Sulfate treatment for the prevention of eclampsia: A brief review. Stroke 2009. Available at: https://www.ncbi.nlm.nih.gov/pmc/articles/PMC2663594/. Accessed February 21, 2022.
19. Building US. Capacity to Review and Prevent Maternal Deaths. Report from nine Maternal Mortality Review Committees 2018. https://www.cdcfoundation.org/sites/default/files/files/ReportfromNineMMRCs.pdf. Accessed February 21, 2022.

The Management of Infectious Pulmonary Processes in the Emergency Department: Pneumonia

Kasey Dillon, DScPAS, PA-C*, Betsy Garnick, PA-S,
Meghan Fortier, PA-S, Belinda Felicia, PA-S, Alison Fulton, PA-S,
Courtney Dumont, PA-S, Brooke Dorval, PA-S,
Katherine Gardella, PA-S

KEYWORDS

- Pneumonia • Bacterial pneumonia • Community-acquired pneumonia
- COVID-19 pneumonia • Viral pneumonia • Fungal pneumonia

KEY POINTS

- Pneumonia is a common disease process, and emergency medicine providers will be required to accurately diagnosis and manage pneumonia.
- The 3 primary types of pneumonia are bacterial, viral, and fungal.
- Since 2019, SARS-CoV-2 has greatly increased the percentage of patients being seen in emergency departments for symptoms consistent with pneumonia.
- Diagnostic and management guidelines have been established for community-acquired bacterial pneumonia, COVID-19 viral pneumonia, and fungal pneumonia.

INTRODUCTION

In the United States, pneumonia accounts for approximately 2.2% of emergency department visits per year. A significant percentage of those patients can be safely managed at home, not requiring admission.[1] Age, male gender, and the presence of complicating comorbidities increase the likelihood of requiring hospitalization, and therefore, increase the disease burden.[1,2] Bacterial, viral, and fungal pathogens can cause infectious pneumonia. The cause, clinical presentation, and treatment recommendations for each class of pathogens are reviewed. Although nosocomial respiratory infections are prevalent, they will not be discussed in this article. In addition, the revised guidelines established in 2019 for the diagnosis and treatment of community-acquired pneumonia (CAP) recommend that the nosocomial pneumonia classification, also known as health care–associated pneumonia or hospital-acquired pneumonia, be

MCPHS University, 1260 Elm Street, Manchester, NH 03110, USA
* Corresponding author.
E-mail address: Kasey.dillon@mcphs.edu

Physician Assist Clin 8 (2023) 123–137
https://doi.org/10.1016/j.cpha.2022.08.005

abandoned and that recommendations for management be based on severity and epidemiologic data alone.[3]

Community-acquired bacterial pneumonia remains a leading cause of death worldwide with a mortality as high as 24.8 per 10,000 cases in the United States and between 1.5 and 14 cases per 1000 people globally.[2,4] Prevalence varies based on season, population characteristics, and geographical factors. Streptococcus pneumoniae and Haemophilus influenzae are the leading causes of bacterial pneumonia worldwide. The most common symptoms of cough, fever, and dyspnea are a result of pathogens being transmitted to the lower-respiratory tract via the pharynx. There is, however, significant heterogeneity within the clinical profile of bacterial pneumonia. Evaluation, treatment recommendations, and guidelines have been established and are considered the standard of care for emergency medicine providers.[2,4]

Viral community–acquired pneumonia has an equal prevalence among children and adults with approximately 100 million cases annually in each group.[5] There is consensus that viral pneumonias are underdiagnosed; however, given the availability and sensitivity of molecular diagnostic tests, the gap may be closing. One in 3 CAP are a result of a viral cause, most commonly rhinoviruses, influenza viruses, and coronaviruses.[5] There is risk of bacterial coinfection, making diagnosis and targeted treatment a challenge. In individual circumstances, neuraminidase inhibitors are recommended for influenza-specific pneumonia; however, a clear consensus does not exist for algorithmic management when concerned about bacterial overlap.[5,6] Although sufficient data exist to support the recommended management of SARS-CoV-2 pneumonia, a provider must approach COVID-19 pneumonia with caution given the relative paucity of data and the frequency of iterations in guidelines and suggestions.[6] Given current global epidemiologic trends, this article dedicates the discussion of viral pneumonias primarily to SARS-CoV-2.

Pneumonias secondary to a fungal pathology are rare in immunocompetent individuals but pose life-threatening risk to those with a compromised immune response. Patients with immunodeficiency disorders, such as HIV/AIDS, or patients receiving immunosuppressive therapy are at higher risk for developing fungal respiratory infections. In developed countries, opportunistic pathogens, such as Candida or Cryptococcus, are increasing in prevalence, as the survival rate of the susceptible population groups increases. Similar to bacterial resistance to antibiotics, there has been an emergence of resistant fungal pathogens to typical treatment, making management of these infections challenging.[7,8] Although not nearly as prevalent as viral or bacterial CAP, it is important that emergency medicine providers consider the possibility of fungal infection in an at-risk patient population so as to ensure early diagnosis and effective treatment.

Community-Acquired Bacterial Pneumonia

Epidemiology
In the United States, CAP accounts for more than 5 million cases of pneumonia per year. Eighty percent of these cases are treated through outpatient management, whereas the remaining 20% of individuals require hospitalization. Incidences of CAP are higher in the male and African American populations. Mortality is greater in women. The incidence rate of CAP increases with the extremes of age, and in the United States, CAP carries a mortality of 7.3%.[3–5]

Cause
CAP is categorized, and treated, based on the cause of "typical" or "atypical" organisms. S pneumoniae, H influenzae, Staphylococcus aureus, and group A streptococci

are 4 of the most common typical organisms causing CAP. Atypical pneumonia can be caused by organisms such as Legionella, *Mycoplasma pneumoniae*, and *Chlamydia pneumoniae*. *S pneumoniae* and *K pneumoniae* are the most common causes of CAP. Methicillin-resistant *Staphylococcus aureus* (MRSA) is the most common cause of health care–associated pneumonia, whereas ventilator-associated pneumonia has a high prevalence of multidrug-resistant bacteria. In recent years, there has been an increase in overall antimicrobial resistance by gram-negative bacteria most commonly found in patients with severe CAP, which substantially increases morbidity, mortality, and health care–associated cost.[4] Bacterial pathogens causing CAP often coexist with viral pathogens, making initial management challenging at best.[3,4]

Clinical presentation
Given the heterogeneity of CAP, the clinical presentation of individuals will vary. The last 10 years, however, have shown substantial expansion of evidence-based data to support the diagnosis and treatment of CAP based on improved and rapid diagnostic testing as well as an increase in understanding of differentiated symptoms based on type of causative agent.[3] The hallmark symptoms of community-acquired bacterial pneumonia include cough, with or without yellow/green sputum production, fever, chills, pleuritic chest pain, and potential confusion in the elderly. Patients may also experience the less-specific symptoms of fatigue, headaches, and feelings of malaise.[9] Progression of bacterial pneumonia can be more rapid than viral or fungal pathogens and, therefore, may produce symptoms representative of systemic involvement, including tachycardia, hypotension, and altered mental status. Atypical pathogens causing CAP are likely to cause extrapulmonary symptoms related to gastrointestinal upset, including nausea, vomiting, or diarrhea.[3,9]

Diagnosis/treatment
Early and accurate diagnosis of CAP is crucial in order to initiate targeted therapy while decreasing unnecessary exposure, and therefore possible resistance or adverse reaction, to antibiotics.[9] Following the physical examination, laboratory diagnostic testing, radiographic imaging, and clinical decision making are crucial components in the diagnosis of CAP.[4,9,10] Clinical decision-making tools are recommended for use in prognosis and to guide the management of patients with pneumonia. They also assist in disposition planning from the emergency department, guiding decision making for individual hospital admission or discharge home. The Pneumonia Severity Index (PSI) is preferential because of the moderate quality of evidence available to support its efficacy over the CURB-65 (confusion, urea level, respiratory rate, blood pressure, and age >65). The PSI demonstrates a higher predictive value as compared with the CURB-65. Clinician judgment must always be integrated into decision making, as predictive tools can oversimplify and do not consistently consider patient variables.[3,9]

   In 2019, the Infectious Diseases Society of America (IDSA) and the American Thoracic Society (ATS) established revised guidelines for the diagnosis and treatment of CAP. Criteria are outlined for determining severe CAP based on the following minor and major symptoms and diagnostic findings[3,4,11]:

- Sputum cultures: Recommended only in patients meeting criteria for severe disease, especially if requiring mechanical ventilation. There is lack of evidence to support the use of sputum cultures in outpatient settings.
- Blood cultures: Recommended in patients meeting criteria for severe disease, those being treated empirically for MRSA or *Pseudomonas aeruginosa*, those with a history of MRSA or *P aeruginosa*, or those hospitalized within the past 90 days. These recommendations do have a low quality of evidence, although

blood cultures continue to remain part of most institutional clinical pathways in the diagnosis of CAP. Given the overlap of CAP and sepsis, utilization of blood cultures is appropriate. Data prove that positive blood cultures within 10 hours of admission have shown an increased risk of mortality; however, only 40% of blood cultures drawn at initial presentation are positive.

- Molecular diagnostic testing/polymerase chain reaction testing: Recommended testing for influenza and SARS-CoV-2 based on local transmissibility data and prevalence. Molecular diagnostic tests have an overall 70% to 80% sensitivity rate and 99% to 100% specificity rate, therefore isolating cases of viral or atypical bacterial cause.
- Legionella and pneumococcal urinary antigen testing (UAT): Recommended only in the patient with severe CAP or in cases of high epidemiologic concern/recent travel (Legionella).
- Imaging: Chest computed tomography (CT) is considered the gold standard in detection of both CAP and viral pneumonia; however, cost, accessibility, and radiation continue to be limiting factors. Chest radiograph alone has a sensitivity of 38% to 76%; however, when combined with molecular testing, sensitivity and specificity increase. Ultrasonography has been shown to have sensitivity rates of 80% to 90% in the detection of pneumonia. The IDSA/ATS guidelines no longer recommend routine use of chest radiograph in follow-up after a pneumonia diagnosis.

In all patients where community-acquired bacterial pneumonia is likely, empiric therapy is recommended. Risk assessment should be used to determine if treatment can be conducted in an outpatient or inpatient setting. As stated, the PSI and CURB-65 clinical assessment tools are effective and recommended guidelines used in beginning treatment decisions. The CURB-65 and PSI help estimate mortality risk in CAP based on various risk factors associated with worse outcomes.[9] Treatment decisions vary greatly owing to differences in risk assessment outcomes indicated, comorbidities, and likelihood of MRSA infection. **Tables 1** and **2** outline the recommended outpatient and in-hospital initial treatments for CAP.[3]

Prognosis

Outcomes of treatment largely depend upon age of onset, hospitalization status with treatment, and the presence of comorbidities. The overall mortality for pneumonia may be up to 30% if left untreated. Overall prognosis, however, is tremendous in a healthy patient. Most individuals respond to treatment within 48 to 72 hours of initial management, both in hospital and at home. Respiratory failure, sepsis, organ failure, coagulopathy, and exacerbation of comorbidities are complications to consider as a result of CAP.[9]

Table 1
Empiric treatment of outpatient community-acquired pneumonia

	Recommended Treatment
No comorbidities/risk factors for MRSA or pseudomonas	Amoxicillin OR doxycycline OR macrolide
With comorbidities	Augmentin or cephalosporin AND macrolide or doxycycline OR monotherapy with respiratory fluoroquinolone

Adapted from Ramirez JA, File, TM, Bond S. UpToDate. Overview of community-acquired pneumonia. Sept 7, 2021. Accessed March 1, 2022.

| Table 2 | | | |
| Empiric treatment of inpatient community-acquired pneumonia | | | |
	Standard	**Prior MRSA**	**Prior Pseudomonas**
Nonsevere inpatient	B-Lactam + macrolide[a] OR respiratory fluoroquinolone[b]	Add MRSA coverage[c]	Add pseudo coverage[d]
Severe inpatient	B-Lactam + macrolide[a]		

[a] Ampicillin and sulbactam, cefotaxime, ceftriaxone, ceftaroline, AND azithromycin or clarithromycin.
[b] Levofloxacin or moxifloxacin.
[c] Per 2016 ATS/IDSA guidelines: vancomycin or linezolid.
[d] Per 2016 ATS/IDSA guidelines: piperacillin-tazobactam, cefepime, ceftazidime, imipenem, meropenem, or aztreonam.
   Adapted from Ramirez JA, File, TM, Bond S. UpToDate. Overview of community-acquired pneumonia. Sept 7, 2021. Accessed March 1, 2022.

Community-Acquired Viral Pneumonia

Epidemiology

As stated, viral pneumonia is discussed, with reference only to pneumonia caused b the SARS-CoV-2 virus. At the time of publication, there have been more than 470 million confirmed cases of COVID-19 globally with more than 6 million deaths reportedy to the World Health Organization (WHO) and to the Centers for Disease Control and Prevention (CDC).[12] Currently, 10 vaccines have been granted an emergency use listing by the WHO. Worldwide vaccination rates are highest in countries like Canada, Chile, and Australia with countrywide vaccination greater than 90%. Sub-Saharan Africa has the lowest overall population vaccination rates at less than 10%, and China does not report vaccination rates. The United States has an overall nationwide vaccination rate of 70%.[13] Vaccination compliance is determined by factors such as availability, vaccination hesitancy, and political or religious affiliation.

Before the COVID-19 pandemic, common viral causes of pneumonia included influenza A and B, human boca viruses, coronaviruses NL63 and HKU1, and respiratory syncytial virus (commonly in children).[5] Although these viral illnesses remain, SARS-CoV-2 pneumonias have contributed to a majority of viral pneumonias worldwide. Vaccination has been proven to decrease mortality in COVID-19 infections and to decrease hospitalization rates of infected individuals, both with and without comorbidities.[12,14,15] Following the evolution of coronavirus variants, delta and omicron, a third vaccination for COVID-19 has shown a 94% and 82% (respectively) prevention rate of an emergency-department encounter following exposure to the virus. Vaccines have proven to be 94% effective in preventing hospitalization from the delta variant and 90% from the omicron variant.[15]

Clinical presentation

Although data are lacking in long-term effects of COVID-19 as well as efficacy of vaccination over time, there is improved understanding within the medical community regarding presenting symptoms of patients infected by SARS-CoV-2. COVID-19 pneumonia has a virulent pathology and is highly transmissible with the inhalation of virus infecting the alveolar and endothelial cells in the pulmonary tissue.[16] The most common method of transmission for this virus is person to person via respiratory particles. Respiratory secretions can spread when one breathes in close proximity to another individual (<6 ft) or when eliciting any phonatory behavior (ie, coughing, singing, speaking, and laughing). It is best understood that the airborne transmission of a viable COVID-19 particle can last up to 16 hours before infecting another host, although likelihood of infection is affected by things like viral load and vaccination status.[17,18]

Current data, including contact tracing, support both asymptomatic and symptomatic spread of SARS-CoV-2. This is due to the similar viral loads detected from nasal and throat swabs from each patient population, with a slightly higher predominance of virus detected via nasal swab.[5,19] COVID-19 infectiousness is highest in the early course of the illness, during the 2 days before symptom onset. This viral nucleic acid shedding pattern of SARS-CoV-2 resembles that of influenza and can make it difficult to control transmission.[19] Specific to immunocompetent individuals, an infected patient is less likely to transmit the virus after day 7.[12,20,21]

Within an emergent setting, patients with COVID-19 infection can present with symptoms ranging in severity from mild to severe. Common complaints include fever, cough, dyspnea, myalgia, loss/alterations of gustatory and olfactory senses, gastrointestinal manifestations (most commonly diarrhea), and headaches.[22] Severe illness is more frequent among older individuals and those with multiple comorbidities. Providers may also note delirium and general health decline especially in the older population, who may have previous neurologic impairments.[23] Acute respiratory distress syndrome (ARDS) is a significant complication of COVID-19 pneumonia and has a high mortality.[16]

Current guidelines recommend laboratory and diagnostic testing in the diagnosis of COVID-19 pneumonia. Recommendations are largely consistent with the initial evaluation of CAP with a few exceptions:

- Procalcitonin: Procalcitonin is a biomarker of bacterial infection. It can be useful in determining bacterial coinfection. Data suggest that procalcitonin is an effective diagnostic tool used upon initial presentation as well as for monitoring treatment and guiding management.[24]
- Laboratory inflammatory markers (erythrocyte sedimentation rate and C-reactive protein): These may be increased in patients presenting with COVID-19 pneumonia, however, are nonspecific and do not assist in specific initial management, although they may be better used to monitor progress and outcome.[23]
- Imaging: Chest radiograph is insensitive in accurately detecting early or mild COVID-19 pneumonia. It is, however, cost-effective and time effective. CT imaging of the chest is more sensitive for early detection as well as for monitoring disease progression.[16] It is common to see ground-glass opacities bilaterally with COVID-19 pneumonia on imaging studies.

Treatment

The management of COVID-19 pneumonia is based on the severity of the illness at time of presentation to the emergency department. Minimizing the risk of health care worker and patient exposure must be considered, and measures such as rapid triage and risk stratification should be implemented.[25] Reliable patients who present with any upper-respiratory symptoms, such as rhinorrhea, loss of taste or smell, diarrhea, and fatigue, and who have minimal to no comorbidities, can be managed at home and often should be evaluated through a telemedicine or primary care visit.[25] With signs of lower-respiratory tract pathologic condition, such as dyspnea or cough, and with patients having multiple comorbidities, hospitalization should be considered. Severe illness is defined by an oxygen saturation below 94%, a respiratory rate greater than 30, and the presence of infiltrates on imaging in greater than 50% of lung tissue.[25]

These patients will be monitored, admitted, and likely need supplemental oxygen. Currently, pharmacologic treatments are recommended based on disease severity.[26] The American Academy College of Emergency Physicians recommends the following specific approach based on severity[26]:

- Mild to moderate signs of COVID-19: These patients may benefit from nonpharmacologic treatment alone. These options include home oxygen therapy, breathing exercises, continual ambulation, adequate sleep, and a consistent healthy diet with adequate hydration.
- Severe signs of COVID-19: Recommendations for oxygen support using a nasal cannula with titration to 6 L, high-flow nasal cannula (HFNC) or high-velocity therapy, noninvasive positive pressure ventilation if HFNC is not available, or a consideration of prone positioning if patient can be monitored closely. Proning of patients is contraindicated in the presence of respiratory distress.
- Endotracheal intubation is considered: If a goal of oxygenation at 92% to 96% cannot be maintained, low-tidal volume, plateau pressures less than 30 cm, higher positive end-expiratory pressure, or if a patient experiences refractory hypoxemia with prone ventilation. Currently, sufficient data do not exist to determine the benefit of extracorporeal membrane oxygenation in the management of severe COVID-19 pneumonia.

Recommendations for pharmacologic management of COVID-19 are not made specific to those patients with or without pneumonia. Recommendations are based on outpatient or inpatient management and therefore on disease severity. Current recommendations as seen in **Tables 3** and **4** and **Fig. 1** are summarized as follows[26,27]:

- Remdesivir is the only antiviral medication approved by the Food and Drug Administration (FDA) for the treatment of COVID-19.
- Ritonavir-boosted nirmatrelvir (Paxlovid) and SARS-CoV-2 monoclonal antibodies have been given an Emergency Use Authorization from the FDA.
- Nonhospitalized patients: All patients with confirmed SARS-CoV-2 who are at risk for progressing to severe disease should receive (in order of preference): paxlovid, sotrovid, remdesivir, and molnupiravir. Systemic corticosteroids are not recommended.
- Hospitalized patients: Remdesivir is recommended in all patients requiring admission for SARS-CoV-2. In addition, dexamethasone is recommended if supplemental oxygen is required. Finally, and dependent on severity of disease and progression, tocilizumab is recommended.
- The National Institutes of Health and CDC update detailed guidelines regularly, including the use of heparin.

Prognosis

The prognosis of COVID-19 pneumonia is variable and ranges widely. Mortality is highest among patients with ARDS. There is no clinical significance in mortalities between COVID-19–related ARDS or non–COVID-19–related ARDS. Data suggest mortalities from 12% to 78% in patients diagnosed with COVID-19 and ARDS. Death from COVID-19 can result from other complications, such as arrhythmias, cardiac arrest, or pulmonary embolism.[28] Rapid symptom progression does not contribute to worsened outcomes. Patient prognosis and outcome are affected by individual comorbidities, patient population and demographics, hospital staffing, and staff experience in treating COVID-19.[28]

Community-Acquired Fungal Pneumonia

Cause/epidemiology

Fungal pneumonia affects 2 different patient populations, neutropenic and nonneutropenic individuals. Risk factors for neutropenic fungal pneumonia include neutropenia greater than 10 days typically following chemotherapy or following a hematopoietic stem cell transplant. Risk factors for nonneutropenic fungal pneumonia include prolonged steroid use, which is further broken down into intermediate risk (<0.3 mg/kg/d prednisone equivalents for >3 weeks) and low risk (<7 days of steroid use). Transplant recipients, and patients with AIDS/HIV infection, chronic obstructive pulmonary disease, diabetes mellitus, liver failure/cirrhosis, renal failure/hemodialysis, severe immunodeficiency (chronic granulomatous disease), and critically ill intensive care unit (ICU) patients are at increased risk for developing fungal pneumonia.[29]

There are several common fungal pathogens leading to pneumonia.[29] Coccidioidomycosis, also known as "valley fever," is endemic to the Southwestern United States (primarily Arizona and California), Mexico, Central America, and South America. The fungal spores of coccidioidomycosis live in soil, which are transmitted via inhalation.[7] *Histoplasma capsulatum* is a dimorphic fungus also transmitted via inhaled spores from soil but is endemic to the Ohio and Mississippi river valleys. Aspergillus species, most commonly *Aspergillus fumigatus*, is a common mold infection found in immunocompromised individuals.[7] Neutropenia is the most common risk factor for invasive aspergillosis.[4,8] *Candida albicans*, *Cryptococcus neoformans*, blastomyces, and *Pneumocystis jiroveci* are additional fungal pathogens found in at-risk patient populations.[2,7]

Clinical presentation

Neutropenic and nonneutropenic individuals with fungal pneumonia will present with varied clinical symptoms. Fever and symptoms consistent with angioinvasion are more prevalent in a neutropenic host. Angioinvasion leads to a higher susceptibility of fungal spread to other organs, most commonly the skin, brain, and eyes. Angioinvasion is not common in a nonneutropenic host. Most nonneutropenic patients are asymptomatic until later stages in the disease.[4,8]

Although variable, patients with fungal pneumonia will typically present with a cough (79%–91%), fever (up to 75%), dyspnea (70%), increased sputum production (up to 65%), or pleuritic chest pain (up to 50%). Generalized symptoms of lightheadedness, malaise, weakness, headache, nausea/vomiting, joint pain, and rash can also be associated with fungal pneumonia but are less common as an initial complaint. The elderly population can present with nonspecific complaints as stated, as well as altered mental status independent of other symptoms. Specifically, coccidioidomycosis can cause fever, cough, headache, rash, muscle aches, and joint pain.[30] *H capsulatum* is commonly asymptomatic but can also mimic mild flulike symptoms, fever, headache, chest pain, dry cough, and night sweats. Inoculum size is a major determinant in the symptomatology of patients.[31] It is important to use appropriate history, physical examination, and laboratory and diagnostic imaging to exclude other disease processes, including bacterial or viral pneumonia.

Diagnosis

Because of the limitations in testing availability within emergency departments, the diagnosis of fungal pneumonia is often limited to the history and physical examination findings that are supported with imaging findings and consistent with patient risk factors[29,32,33]:

- Complete blood Count: Recommended to determine the presence of neutropenia and/or lymphopenia. This allows for a more targeted approach to management.

Table 3
Nonhospitalized patient guidelines for COVID-19[27]

Patient Disposition	Panel's Recommendations
Does not require hospitalization or supplemental oxygen	All patients should be offered symptomatic management (*AIII*)
	For patients who are at high risk of progressing to severe COVID-19[a] (treatments are listed in order of preference based on efficacy and convenience of use):
	• Ritonavir-boosted nirmatrelvir (Paxlovid)[b,c] (AIIa)
	• Sotrovimab[d] (AIIa)
	• Remdesivir[c,e] (BIIa)
	• Molnupiravir[c,f] (CIIa)
	The panel *recommends against* the use of *dexamethasone or other systemic corticosteroids* in the absence of another indication (*AIIa*)[g]
Discharged from hospital inpatient setting in stable condition and does not require supplemental oxygen	The panel *recommends against* continuing the use of *remdesivir (AIIa)*, *dexamethasone*[g] *(AIIa)*, or *baricitinib*[g] *(AIIa)* after hospital discharge
Discharged from hospital inpatient setting and requires supplemental oxygen *For those who are stable enough for discharge but who still require oxygen*[h]	There is insufficient evidence to recommend either for or against the continued use of remdesivir or dexamethasone
Discharged from ED despite new or increasing need for supplemental oxygen *When hospital resources are limited, inpatient admission is not possible, and close follow-up is ensured*[i]	The panel recommends using *dexamethasone* 6 mg PO once daily for the duration of supplemental oxygen (dexamethasone use *should not* exceed 10 days) with monitoring of AEs (*BIII*) Because remdesivir is recommended for patients with similar oxygen needs who are hospitalized,[j] clinicians may consider using it in this setting. Given that remdesivir requires intravenous infusions for up to 5 consecutive days, there may be logistical constraints to administering remdesivir in the outpatient setting

Rating of Recommendations: A = strong; B = moderate; C = Optimal.
  Rating of Evidence: I = one or more randomized trials without major limitations; IIa = other randomized trials or subgroup analyses of randomized trials; IIb = nonrandomized trials or observational cohort studies; III = expert opinion.

- Blood and sputum cultures: There are limited data to support the benefit of blood and sputum cultures in the emergency department. Both cultures are useful for long-term management of patients and are often obtained upon presentation, especially if the patient is presenting with signs and symptoms of severe disease.
- Serologic testing: Not commonly recommended in the emergent setting. Both acute and convalescent serum titers are necessary and are less likely to be available in this environment. IDSA/ATS guidelines state that serologic testing is only recommended in certain circumstances, such as ICU admission, failure of outpatient antibiotic management, presence of cavitary infiltrates, active alcohol

Table 4
Fungal pneumonia—comparison of 2007 American Thoracic Society/Infectious Diseases Society of America guidelines with 2019 guidelines[3]

Recommendation	2007 ATS/IDSA Guideline	2019 ATS/IDSA Guideline
Sputum culture	Primarily recommended in patients with severe disease	Now recommended in patients with severe disease as well as in all inpatients empirically treated for MRSA or *P aeruginosa*
Blood culture	Primarily recommended in patients with severe disease	Now recommended in patients with severe disease as well as in all inpatients empirically treated for MRSA or *P aeruginosa*
Macrolide monotherapy	Strong recommendation for outpatients	Conditional recommendation for outpatients based on resistance levels
Use of procalcitonin	Not covered	Not recommended to determine need for initial antibacterial therapy
Use of corticosteroids	Not covered	Recommended not to use. May be considered in patients with refractory septic shock
Use of health care-associated pneumonia category	Accepted as introduced in the 2005 ATS/IDSA hospital-acquired and ventilator-associated pneumonia guidelines	Recommend abandoning this categorization. Emphasis on local epidemiology and validated risk factors to determine need for MRSA or *P aeruginosa* coverage. Increased emphasis on deescalation of treatment if cultures are negative
Standard empiric therapy for severe CAP	β-Lactam/macrolide and β-lactam/fluoroquinolone combinations given equal weighting	Both accepted but stronger evidence in favor of β-lactam/macrolide combination
Routine use of follow-up chest imaging	Not addressed	Recommended not to obtain. Patients may be eligible for lung cancer screening, which should be performed as clinically indicated

Patient Disposition	Recommendations for Antiviral or Immunomodulator Therapy		Recommendations for Anticoagulant Therapy
	Clinical Scenario	Recommendation	
Hospitalized for Reasons Other Than COVID-19	Patients with mild to moderate COVID-19 who are at high risk of progressing to severe COVID-19[a]	See Therapeutic Management of Nonhospitalized Adults With COVID-19.	For patients without an indication for therapeutic anticoagulation:
Hospitalized but Does Not Require Oxygen Supplementation	All patients	The Panel **recommends against** the use of **dexamethasone (AIIa)** or other **systemic corticosteroids (AIII)** for the treatment of COVID-19.[b]	
	Patients who are at high risk of progressing to severe COVID-19[a]	**Remdesivir**[c] **(BIII)**	**Prophylactic dose of heparin**, unless contraindicated **(AI)**; **(BIII)** for pregnant patients
Hospitalized and Requires Conventional Oxygen[d]	Patients who require minimal conventional oxygen	**Remdesivir**[e] **(BIIa)**	For nonpregnant patients with D-dimer levels above the ULN who do not have an increased bleeding risk:
	Most patients	Use **dexamethasone plus remdesivir**[e] **(BIIa)**. If remdesivir cannot be obtained, use **dexamethasone (BI)**.	**Therapeutic dose of heparin**[g] **(CIIa)** For other patients:
	Patients who are receiving dexamethasone and who have rapidly increasing oxygen needs and systemic inflammation	Add **PO baricitinib**[f] or **IV tocilizumab**[f] to 1 of the options above **(BIIa)**.	**Prophylactic dose of heparin**, unless contraindicated **(AI)**; **(BIII)** for pregnant patients
Hospitalized and Requires HFNC Oxygen or NIV	Most patients	Promptly start 1 of the following, if not already initiated:	For patients without an indication for therapeutic anticoagulation:
		Dexamethasone plus PO baricitinib[f] **(AI)**	**Prophylactic dose of heparin**, unless contraindicated **(AI)**; **(BIII)** for pregnant patients For patients who are started on a therapeutic dose of heparin in a non-ICU setting and then transferred to the ICU, the Panel recommends switching to a **prophylactic dose of heparin**, unless there is another indication for therapeutic anticoagulation **(BIII)**.
		Dexamethasone plus IV tocilizumab[f] **(BIIa)**	
		If **baricitinib, tofacitinib, tocilizumab**, or **sarilumab** cannot be obtained:	
		Dexamethasone[h] **(AI)** Add **remdesivir** to 1 of the options above in certain patients **(CIIa)**.[i]	
Hospitalized and Requires MV or ECMO	Most patients	Promptly start 1 of the following, if not already initiated:	
		Dexamethasone plus PO baricitinib[f] **(BIIa)**	
		Dexamethasone plus IV tocilizumab[f] **(BIIa)**	
		If **baricitinib, tofacitinib, tocilizumab**, or **sarilumab** cannot be obtained:	
		Dexamethasone[h] **(AI)**	

Fig. 1. Hospitalized patient guidelines for treating COVID-19.[27]

abuse, severe or structural lung disease, positive Legionella UAT, positive pneumococcal UAT, and presence of pleural effusion.

- Imaging: Chest radiograph is an appropriate and recommended initial diagnostic test. Findings may include lobar consolidation, cavitary lesions, or pleural effusions. As with bacterial and viral pneumonia, CT imaging may be required for further diagnostic accuracy. Bedside ultrasound is sensitive and specific in identifying pleural pulmonary lesions.

Treatment

For patients that have not been previously treated for pneumonia, empiric antibiotics are recommended and based on patient's exposure history, risk factors, and severity of disease. Severity of disease and short-term risk assessment can be determined using the CURB-65 and PSI criteria to establish inpatient versus outpatient management. Failure to improve with initial antibiotic management should raise suspicion for fungal infection.[29,32–34]

Treatment of fungal infection is often targeted and based on blood and/or sputum culture results:

- Aspergillosis: Initial therapy with voriconazole is recommended for most patients. The preferred alternative for patients that cannot tolerate the recommended initial therapy is a combination of posaconazole and isavuconazole.[35]
- *P jiroveci*: Initial therapy with trimethoprim/sulfamethoxazole is recommended.[30]
- *H capsulatum*: If less than 4 weeks of an acute lung infection, no treatment is recommended. If greater than 4 weeks of an acute lung infection, a 3-month course of itraconazole is recommended.[31]

Because of the rise in cases of COVID-19, and with the increased need for long-term intubation, there is a concomitant rise in *A fumigatus* infections.[5] Any patient with a recent COVID-19 infection, particularly in the circumstance of a recent history of hospitalization requiring intubation, has a higher risk of developing fungal pneumonia.[3,35] The ATS/IDSA guidelines were revised in 2019 and are accepted as the standard of care (see **Fig. 1**).

DISCUSSION

Pneumonia remains a common condition evaluated and treated in the emergency department. With the emergence of the SARS-CoV-2 virus and COVID-19–associated pneumonia, hospital admission rates for severe pneumonia have increased, leading to increased overall mortality. It is imperative that emergency medicine providers easily identify patients displaying signs and symptoms of both typical and atypical pneumonia and are familiar with the guidelines established for diagnosis and management of pneumonia, including recommended diagnostic testing. Guidelines for the management of bacterial, viral, and fungal pneumonias are created collaboratively by organizations like the IDSA, CDC, and ATS and revised regularly. The prevalence and cause of pneumonia are demographically and seasonally determined; therefore, providers must be aware of guiding treatment based on these factors. Individual patient risk factors must also be considered.

CLINICS CARE POINTS

- *Streptococcus pneumoniae, Haemophilus influenzae, Staphylococcus aureus*, and group A streptococci are 4 of the most common typical organisms causing community-acquired bacterial pneumonia. Geographical susceptibility, in addition to current guidelines, must be considered when selecting the appropriate treatment.

- Empiric therapy is recommended in all patients with suspected community-acquired bacterial pneumonia.

- Standard empiric therapy for severe community-acquired bacterial pneumonia includes a B-lactam/macrolide combination.

- Because of the significant overlap in presentation of community-acquired bacterial pneumonia and sepsis, blood cultures are recommended in patients with severe disease or in those at risk for methicillin-resistant *Staphylococcus aureus* and/or pseudomonas.

- Acute respiratory distress syndrome is a significant complication of COVID-19 pneumonia and has a high mortality, making rapid diagnosis critical.

- Remdesivir is recommended in all patients requiring admission for SARS-CoV-2. In addition, dexamethasone is recommended if supplemental oxygen is required.

- Failure to improve with initial antibiotic management should raise suspicion for fungal infection.

DISCLOSURE

These authors declare that they have no conflicts of interest. These authors declare that they have no competing monetary interests or personal relationships that could have influenced the work reported here.

REFERENCES

1. Self WH, Grijalva CG, Zhu YZ, et al. Rates of emergency department visits due to pneumonia in the United States, July 2006-June 2009. Acad Emerg Med 2013; 20(9):957–60.
2. Regunath H, Oba Y. Community-acquired pneumonia. StatPearls. Updated August 18, 2021. Available at: https://www.ncbi.nlm.nih.gov/books/NBK430749/.
3. Metlay JP, Waterer GW, Long AC, et al. Diagnosis and treatment of adults with community-acquired pneumonia. An official clinical practice guideline of the American Thoracic Society and Infectious Diseases Society of America. Am J Respir Crit Care 2019;200(7).
4. Martin-Loeches I, Torres A. New guidelines for severe community-acquired pneumonia. Curr Opin Pulm Med 2021;27(3):210–5.
5. Ruuskanen O, Lahti E, Jennings LC, et al. Viral pneumonia. Lancet 2011; 377(9773):1264–75.
6. Ng TM, Ong SWX, Loo AYX, et al. Antibiotic therapy in the treatment of COVID-19 pneumonia: who and when? Antibiotics 2022;11(2):184.
7. Arastehfar A, Gabaldon T, Garcia-Rubio R, Jenks JD, Hoenigl M, Salzer HJF, Ilkit M, Lass-Florl C, Perlin DS. Drug-resistant fungi: an emerging challenge threatening our limited antifungal armamentarium. Antib 2020;9(12).
8. Li A, Lu G, Meng G. Pathogenic fungal infection in the lung. Front Immunol 2019; 10(1524).
9. Sattar SA, Sharma S. Bacterial pneumonia. StatPearls. Updated December 28, 2021. Available at: https://www.ncbi.nlm.nih.gov/books/NBK513321/
10. Ramirez JA, File, TM, Bond S. UpToDate. Overview of community-acquired pneumonia. 2021. Available at: https://www.uptodate.com/contents/overview-of-community-acquired-pneumonia-in-adults?search=diagnosis%20of%20community

%20acquired%20pneumonia&source=search_result&selectedTitle=2-
~150&usage_type=default&display_rank=2. Accessed March 1, 2022.

11. Karimi E. Comparing sensitivity of ultrasonography and plain chest radiography in detection of pneumonia: a diagnostic value study. Arch Acad Emerg Med 2019;7(1):8.

12. McIntosh K, Hirsch MS, Bloom A. UpToDate. COVID-19: Epidemiology, virology, and prevention. 2022. Available at: https://www.uptodate.com/contents/covid-19-epidemiology-virology-and-prevention?sear ch=COVID%20PNA&topicRef=128323&source=. Accessed March 4, 2022.

13. Vaccination rates, approvals, and trials by country. COVID-19 Vaccine Tracker. 2022. Available at: https://covid19.trackvaccines.org/trials-vaccines-by-country/. Accessed March 18, 2022.

14. 10. CDC. COVID Data Tracker. Updated daily by 8 pm EST. Available at: https://covid.cdc.gov/covid-data-tracker/#vaccine-effectiveness.

15. CDC. Effectiveness of a third dose of MRNA vaccines against COVID-19–associated emergency department and urgent care encounters and hospitalizations among adults during periods of delta and omicron variant predominance — VISION network, 10 states, August 2021–January 2022. Morbidity Mortality Rep 2022;71(4):139–45. Available at: https://www.cdc.gov/mmwr/volumes/71/wr/mm7104e3.htm#:~:text=During%20both%20 Delta%2D%20and%20Omicron,and%2090%25%2C%20respectively.

16. Guarnera A, Podda P, Santini E, Paolantonio P, Laghi A. Differential diagnosis of COVID-19 pneumonia: the current challenge for the radiologist – a pictorial essay. *In*. Img 2021;34.

17. Samet J, Prather K, Benjamin G, et al. Airborne transmission of severe acute respiratory syndrome coronavirus 2 (SARS-CoV-2): what we know. Clin Infect Dis 2021;73(10):1924–6. https://doi.org/10.1093/cid/ciab039. Available at: https://escholarship.org/uc/item/1dx8f89w.

18. Ahn JY, An S, Sohn Y, et al. Environmental contamination in the isolation rooms of COVID-19 patients with severe pneumonia requiring mechanical ventilation or high-flow oxygen therapy. J Hosp Infect 2020;106(3). https://doi.org/10.1016/j.jhin.2020.08.014.

19. Zou L, Ruan F, Huang M, et al. SARS-CoV-2 viral load in upper respiratory specimens of infected patients. N Engl J Med 2020;382(12):1177–9. https://doi.org/10.1056/NEJMc2001737.

20. He X, Lau EHY, Wu P, et al. Temporal dynamics in viral shedding and transmissibility of COVID-19. Nat Med 2020;26:672–5.

21. Jones TC, Biele G, Muhlemann B. Estimating infectiousness throughout SARS-CoV-2 infection course. Science 2021;373(655). https://doi.org/10.1126/science.abi5273.

22. Pagliano P, Sellitto C, Conti V, et al. Characteristics of viral pneumonia in the COVID-19 era: an update. Infection 2021;49:607–16.

23. McIntosh, K. COVID-19: Clinical Features. UpToDate. Updated Jan 10, 2022. Available at: https://www.uptodate.com/contents/covid-19-clinical-features. Accessed March 18, 2022.

24. Wonhee S, Simon MS, Choi JJ, et al. Characteristics of procalcitonin in hospitalized COVID-19 patients and clinical outcomes of antibiotic use stratified by procalcitonin levels. Inter Emerg Med 2022;17(5):1405–12.

25. Schalekamp S, Bleeker-Rovers CP, Beenen LFM. Chest CT in the emergency department for diagnosis of COVID-19 pneumonia: Dutch experience. Radiology 2020;298:2.

26. Pantazopoulos I, Tsikrika S, Kolokytha S, et al. Management of COVID-19 patients in the emergency department. J Pers Med 2021;11(10):961.
27. Coronavirus Disease 2019 (COVID-19) Treatment guidelines. National Institutes of Health. 2022. Available at: https://www.covid19treatmentguidelines.nih.gov/. Accessed March 18, 2022.
28. Emergency department Covid-19 management tool. 2022. Available at: https://www.acep.org/globalassets/sites/acep/media/covid-19-main/acep-covid-19-ed-managem ent-tool.pdf. Accessed March 12, 2022.
29. Mertersky   Mark.   https://www.dynamed.com/condition/community-acquired-pneumonia-in-adults. Accessed 18 March 2022.
30. Center for Disease Control. Pneumocystis pneumonia: fungal diseases. 2021. Available   at: https://www.cdc.gov/fungal/diseases/pneumocystis-pneumonia/index.html. Accessed March 6, 2022.
31. Akram SM, Koirala J. Histoplasmosis. StatPearls. Available at: http://www.ncbi.nlm.nih.gov/books/NBK448185/. Accessed March 6, 2022.
32. Patterson TF, Kauffman CA, Hall KK. UpToDate. Available at: https://www.uptodate.com/contents/treatment-and-prevention-of-invasive-aspergillosis?search=aspergillus%20pneumonia&source=search_result&selectedTitle=2~150&usage_type=default&display_rank=2#H5.   Accessed March 6, 2022.
33. Woolfrey KGH. Pneumonia in adults: the practical emergency department perspective. Emerg Med Clin North Am 2012;30(2):249–70.
34. Kosmidis C, Denning DW. The clinical spectrum of pulmonary aspergillosis. Thorax 2015;70(3):270–7.
35. Khan AA, Farooq F, Jain SK, et al. Comparative host-pathogen interaction analyses of SARS-CoV2 and aspergillus fumigatus, and pathogenesis of COVID-19-associated aspergillosis. Microb Ecol 2021;(Nov 4):1–9.

The Approach to Altered Mental Status

Amanda Smith, DMSc, PA-C, CAQ-EM*, Mary Masterson, MPAS, PA-C, CAQ-EM, DFAAPA

KEYWORDS

- Altered mental status • Delirium • Dementia • Confusion
- Altered level of consciousness • Change in mental status

KEY POINTS

- Define altered mental status, delirium, and dementia.
- Review underlying causes of AMS.
- Identify a systematic approach to patients presenting with altered mental status in the emergency department.

INTRODUCTION TO ALTERED MENTAL STATUS

Altered mental status (AMS) is a challenging chief complaint to address in the emergency department (ED). This article defines AMS, provides a framework for how to systematically assess this clinical presentation, and identifies some diagnoses that can present in this manner.

AMS is not a singular diagnosis but rather a clinical sign that is representative of an extensive list of differential diagnoses ranging from benign to life threatening and causes that are reversible versus not reversible.[1] In broad terms, AMS indicates a change in the level of consciousness and/or orientation from a patient's baseline mental status.[2] However, other clinical signs, such as confusion, somnolence, agitation, or belligerence, are commonly referred to as AMS.[1–3]

CONSIDERATIONS

ED visits for AMS are prevalent. In 2018, the National Hospital Care Survey estimated that there were 130 million ED visits for AMS representing an estimated 5% to 10% of ED visits.[2,4,5] Patients across the lifespan may present with AMS, although the most common underlying causes vary across different age groups. It is an especially common presentation in the geriatric population accounting for up to 40% of ED visits in this demographic.[2]

The authors have no financial conflicts of interest to disclose.
Department of Emergency Medicine, Johns Hopkins Bayview Medical Center, 4940 Eastern Avenue, Suite A-150, Baltimore, MD 21224, USA
* Corresponding author.
E-mail addresses: asmit124@jhmi.edu (A.S.); mmaster1@jhmi.edu (M.M.)

AMS is also a high-risk complaint. Patients presenting with AMS have significantly increased need for hospital admission. Their mortality is also the highest among common emergency medicine chief complaints, such as chest pain, generalized weakness, abdominal pain, and headache.[4] In patients with delirium, one of the most common and often reversible causes of AMS, this increased mortality risk extends beyond the initial hospitalization continues into the months to years following.[6,7]

DELIRIUM VERSUS DEMENTIA

Although the terms delirium and dementia are often used interchangeably, this is not accurate. They are two separate and different disease processes. Dementia is a gradual loss of cognitive function over months to years. Delirium, as defined in the Diagnostic and Statistical Manual of Mental Disorders, Fifth Edition, is a disturbance in attention and awareness that develops over a short period of time, tends to fluctuate in severity, and is not explained by another preexisting neurocognitive disorder.[8] Presentations of delirium can vary widely based on the subtype. Unfortunately, delirium is often unrecognized by emergency providers.[9–11]

Subtypes of delirium include hyperactive, hypoactive, and mixed-type presentations. Hyperactive delirium is the easiest to detect, but the least common subtype. Patients may be restless, agitated, and/or combative in addition to having the disturbances in attention and awareness. Those with hypoactive delirium may be lethargic or somnolent and have psychomotor retardation. Because these symptoms may be subtle, hypoactive delirium is often missed and the clinical signs may be attributed to other pathologies. Mixed-type presentations show characteristics of hyperactive and hypoactive delirium.[2]

Differentiating between dementia and delirium is difficult, but several key characteristics can assist in recognizing the appropriate diagnosis (Table 1).[13,14] The onset of delirium is over hours to days, whereas dementia typically has a progressive onset of cognitive deficits over months to years.[12] Alertness and attention are also key differentiating factors. Patients with dementia usually have a constant level of alertness and normal ability to focus. Patients with delirium have a waxing and waning level of alertness and fluctuating ability to focus. The speech and thought patterns of patients with dementia are typically coherent, unless the disease is in the end-stage when it is more similar to patients with delirium who often have disorganized thoughts and incoherent speech.[5,13,14] Dementia and delirium may coexist in patients. In fact, dementia is a significant predisposing factor for delirium especially in those of advanced age.

EVALUATION
Initial Approach

Systematically approaching the patient with AMS helps the clinician to identify and treat the underlying cause as expeditiously as possible. Mortality rates are reduced by quick identification and remediation of the underlying cause.[4] As with all ED patients, initial assessment of the "A, B, C's" is the same in the patient presenting with AMS. However, "D, E, and F" are included in the initial evaluation of the patient with AMS.[15]

Airway: Is the airway patent? Is the patient able to speak? Is the patient able to protect their airway? Are there secretions, blood, emesis, or obvious foreign body that can be suctioned or removed?

Breathing: Is the chest rise symmetric? Are there audible breath sounds bilaterally? Is the patient bradypneic or tachypneic? Is the patient hypoxic on pulse oximetry?

Table 1
Characteristics of delirium versus dementia[5,13,14]

Characteristic	Delirium	Dementia
Typical onset	Acute onset, typically hours to days	Insidious onset, typically over months to years
Course	Waxing and waning	Constant
Consciousness/arousal	Reduced or fluctuating	Generally intact[a]
Attention	Reduced	Generally intact[a]
Speech and thought	Incoherent, disorganized	Generally intact[a]
Perceptual disturbances and hallucinations	May be present	Typically absent[a]
Sleep disruption	Present	Typically absent
Reversible cognitive decline	Usually reversible	Rarely reversible
Precipitated by underlying medical illness	Likely	Unlikely
Percentage of older ED patients affected	10%–17%	20%–38%

[a] End-stage dementia patients can exhibit delirium-like symptoms that are difficult to diagnose. Additionally, patients with dementia can develop delirium, especially in the setting of an underlying acute illness.

Circulation: Are the distal pulses present? Is the patient bradycardic or tachycardic? What is the cardiac rhythm? Is the patient hypotensive or hypertensive? Are the extremities warm and well-perfused? Is the skin dry or is the patient diaphoretic?

Disability: Check for level of consciousness; such tools as the Glasgow Coma Scale or Alert Verbal Painful Unresponsive can direct a rapid assessment.[2] Is the patient alert and oriented? Are the pupils equal and reactive? Can the patient follow directions and move all extremities grossly? Is a sensory deficit present? Is the patient actively seizing or appear to be postictal?

Exposure: Fully expose the patient. Are there any signs of trauma? Are there any medication patches (transdermal, insulin pump) or catheters/wires? Are there any apparent sources of infection, such as a wound draining purulent material?

Fingerstick glucose: Is the patient hypoglycemic or hyperglycemic?

As you move through the initial assessment, abnormalities should be addressed before moving on to the next portion of the evaluation. For example, if the airway was found to be patent, but subsequently the patient is noted to be hypoxic this must be addressed before moving onto the circulation portion of the assessment.

It is important to assess for other easily reversible life-threatening conditions and for those that require time-sensitive treatment while completing the initial assessment. Examples of conditions that may be life-threatening that are easily reversible include hypoglycemia and opioid overdose.[16,18] An example of conditions that required time-sensitive treatment include ischemic stroke.[19]

Hypoglycemia should be recognized during the fingerstick glucose test, which can be performed at the bedside and is rapid. If hypoglycemia is identified, immediate treatment should be initiated. For those patients who are able to swallow, 15 g of rapidly absorbed oral glucose should be provided. Examples of 15 g of oral glucose include 6 oz of regular soda, 6 oz of fruit juice, or 8 oz of skim milk. For those patients unable to swallow, 25 mL of 50% dextrose should be administered. Infusions of 5%, 10%, or 20% dextrose may need to be initiated until glucose levels are stabilized.

Serial glucose checks should be performed to ensure that episodes of hypoglycemia do not recur.[16]

Patients with opioid overdose often have small or pinpoint pupils, bradypnea, and may have sequelae of intravenous drug use on their skin. Naloxone should be administered in a dose between 0.4 mg and 2 mg and may be given in the intranasal, intramuscular, or intravenous routes.[17] With increasing prevalence of fentanyl, escalating doses of naloxone may be required.[18]

Patients with new lateralizing focal neurologic deficits and/or speech disabilities need to be evaluated for ischemic stroke.[19] Noncontrast computed tomography (CT) and CT angiography of the head and neck should be completed to assess for this cause.[2] It is essential to identify acute ischemic stroke in a timely fashion to ensure that patients who are in the window for thrombolytic therapy and/or clot retrieval are able to receive treatment. Timeliness of diagnosis also improves morbidity and mortality of these patients.[19]

Secondary Approach

Once the initial assessment has been completed and immediately life-threatening conditions have been addressed, completing a comprehensive history and physical is essential.

The information gathered from these assessments aids in guiding further evaluation with laboratory and imaging studies that allow you to rule in or rule out suspected diagnoses.[2] Although it may be necessary in some cases, it is best practice to avoid broad, nondirected laboratory and imaging assessments.[15]

The history should characterize details of the acute presentation and of the patient's past medical history. When describing the acute presentation, details regarding the timing and symptoms are essential. Chronic medical conditions, surgical history, social history, sexual history, and medications are essential elements to establishing a comprehensive medical history.[2] Examples include the following:

Timing: When did the symptoms start? Did the symptoms start gradually or suddenly?

Symptoms: What symptoms are present? How is this different than the patient's baseline mental status? Were there any events preceding the AMS event? Are there any associated symptoms, such as fever, palpitations, neck pain, or stiffness?

Medical and surgical history: What kinds of medical problems does the patient have? Are they well managed or difficult to control?

Social and sexual history: Does the patient drink alcohol or use drugs? If so, which and via what modalities? Does the patient have a history of sexually transmitted infection? Has the patient had syphilis? Has it been completely treated?

Medications: What prescription medications, over-the-counter medications, or supplements does the patient take (**Box 1**)? Is the patient compliant with taking their medications? Does the patient self-manage their medications or does someone else? Any recent dose changes?

Some patients may be too altered to accurately provide a detailed history of present illness for themselves. In these situations, it is important to obtain information from collateral sources so that an accurate diagnosis is made quickly and appropriate treatment are initiated.[23] Collateral sources can include family members, caregivers, friends, and neighbors. If the patient has been transported from a nursing home or subacute nursing facility, it is essential to contact the care staff who regularly care for the patient to establish details of present illness, provide context regarding relevant

Box 1 **Common medications that can cause delirium**[20–22]
Amphetamines
Anticholinergics (atropine, benztropine, dicyclomine)
Antidepressants (tricyclic antidepressants, selective serotonin uptake inhibitors)
Antihistamines (diphenhydramine)
Antipsychotics
Benzodiazepines
β-Blockers
Calcium-channel blockers
Digoxin
Diuretics
Dopaminergic medications (levodopa, dopamine agonists)
H_2-Blockers (cimetidine, ranitidine, famotidine)
Isonicotinic acid hydrazide (INH)
Lithium
Narcotics
Neuroleptics
Nonsteroidal anti-inflammatory drugs
Salicylates
Steroids
Theophylline

circumstances, and to confirm the patient's baseline mental status.[2] For those patients transported via ambulance, emergency medical system providers often obtain a history from bystanders and describe the scene in which they found the patient. This information may provide clues to the underlying cause.[24]

In addition to close contacts that may provide collateral information, reviewing the electronic health record systems may provide insight into the patient's past medical history and baseline mental status. Beyond the institutional electronic health record level, the state or regional medical record repositories are an extremely useful resource and expeditious way to identify the patient's past medical history.[23]

Collecting additional history especially from those not present in the ED is time consuming, but is necessary. With vast possibilities for differential diagnoses and the impact of initiating appropriate treatment on morbidity and mortality, this step is critical to come to the correct diagnosis.[19]

CAUSES OF ALTERED MENTAL STATUS

In the following section, several causes of AMS are reviewed. It is critical to note that this is not a comprehensive list of differential diagnoses. Those highlighted next may have notable physical examination or historical characteristics that may be helpful for their identification. Mnemonics that broadly address causes of AMS and life-threatening causes of delirium are included in **Boxes 2** and **3**. Presence of one pathology does not preclude another. For example, a patient with a past medical history for cirrhosis who was brought into the ED after a fall may have concurrent hepatic encephalopathy and a subdural hematoma that could contribute to their AMS. Remember to keep your differential diagnoses wide and avoid early diagnostic closure.

Trauma

Trauma should be considered as the cause of AMS for patients unable to provide a history of present illness and for those with history of traumatic incident preceding the change in mental status. Patients with traumatic injury can present with or without outward signs of trauma.

Outward signs of traumatic injury include lacerations, wounds, bruising, and/or swelling on the head and body.[2,15] Providers should have increased clinical suspicion of traumatic cause in patients using anticoagulation or antiplatelet therapy and those with substance intoxication because they are at higher risk of intracranial hemorrhage secondary to increased risk of bleeding and falls, respectively.[25]

In patients with AMS, a thorough head, eyes, ears, nose, and throat examination is required. It is important to specifically evaluate for raccoon eyes (periorbital ecchymoses), Battle sign (ecchymosis behind the ears), hemotympanum, epistaxis, or clear nasal drainage indicating possible cerebral spinal fluid leak because these clinical signs may indicate basilar skull fractures and resultant intracranial hemorrhages. Traumatic brain injury and intracranial hemorrhage cannot be completely eliminated on physical examination alone. Noncontrast CT imaging of the head may be required to fully assess for traumatic causes of AMS. All types of intracranial hemorrhage to include epidural, subdural, intraparenchymal, and subarachnoid hemorrhages can cause AMS.[2]

Hepatic Encephalopathy

Hepatic encephalopathy is a complication of severe acute or chronic liver insufficiency. This diagnosis is one of exclusion. All other causes should be eliminated before assigning this diagnosis. Other causes that should specifically be considered for patients with hepatic impairment are intracranial hemorrhage secondary to coagulopathy, electrolyte abnormalities, thiamine deficiency, and sepsis.[28]

When evaluating patients with AMS, past medical history of cirrhosis should increase suspicion for hepatic encephalopathy. In patients who are unable to provide past medical history, physical examination findings to include jaundice, spider angiomata, nodular liver, ascites, splenomegaly, and palmar erythema may be indicative of cirrhosis.[29]

When assessing for hepatic encephalopathy, history of present illness elements and physical examination findings may assist in identification of this diagnosis. Typical historical features include personality changes, episodes of abnormal cognition, changes in level of consciousness, sleep disturbances, cognitive impairment, and motor impairment.[28,30] On physical examination findings may include abnormal cognition, hyperreflexia, asterixis, and gait ataxia.[30]

Uremic Encephalopathy

Uremic encephalopathy is an acute, or sometimes subacute, toxic syndrome that is attributed to the accumulation of solutes in plasma from severely reduced kidney function. It usually occurs when the glomerular filtration rate is less than 15 mL/min/1.73 m^2 or in patients with kidney failure who are not receiving adequate dialysis or have missed dialysis sessions.[31]

Like hepatic encephalopathy, uremic encephalopathy is a diagnosis of exclusion and other causes of the AMS should be evaluated. Patients with end-stage renal

---

Box 2
AEIOU TIPS: a mnemonic for causes of altered mental status[12,15,25]

A: Alcohol intoxication

E: Electrolyte derangements (hyponatremia, hypernatremia, hypocalcemia, hypercalcemia, hypomagnesemia, hypermagnesemia), endocrine (thyroid disease, hyperglycemia, hypoglycemia), epilepsy, encephalopathy (Wernicke syndrome, anti-N-methyl-D-aspartate receptor)

I: Insulin, inborn errors of metabolism

O: Opiates, opioid overdose, oxygen (hypercarbia, hypoxemia)

U: Uremia

T: Trauma (concussion, traumatic brain injury, epidural hemorrhage), temperature (hypothermia, hyperthermia)

I: Infection (encephalitis, meningitis, sepsis)

P: Poisons (carbon monoxide, lead, iron), psychiatric (psychosis, conversion disorder, pseudoseizure), porphyria

S: Stroke (hemorrhagic, ischemic), shock (septic, cardiogenic, neurogenic)

---

disease often have AMS secondary to sleep disorders, malnutrition, dialysis complications, and uremia.[31]

Patients presenting with uremic encephalopathy may have a loss of memory, impaired cognition, insomnia, delusions, and/or psychosis. They may also complain about pruritis or muscle twitching.[32] On physical examination, patients may demonstrate cognitive impairment, hyperreflexia, and asterixis. Those patients with advanced uremic encephalopathy can show additional signs of anorexia and upper motor neuron dysfunction causing gait and speech disturbances.[31]

Anti-N-Methyl-D-Aspartate Receptor Encephalitis

Although anti-N-methyl-D-aspartate receptor encephalitis has likely been present since 1895, it was presented in 2005 as a new category of paraneoplastic encephalitis linked to ovarian teratomas.[33] However, growing evidence suggests that underlying pathophysiology is more likely a neuroautoimmune syndrome, which is seen across the lifespan and in both sexes.[33,34]

Box 3
WHHHHIMPS: life-threatening causes of delirium[12,26,27]

W: Wernicke encephalopathy, alcohol withdrawal

H: Hypoxia, hypercarbia

H: Hypoglycemia, hyperglycemia

H: Hypertensive encephalopathy

H: Hyperthermia, hypothermia

I: Intracerebral hemorrhage

M: Meningitis/encephalitis, metabolic

P: Poisons (exogenous or iatrogenic), porphyria

S: Status epilepticus, sepsis

This syndrome follows a typical progression of prodromal psychotic, unresponsive, and hyperkinetic phases. In 70% of patients, a viral illness–like prodrome precedes the AMS. During the viral illness, symptoms may include fever, headache, nausea, vomiting, diarrhea, and malaise. In the psychotic phase, patients may have emotional and behavioral disturbances, such as decreased cognitive skills, delusions, hallucinations, ataxia, fear, and depression. They are often admitted to psychiatric units with a diagnosis of acute psychosis or schizophrenia. Generalized tonic-clonic seizures may occur in the psychotic phase. During the unresponsive phase, patients may have their eyes open, but no longer follow commands or respond to visual threats. Although they are typically mute during this phase, mumbling may be noted. Lastly, this phase is followed by a hyperkinetic phase. Muscle tone is increased and dystonic or cataleptic posturing may be noted. Dyskinesias and extrapyramidal signs are observed to include jaw clenching, lip-smacking, and grimacing. Additionally, autonomic instability is seen in blood pressure and temperature fluctuations and cardiac arrhythmias, such as tachycardia, bradycardia, or cardiac pauses.[34,35]

Because this condition has recently been recognized, the knowledge base is still growing. Symptoms, diagnostic criteria, and treatments recommendations are still evolving. There is much more to learn about anti-*N*-methyl-D-aspartate receptor encephalitis and how to manage it in the clinical setting.

TREATMENT

Identifying and treating the underlying causes of the AMS is the cornerstone of managing the patient with AMS. Approaching these patients in a systematic way by identifying possible life-threatening causes, followed by meticulous history taking, including obtaining collateral history, performing an extensive physical examination, and using laboratory work and imaging in a methodical manner helps to avoid early closure, keep a wide differential, and initiate appropriate treatment.[2]

In addition to diagnosis-directed management, using nonpharmacologic treatment should be a mainstay in treating patients with AMS. Being cognizant of the hospital environment is essential. Lights should be dimmed or turned off at night and on during the day to preserve normal light-dark cycles. Auditory disruption to include monitor alarms and beeping of intravenous pumps should be minimized. Unless necessary to the patient's care, removing medical equipment that may tether the patient is important. Examples of these medical devices include oxygen tubing, intravenous tubing, urinary catheters, and cardiac monitoring wires. To make the environment more comfortable and familiar, it may be helpful to have objects from home in their room and/or have family members remain at bedside with the patient.[5] Maintaining appropriate hydration and nutritional status is important to decrease the likelihood of worsening mental status. Decreasing or eliminating periods of nil per os (NPO) time are an essential component to this.[36]

In cases where nonpharmacologic interventions are incompletely effective or if the patient is agitated or combative, additional interventions should be attempted before pharmacologic management. Verbal de-escalation strategies, such as reassurance, respecting the patient's personal space, and redirection in a calming voice using simple language, should be attempted.[2] It is also important to reassess the patient for discomfort or pain, because patients with AMS may be unable to communicate these sensations directly with their health care team and may become agitated or distressed as a result. Multimodal pain management is recommended, although opioids should be avoided because they may worsen delirium.[36]

Additional pharmacologic intervention may be required for patients that are agitated or combative when the previously mentioned methods are unsuccessful. Oral antipsychotics are the first-line interventions. If the patient has previously been on antipsychotics, those medications should be initiated. If the patient has not been on antipsychotics in the past, such agents as haloperidol, olanzapine, risperidone, quetiapine, or ziprasidone are used. If the agitation or combative behavior continues after oral therapy, intramuscular or intravenous antipsychotic medication should be used. In all cases, dosages should start low with the understanding that the medications may need to be redosed to obtain the desired result and maintain the safety of the patient and staff.[36] Benzodiazepines and diphenhydramine are often used for sedation in the ED, but these agents should be avoided in the delirious patient because they are known to cause delirium and are associated with increased agitation.[5,36]

SUMMARY

Altered mental status is a prevalent ED complaint with a high association for morbidity and mortality.[2,4,5] AMS is a clinical sign and not a single diagnosis. The cause of the patient's AMS can be one or more disease processes.[1] Delirium and dementia are important to understand when discussing AMS and that these diagnoses may coexist in the same patient.[7,8] It is essential to have a systematic approach to evaluate patients presenting with AMS that allows immediate life-threatening causes to be quickly identified and treated, and help to work your way through an extensive differential diagnosis list.[2,15] Although it does not review all the potential causes of AMS or possible management plans, this article should help providers to establish a focused, stepwise approach to these often-complicated patients.

CLINICS CARE POINTS

- Altered mental status (AMS) is a prevalent and high-risk ED complaint in the US.
- AMS is a clinical sign that is representative of an extensive list of differential diagnoses ranging from benign to life-threatening causes that are reversible vs. irreversible.
- Delirium and dementia are often used interchangeably; however, it is important to distinguish the difference (Table 1).
- Initial approach to patients presenting with AMS should begin with ABCDEF (Airway, Breathing, Circulation, Disability, Exposure, Fingerstick glucose) addressing life-threatening issues immediately during this primary survey.
- Secondary survey includes identifying symptoms, timing of symptom onset, the patient's past medical and surgical history, social and sexual history, and a complete medication history.
- History-taking can be difficult in the patient with AMS and all resources must be used, including care facility staff, EMS personnel, family members, caretakers, neighbors, and electronic medical records.
- Keep your differential diagnoses wide and avoid early diagnostic closure.
- Mnemonics such as AEIOU TIPS and WHHHHIMPS may be helpful to determine the underlying cause of AMS.
- Treatment of AMS relies on identifying the underlying cause(s).

REFERENCES

1. Xiao H, Wang Y, Xu T, et al. Evaluation and treatment of altered mental status patients in the emergency department: life in the fast lane. World J Emerg Med

2012;3(4):270–7. Available at: https://www.ncbi.nlm.nih.gov/pmc/articles/PMC4129809/.

2. Smith AT, Han JH. Altered mental status in the emergency department. Semin Neurol 2019;39(01):5–19. Available at: https://www.thieme-connect.com/products/ejournals/pdf/10.1055/s-0038-1677035.pdf.

3. Gimelshteyn Y, Rabins P. Altered mental status. Johns Hopkins Psychiatry Guide Web site. 2018. Available at: https://www.hopkinsguides.com/hopkins/view/Johns_Hopkins_Psychiatry_Guide/787028/5/Altered_Mental_Status. Accessed January 15, 2022.

4. Simkins T, Bissig D, Moreno G, et al. A clinical decision rule predicting outcomes of emergency department with altered mental status. J Am Coll Emerg Physicians Open 2021;2(5):e12522. Available at: https://www.ncbi.nlm.nih.gov/pmc/articles/PMC8432088/#emp212522-bib-0001.

5. Han JH, Wilber ST. Altered mental status in older emergency department patients. Clin Geriatr Med 2013;29(1):101–36. Available at: https://explore.openaire.eu/search/publication?articleId=od_____267::570fbadf9a961df2286bc96db077c882.

6. McCusker J, Cole M, Abrahamowicz M, et al. Delirium predicts 12-month mortality. Arch Intern Med 2002;162(4):457–63. Available at: https://jamanetwork.com/journals/jamainternalmedicine/fullarticle/211205.

7. Dani M, Owen L, Jackson T, et al. Delirium, frailty, and mortality: Interactions in a prospective study of hospitalized older people. Journals Gerontol 2018;73(3):415–8. Available at: https://academic.oup.com/biomedgerontology/article/73/3/415/4584142.

8. Diagnostic and statistical manual of mental disorders DSM-5. 5th edition. Arlington, VA: American Psychiatric Publishing; 2013. Available at:.

9. Hustey FM, Meldon SW. The prevalence and documentation of impaired mental status in elderly emergency department patients. Ann Emerg Med 2002;39(3):248–53.

10. Elie M, Rousseau F, Cole M, et al. Prevalence and detection of delirium in elderly emergency department patients. Can Med Assoc J 2000;163(8):977–81. Available at: ncbi.nlm.nih.gov/pmc/articles/PMC80546.

11. Han JH, Shintani A, Eden S, et al. Delirium in the emergency department: an independent predictor of death within six months. Ann Emerg Med 2010;56(3):244–52.e1. Available at: https://explore.openaire.eu/search/publication?articleId=od_____267::5ce13a95c29bc26e3ceebe2fadd4c9b5.

12. Saint S, Chopra V, Burke J. Altered mental status. In: Sanjay S, Chopra V, Burke J, editors. The saint-chopra guide to inpatient medicine. New York: Oxford University Press; 2018. p. 463. Available at:.

13. Han Jin H, MSc MD, Suyama J, et al. Delirium and dementia. Clin Geriatr Med 2018;34(3):327–54. Available at: https://www.clinicalkey.es/playcontent/1-s2.0-S0749069018309820.

14. Fong TG, Davis D, Growdon ME, et al. The interface between delirium and dementia in elderly adults. Lancet Neurol 2015;14(8):823.

15. Alvarez A, Morrissey T. Approach to altered mental status. Society for Academic Emergency Medicine Web site. 2019. Available at: https://www.saem.org/about-saem/academies-interest-groups-affiliates2/cdem/for-students/online-education/m4-curriculum/group-m4-approach-to/approach-to-altered-mental-status. Accessed January 15, 2022.

16. Hulkower R, Pollack R, Zonszein J. Understanding hypoglycemia in hospitalized patients. Diabetes Management 2014;4(2):165–72. Available at: https://www.ncbi.nlm.nih.gov/pmc/articles/PMC4153389/.

17. Friedman Matt S, Manini Alex F. Validation of Criteria to Guide Prehospital Naloxone Administration for Drug-Related Altered Mental Status. Journal of Medical Toxicity 2016;12(3):270–5. https://doi.org/10.1007/s13181-016-0549-5. In press.

18. Faul M, Lurie P, Kinsman JM, et al. Multiple naloxone administrations among emergency medical service providers is increasing. Prehosp Emerg Care 2017;21(4):411–9. Available at: https://www.tandfonline.com/doi/abs/10.1080/10903127.2017.1315203.

19. Jamieson D. Diagnosis of ischemic stroke. Am J Med 2009;122(4):S14–20. Available at: https://www.sciencedirect.com/science/article/pii/S0002934309001405.

20. Alagiakrishnan K. An approach to drug induced delirium in the elderly. Postgrad Med J 2004;80(945):388. https://doi.org/10.1136/pgmj.2003.017236.

21. Wills B, Reynolds P, Chu E, et al. Clinical outcomes in newer anticonvulsant overdose: a poison center observational study. J Med Toxicol 2014;10(3):254–60. Available at: https://link.springer.com/article/10.1007/s13181-014-0384-5.

22. Berman BD. Neuroleptic malignant syndrome. Neurohospitalist 2011;1(1):41–7. Available at: https://journals.sagepub.com/doi/full/10.1177/1941875210386491.

23. Fitzpatrick D, Doyle K, Finn G, et al. The collateral history: an overlooked core clinical skill. Eur Geriatr Med 2020;11(6):1003–7. Available at: https://link.springer.com/article/10.1007/s41999-020-00367-2.

24. Jones T. Chapter 1. approach to the emergency department patient. In: CURRENT diagnosis & treatment emergency medicine. 7e ed. McGraw Hill; 2011. p. 1–4.

25. Sanello A, Gausche-Hill M, Mulkerin W, et al. Altered mental status: current evidence-based recommendations for prehospital care. WestJEM 2018;19(3):527. https://doi.org/10.5811/westjem.2018.1.36559.

26. Caplan JP, Stern TA. Mnemonics in a mnutshell: 32 aids to psychiatric diagnosis. Curr Psychiatry 2008;7(10). Available at: https://www.mdedge.com/psychiatry/article/63313/mnemonics-mnutshell-32-aids-psychiatric-diagnosis.

27. Caplan JP, Cassem NH, Murray GB, et al. Massachusetts General Hospital handbook of general hospital psychiatry. 6th edition. Philadelphia: Saunders Elsevier; 2010. p. 93–104.

28. Weissenborn K. Hepatic encephalopathy: definition, clinical grading and diagnostic principles. Drugs 2019;79(Suppl 1):5–9. Available at: https://link.springer.com/article/10.1007/s40265-018-1018-z.

29. Schuppan D, Nezam A. Liver cirrhosis. The Lancet 2008;371(9615):838–51. Available at: https://www.sciencedirect.com/science/article/pii/S0140673608603839.

30. Shawcross DL, Dunk AA, Jalan R, et al. How to diagnose and manage hepatic encephalopathy: a consensus statement on roles and responsibilities beyond the liver specialist. Eur J Gastroenterol Hepatol 2016;28(2):146–52. Available at: https://www.narcis.nl/publication/RecordID/oai:repub.eur.nl:96754.

31. Seifter JL, Samuels MA. Uremic encephalopathy and other brain disorders associated with renal failure. Semin Neurol 2011;31(2):139–43.

32. Rosner MH, Husain-Syed F, Reis T, et al. Uremic encephalopathy. Kidney Int 2022;101(2):227–41.

33. Dalmau J, Tüzün E, Wu H, et al. Paraneoplastic anti-*N*-methyl-ᴅ-aspartate receptor encephalitis associated with ovarian teratoma. Ann Neurol 2007;61(1):25–36. Available at: https://api.istex.fr/ark:/67375/WNG-V4QRDDLL-B/fulltext.pdf.

34. Peery HE, Day GS, Dunn S, et al. Anti-NMDA receptor encephalitis. the disorder, the diagnosis and the immunobiology. Autoimmun Rev 2012;11(12):863–72. Available at: https://www.clinicalkey.es/playcontent/1-s2.0-S1568997212000614.

35. Chapman MR, Holly E, Vause DNP, , P M H N, P-C. Appi.ajp.2010.10020181. Clinical Case Conference Am J Psychiatry. 2011;168.

36. Lee S, Angel C, Han JH. Succinct approach to delirium in the emergency department. Curr Emerg Hosp Med Rep 2021;9(2):11–8. Available at: https://link.springer.com/article/10.1007/s40138-021-00226-9.

Pain Management and Analgesia Procedures and Strategies in the Emergency Department

Jason Ausmus, MS, PA-C

KEYWORDS

- Analgesia • Nonsteroidal anti-inflammatory drugs • Acetaminophen • Opiates
- Dissociative agents • Systemic local agents • Gabapentin
- Ultrasound-guided nerve block

KEY POINTS

- Although common in practice, the use of pain scales is not very effective in the assessment of pain.
- Effective pain management includes a balanced or multimodal approach.
- Lidocaine with epinephrine can be safely used for digital blocks in most cases.
- While ultrasound-guided nerve blocks are effective in decreasing accumulative doses of analgesics, providers experienced in the technique should perform them.

INTRODUCTION

Pain is a common component of most patient presentations to the emergency department,[1] representing up to 75% of complaints.[2,3] Pain can be present in many forms and can affect a patient's personal and professional lifestyle. This could lead to long-term effects on behavioral, physiologic, and social interactions. While many patients often look for oligoanalgesia,[3–6] this can be a difficult discussion without identifying the cause of the pain. The use of pain scales to assess response to analgesia is common in emergency departments, but their validity is questionable as they are subjective in nature. Too often, the initial approach to pain management includes additional doses of the same class of medication without considering a more balanced or multimodal approach to pain management.[2,4,7,8] Regional and ultrasound-guided nerve blocks can reduce the need for additional dosing of medications that can have but intermediate and long-term adverse effects.

Tacoma Emergency Care Physicians, 315 MLK Jr Way, Tacoma WA, 98405, USA
E-mail address: jason.ausmus@wecphealth.org

Physician Assist Clin 8 (2023) 151–165
https://doi.org/10.1016/j.cpha.2022.08.013
2405-7991/23/© 2022 Elsevier Inc. All rights reserved.

Pain can be classified as acute, chronic, acute chronic and neuropathic.[3,4,8,9] Acute pain is typically less than 30 days in duration and typically has a known cause. There are often associated signs of tachypnea, tachycardia, hyper or hypotension, and diaphoresis.[3] These symptoms typically resolve when adequate analgesia is provided. Chronic pain can persist from months to years without evidence of abnormal vital signs.[3,4] One of the most common causes of chronic pain is back pain, but may be related to a number of factors such as age or multiple comorbidities.[3,9] Patients with previously known chronic pain syndromes may present with an acute exacerbation of their condition. Typical examples include the exacerbation of low back pain and sickle cell disease.[3,9] Neuropathic pain is typically described as burning or tingling and can be exacerbated by repetitive activity.[3,9] This type of pain is present in conditions such as diabetes, trigeminal neuralgia, multiple sclerosis, or with postamputation pain.[3,9]

EVALUATION OF PAIN

Although pain is identified as the fifth vital sign, there are unfortunately very few reliable tools for the assessment of pain.[5,8,10] The Numerical Rating Scale (NRS) and the Visual Analog Scale (VAS) are 2 of the most commonly used pain scales in emergency medicine.[3,6,10–12] Both scales are unfortunately limited in their utility by the quantitative and unimodal characteristics.[3,6,11,12] The NRS and VAS scales uses a series of numbers to subjectively score the severity of the patient's current pain level. These scales are most effective when repeated often during patient management.[6] In the pediatric population the Wong-Baker Pain Rating Scale uses a series of faces to describe the current state of pain with a corresponding description of no hurt, to hurt worst.[3,6,10] Challenges to the evaluation of pain in children include barriers in language and cogitative development. Also, patients in this group may appear to be in distress, but their symptoms may be more related to anxiety.[10] Two additional tools for use in pediatric patients to assess their pain level are the Face, Legs, Activity, Cry, Consolability (FLACC) scale and Children's Hospital of Eastern Ontario Pain Scale (CHEOPS).[6,10–13]

Additional patient populations that can have barriers to pain assessment are patients with dementia and those who are under sedation. The Pain Assessment in Advanced Dementia (ADD) objectively evaluates levels of discomfort, comfort of breathing, vocalization, facial expression, and body language.[10] In sedated patients, vital signs such as tachycardia and hypertension can be used, but are often unreliable in the true assessment of pain. The Critical-Care Pain Observation Tool (CPOT) and the behavior pain scale have proved the most reliable in assessing pain in this patient population, but have their own limitations as subtle changes can be missed without frequent reassessment.[10,14]

Nonsteroidal Anti-inflammatory Drugs

The most commonly prescribed class of analgesic prescribed in the emergency department are nonsteroidal anti-inflammatory drugs (NSAIDS)[1] and are available in topical, oral, rectal, and parenteral forms. NSAIDS act centrally by binding to the cyclooxygenase (COX) receptor located in the spinal cord.[10] Peripherally, they inhibit the COX 1 and 2 isoform enzymes thereby limiting the production of prostaglandins and thromboxane mediators.[2,4,10,15] The COX 1 isoforms are involved with organ systems involved with gastric function, platelet aggregation, vascular hemostasis, and renal hemodynamics. Selective COX 2 inhibitors provide the anti-inflammatory effects of NSAIDS while minimizing the adverse effects of blocking COX 1.[10]

Most NSAIDS administered in the emergency department are typically above their therapeutic ceiling. For example, Ibuprofen has a therapeutic ceiling of 400 mg (1200 mg/24 h) orally and Toradol 10 mg (10 mg/24 h) intravenous.[2,4,10,15] Topical preparations provide adequate analgesic effect with no systemic or significant local side effects. They can provide direct treatment to various musculoskeletal injuries at greater concentrations than oral treatment.[2,15] Patients who cannot tolerate oral NSAIDS can be provided topical preparations which can provide isolated concentrations 4–7 times oral doses.[2,10,14] Diclofenac is the most common topical NSAID in the world[2,15,16] and is available as a 1% gel and absorption can with peak concentrations within 48 hours.[16] The most common oral NSAID agents are aspirin, ibuprofen, and Naprosyn. Indications for administration include renal colic, dental and musculoskeletal pain. Aspirin has a therapeutic ceiling of 1000 mg a day.[10,15] The analgesic properties of ibuprofen have a ceiling limit of 400 mg orally every eight hours.[2,4,10,15] Typical doses of Ibuprofen provided in the emergency department are above this limit. Naprosyn is available in 250 mg and 500 mg dosages but should be limited to 1000 mg a day.[15] Ketorolac (Toradol) is the most common parenteral NSAID used in emergency departments. The preferred route of administration is intravenous, as pain can be experienced during intramuscular administration.[2] Similar to oral doses of NSAIDS, intravenous administration is typically 15–30 mg, although the analgesic ceiling is 10 mg every six hours.[2,4,15,17]

Medication	Average Dose	Duration of Effect	Max Dosing	Side Effects
Ibuprofen	400 mg PO	8 hours	1200 mg/day	GI disturbance,
Naprosyn	250 mg PO q8hr	8–12 hours	1000 mg/day	hemorrhage,
	500 mg PO q12 hr			renal dysfunction,
Ketorolac	10–15 mg IV	6 hours	60 mg day	bronchospasm,
Diclofenac 1% gel	2 g	4–6 hours	8 g/day upper extremity; 16 g/day lower extremity	delayed wound healing
Aspirin	325–650 mg PO	4–6 hours	4g/day	

There are many considerations when using NSAIDS. The most common side effects include gastric irritation[2,4,6,9,10,12,15–17] by the inhibition of prostaglandin synthesis and therefore the inhibition of the protective role of the gastric mucosa.[10] The renal effects of NSAID include impeding the dilatation of the afferent glomerular arteriole, which can decrease renal perfusion pressure and the glomerular filtration rate (GFR).[10] These effects can be more profound in patients with underlying renal disease, hypervolemia, those taking ACE inhibitors, or those with advanced age.[10] The cardiac effects of NSAIDS may increase the risk of myocardial infarction, CVA, HTN and heart failure by suppressing cardio-protective prostaglandins by blocking the COX 2 enzyme.[10] Additionally NSAIDS inhibit prostaglandin stimulation essential for bone formation and should be avoided in the treatment of fractures.[10] Contraindications to the oral administration of NSAIDS include allergy, active peptic ulcer disease (PUD), poor renal function, previous bleeding disorder, severe hypertension (HTN), hyperkalemia, hepatic insufficiency, prior myocardial infarction or cardiovascular accident (CVA), congestive heart failure (CHF), recent major cardiac or vascular surgery and pregnancy.[2,4,10,15]

Acetaminophen (APAP, paracetamol) is an acceptable first-line agent for mild pain and is available in oral, rectal, and intravenous preparations. The analgesic effect of acetaminophen is achieved by inhibiting the COX 1, COX 2, and COX 3 isoforms, which decrease prostaglandin and thromboxane inflammatory mediators and subsequently pain.[4,10,15] Acetaminophen does not inhibit proclotting thromboxanes and therefore does not prevent platelet aggregation.[10] Typical oral or rectal dosing of acetaminophen is 325–1000 mg orally every 4–6 hours with an analgesic ceiling of 1000 mg and an upper limit of 4000 mg daily.[2,4,15] **Table 1** reviews the common dosing and side effects of acetaminophen. While available in the United States, IV paracetamol has been demonstrated to be no more effective than oral or rectal doses.[2,4,10,15,18] Acetaminophen has a fairly safe medication profile and considered the first line analgesic in pregnancy although caution should be used in patients with the history of liver disease and the elderly.[15]

Opiates

Opiates are another common class of medication used in the emergency department. Medications in this class bind to the opiate receptors with the μ-opioid receptor.[2,4,15] This binding mediates blockade of neurotransmitter release and pain transmission which produce both an analgesic and euphoric effect.[2] This combined effect has led to a public health crisis with medications in this class that often lead to abuse, misuse, and diversion. The most commonly used preparations in emergency medicine are morphine, oxycodone, hydromorphone, fentanyl, and tramadol. Diligence is required when providing opiates in the emergency department. The use of state prescription monitoring programs can assist in identifying those at potential risk of abuse.[7,8] Typical side effects include respiratory depression, hypotension, bradycardia, miosis, pruritus, urinary retention, and gastrointestinal distress such as nausea and constipation. The most preventable side effect in the emergency department is respiratory depression which is not proportional to the level of analgesia. Additionally, fentanyl has been known to cause muscle wall rigidity.[15]

Morphine is the most common parenteral opiate provided in the emergency department and considered the benchmark to which other opiates are compared to.[2,15] Typical doses are titrated at 0.1 mg/kg intravenous or 10–15 mg orally every 3–6 hours. Increasing the dosing to 0.15 mg/kg may provide adequate analgesia in the majority of patients. Reassessment every 20–30 minutes is advised to adequately assess patient response.[2,8] If intravenous access cannot be obtained, morphine can be administered in other ways. Dosing of 10 mg IM, SQ, or 10–20 mg rectally every four hours can be used to achieve adequate analgesia in most patient populations. Morphine nebulized at 10–20 mg every 10 minutes for a total of 3 doses can have a similar effect to intravenous morphine.[2]

Hydromorphone is approximately seven times more potent than morphine.[2] Typical dosing in opiate naive patients is 0.25–0.5 mg intravenous, but typically patients require additional doses.[2] Patients who are not opiate naive typically receive an initial 1 mg dose followed by an additional 1 mg at 15 minutes.[2] Administration should be

Table 1
Acetaminophen dosing and related side effects

Medication	Average Dose	Duration of Effect	Max Dosing	Side Effects
Acetaminophen	PO:500–1000 mg PR: 650 mg IV:1000 mg	4–6 hours	4000 mg/day (3000 mg/day for the elderly and those with liver disease)	Liver toxicity and necrosis, nausea, and vomiting

provided over 1–2 minutes to prevent adverse events. Patients provided over 2 mg intravenous should be monitored for hypoxia.[2]

The opiate fentanyl is 100 times more potent than morphine.[2] Fentanyl provides a quicker onset and shorter duration than other forms of opiates and can be safely used in patients who are hemodynamically compromised.[15] Typical dosing is 0.5 mg/kg intravenously every 30 minutes. Fentanyl can also be administered nebulized at 1.5 to 3mcg/kg in all patient populations and intranasal at 1–2mcg/kg with similar efficiency as intravenous doses,[2] but variability in effectiveness has been noted.

Oxycodone and hydrocodone are the most common oral opiates provided in the emergency department. Oxycodone can be provided individually or in combination with acetaminophen, whereas hydrocodone is administered with acetaminophen.[2] Typical opiate doses are 5–10 mg with 325 mg of acetaminophen with dosing every 6–8 hours. Because of the convenience of oral dosing, they are the most commonly prescribed oral opiates.[1,2] This unfortunately has had the unintentional effect of potential addiction and/or abuse. Because of this prescriptions should be limited to a few days.[8] Patients who require opiates for longer durations should be referred for definitive management evaluated in person and a referral to pain management should be considered.[8]

Medication	Average Dose	Duration of Effect	Side Effects
Morphine	IV: 0.05–0.1 mg/kg or 5–10 mg PO:10 mg	4–6 hours	Hypotension, respiratory depression, constipation, renal dysfunction
Hydromorphone	IV: 0.01 mg/kg or 0.2–0.5 mg	4–6 hours	Hypotension, respiratory depression, constipation
Fentanyl	IV: 0.5–1.0mcg/kg	1–2 hours	Constipation, hepatic dysfunction
Oxycodone	PO: 5–10 mg	IR: 4–6 hours ER: 12 hours	Sedation, constipation

Dissociative Agents

Ketamine is a phencyclidine analog or noncompetitive N-methyl-D-aspartate (NMDA) and glutamine receptor antagonist[4,15] that has analgesic, amnesic, and dissociative properties that do not cause hypotension or respiratory depression.[10] Typical doses of intravenous or subcutaneous are 0.1–0.3 mg/kg. Doses of 0.3 mg/kg intravenously have been shown to be just as effective as morphine at 0.1 mg/kg and doses of 0.15 mg/kg provide better analgesia as compared to morphine,[2,4] but with higher incidence of minor side effects. These may include nausea, dizziness, nystagmus, and hypersalivation in what is defined as emergence phenomena. Slower administration of ketamine and coadministration of antiemetics can reduce these effects.[2,15] Intravenous infusions of ketamine have proven effective for multiple conditions including those with opiate tolerance, but the effects are variable.[19] Intranasal administration of Ketamine is well tolerated in the pediatric patient population, especially if intravenous access is difficult to obtain.[2,19]

Local Agents

Lidocaine, bupivacaine, and procaine are sodium channel blockers that provide analgesia through noncompetitive inhibition of nerve signal propagation.[15] This class of medications is typically used during common bedside procedures, but can also be used topically. Transdermal lidocaine at 4–5% is a superior agent for musculoskeletal and neuropathic pain. Typical dosing is to apply a patch to the target area for a period of 12 hours. Intravenous lidocaine has been used to treat regional pain syndromes and radiculopathies. Clinical trials have shown that dosages of 2% 1.5 mg/kg intravenously with a maximum of 200 mg or infused at 0.05–3 mg/kg/hr are effective for renal colic and lumbar radiculopathy.[15] This route and indication are not typical for Emergency Room use. Caution should be used if providing lidocaine by continuous infusion. Doses can accumulate quickly when infused intravascularly and can cause confusion, headaches, drowsiness, hypotension, seizures, and cardiac dysrhythmias.[2,4,8,10,15]

Gabapentin

Gabapentin works by inhibiting the alpha 2-delta subunit of the presynaptic voltage-dependent calcium channels, which inhibit nerve excitability.[2,4,15] It is a common misconception that gabapentin binds to the GABA receptors.[15] Typically, the effects of gabapentin are not seen immediately. Despite this, it can be a superior adjunct for neuropathic pain. Dosing in the emergency department begins at 100 mg three times a day but can be titrated up to 1200 mg.[15] Caution should be used with patients who are taking opiates, as there can be intensified euphoric effects of the opiates along with increased CNS and respiratory depression while taking Gabapentin.[15]

Medication	Average Dose	Duration of Effect	Max Dosing	Side Effects
Ketamine	IV: 0.1–0.3 mg/kg Infusion: 0.15 mg/kg/hr IM: 4.5 mg/kg IN: 0.7–1.0 mg/kg	30–45 minutes depending on route/dose	N/A	Emergence reaction, dizziness agitation, nystagmus
Lidocaine	IV: 1.5 mg/kg 0.05–3 mg/kg/hr	1–2 hours	200 mg (5 mg/kg)	Confusion, headaches, drowsiness, hypotension, seizures, and cardiac dysrhythmias
Gabapentin	PO: 300 mg titrated to 1200 mg TID	24 hours	3600 mg/day	Dizziness, fatigue, ataxia, nystagmus, leukopenia, rhabdomyolysis, weight gain

Digital Blocks

One of the most common regional blocks performed in the Emergency Department is the digital block. This block is effective for the management of lacerations, orthopedic injuries, trepanation of the nail bed, nail removal, and management of infections.[20,21] An advantage of performing a digital block in wound management over local infiltration is that the digital block does not distort the wound edges.[22] Typical equipment includes the use of a 5 mL or 10 mL syringe with a 27–30-gauge needle attached along with 3mL–5 mL of anesthetic.[21,23,24] There are 2 common approaches to digital blocks.[22,25] The traditional approach to digital blocks involves a dorsal approach at the webspace, placing anesthesia intradermal along one side of the digit then directing the needle toward the palmar surface and around the bone. This technique is then repeated on the opposite side of the digit. Another approach to digital blocks is the modified transthecal block.[22,23] This is performed along the volar aspect of the digit injecting the anesthetic into the flexor tendon sheath at the metacarpal phalangeal joint.

The typical anesthetic used for digital blocks is Lidocaine. Traditional medical practice has been that Lidocaine with Epinephrine should be avoided, but recent research to has proven that sustained vasoconstriction is not as much of a common occurrence as what is traditionally discussed in medical literature but can still occur.[21,23,25] Caution should be used in those patients with known peripheral vascular disease or poor circulation of the digit such as Raynaud's syndrome while using Lidocaine with Epinephrine. Other conditions include uncontrolled hypertension, diabetes, hyperthyroidism, and pheochromocytoma.[23] The amount of anesthetic and duration of action depends on the technique used. Typically, the traditional digital block requires a lower volume of anesthetic and has a longer duration of action.[22,26] **Fig. 1.**

Dental Blocks

Dental blocks are another common regional block that can be useful in the emergency department. Anesthesia can be provided as either general infiltration to an area or specific block of a region. In performing a dental block, the understanding of specific landmarks can assist in the isolation of these nerves.[26,27] The maxillary and mandibular branches of the trigeminal nerve innervate the hard and soft palate.[28] Typically infiltration is used with the maxilla while blocks are used with the mandible.[29] Buccal infiltration involves the insertion of the needle into the buccal sulcus next to the target area. The needle is inserted 2 to 3 mm into the sulcus and provides anesthesia to the buccal gingiva, periodontium, and adjacent tooth.[29] This type of infiltration is typically reserved for the maxilla due to the porous structure of the bone, which allows for easier distribution.[30] The palatal gingiva can be anesthetized by providing anesthesia to the nerve endings of the nasopalatine and greater palatine nerve roots.

The anterior superior alveolar block anesthetizes the canines, maxillary incisors, periodontium, and buccal soft tissues and the middle superior alveolar block anesthetizes the maxillary premolars, the root of the first molar, periodontium, and adjacent soft tissues.[26,27] The posterior superior alveolar block is used for the maxillary molars, but does not cover the first molar.[26,27] One ml of anesthetic is used for each of these regions with the insertion of the needle 5 mm to 15 mm into the buccal vestibule over the desired area.[27]

Mandibular blocks include the inferior alveolar nerve, mental, incisive, and buccal nerves. The inferior alveolar nerve innervates the ipsilateral mandibular teeth, lower lip, chin, periosteum, and buccal soft tissues from the premolars to the midline.[27] During this block it is common to also anesthetize the lingual nerve, which innervates the ipsilateral tongue, lingual soft tissues and floor of the mouth.[31] To perform this block, the needle is positioned above the contralateral molars and inserted toward the pterygotemporal depression located between the pterygomandibular raphe and coronoid notch of the mandibular ramus into the pterygomandibular space.[26,31] The coronoid notch is identified as the most concave point on the anterior ramus and can be palpitated with the nondominant hand during the procedure.[31] **Fig. 2**

Two variations in approach to the mandibular block are the Gow-Gates and Vazirani-Akinosi techniques.[26,27] The Gow-Gates technique provides anesthesia to the mandibular nerve and subsequent divisions of the auriculotemporal, inferior alveolar, mylohyoid, lingual and buccal nerves.[26] This effectively provides anesthesia to the ipsilateral mandibular soft and hard palate, the anterior two-thirds of the tongue, floor of the mouth along with the zygoma and temporal dermis.[32] To perform this block, the patient fully opens their mouth to allow for the forward projection and rotation of the condyle. This technique is performed by palpating the condyle, then retracting the cheek with the nondominant hand then approaching from the contralateral mandibular canine, inserting the needle at the level of the upper second molar just

Digital Nerve Blocks

Dorsal Approach

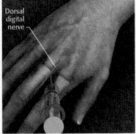

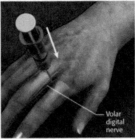

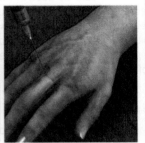

1. Insert the needle at the web space, just distal to the knuckle at the edge of the bone. Once the needle tip is subdermal, inject 0.5 to 1 mL of anesthetic to block the dorsal digital nerve.

2. Advance the needle along the bone toward the palmar surface until the palmar skin begins to tent. Inject another 0.5 to 1 mL of anesthetic to block the volar digital nerve.

3. Repeat steps 1 and 2 on the opposite side of the finger. The result is a circumferential band of anesthetic around the base of the finger. Firmly massage the area for 30 seconds to enhance diffusion of the anesthetic.

A

Dorsal Approach—Alternative Method

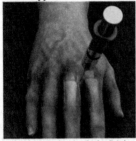

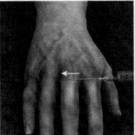

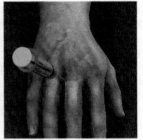

1. Block both the dorsal and volar digital nerves on one side of the finger as described above. *Do not* fully remove the needle after blocking the volar nerve.

2. *Without removing the needle*, redirect it across the top of the finger to anesthetize the skin on the opposite side. After injecting the opposite side, remove the needle.

3. Insert the needle at the site that was anesthetized in step 2, and block the other side of the finger. The presumed benefit of this technique is that it minimizes pain at the second skin puncture site.

B

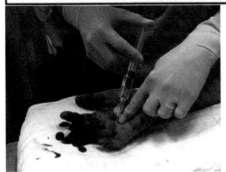

Fig. 1. Digital and transthecal digital nerve blocks. (*From* Roberts and Hedges Procedures in Emergency Medicine and Acute Care. Seventh Edition. Philadelphia, PA: Elsevier; 2018.54, 732–744.e2; with permission (figures 31.12 and 31.14 in original).)

below the insertion of the lateral pterygoid muscle[26] until you contact the osseous structures.[31]

The Vazirani-Akinosi technique is helpful in patients who present with landmarks that are not easily identified or with trismus.[31] During this block, the patient's mouth

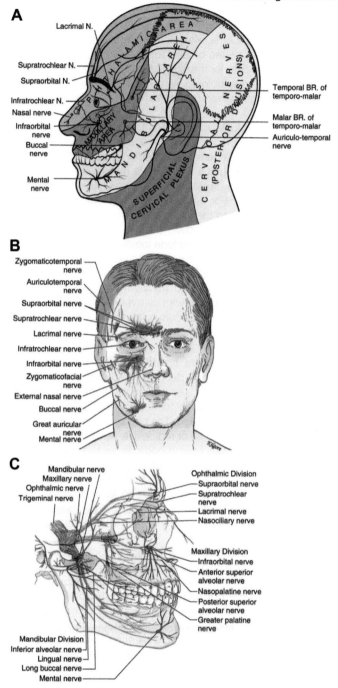

Fig. 2. (*A*), Distribution of the areas innervated by the 3 major branches of the trigeminal nerve. (*B*), Cutaneous branches of the trigeminal nerve and their exit points from the skull. (*C*), Branches of the trigeminal nerve. BR, Branch; n, nerve. (*A*, Borrowed from Henry Vandyke Carter-Henry Gray Anatomy of the human body 1918, Gray's anatomy, Plate 784. (*B* and *C*). Adapted from Eriksson E, editor: Illustrated handbook in local anesthesia. Philadelphia, 1980, Saunders.) (*From* Roberts and Hedges Procedures in Emergency Medicine and Acute Care. Seventh Edition. Philadelphia, PA: Elsevier; 2018.54, 732–744.e2; with permission (figure 30.1 in original).)

remains closed which allows for the relaxation of the muscles. The coronoid process is palpated and the needle is inserted parallel to the coronoid process and maxillary tuberosity at the level of the posterior maxillary teeth.[31] The needle should be advanced toward the ramus with the bevel pointed away from the ramus and half the distance of the anterioposterior width of the ramus. Contact with bone means that the approach was too lateral.[31]

Mental and incisive nerve blocks can be useful to provide anesthesia to the incisors, canines, anterior mandibular premolars, and surrounding lower lip and chin bilaterally.[26,27] Buccal nerve blocks are useful in providing anesthesia to the buccal gingiva and mandibular molars.[26] For mental and incisive blocks, the needle is inserted with the bevel facing the bone to a depth of 5 to 6 mm.[26] Gentle massaging of region will provide greater coverage. For the buccal nerve block, the needle is advanced into the buccal vestibule distal to the second or third molar typically at a depth of 1 to 3 mm until contact with bone is made.[26]

Complications to dental blocks can include localized hematoma, localized soft tissue trauma, associated nerve injury or palsy, needle fracture due to sudden patient movement, intravascular injection of the local anesthetic, and ocular complications such as diplopia, ptosis, mydriasis, and transient vision loss, opthalmoplegia[33,34] Another ocular complication can occur with inadvertent retrograde flow of the anesthetic that can lead to anesthesia of the oculomotor, abducens and trochlear nerves.[33]

Ultrasound-guided Nerve Blocks

Ultrasound-guided regional anesthesia provides substantial relief, reduced opiate use, increase patient satisfaction, and decrease department resources and patient length of stay.[4,34–37] Most importantly, nerve blocks should not be performed without adequate training and supervision by a trained medical provider. Additionally, the most distal and local infiltration is advised. The principal concept is to target the nerve intervention for a particular dermatome or region. Nerve blocks can be a safe and useful option for wound management, foreign body removal, laceration repair, fracture, and joint reduction. Patients who receive nerve blocks under ultrasound guidance typically utilize less analgesics overall and therefore the unintentional side effects.[4,34–37] Contraindications are either allergic to local analgesia or those with a known neurological deficit in the affected area.[35–37] While there is a low possibility of developing peripheral nerve injury, it is imperative to differentiate this from a known deficit.

Preparation for an ultrasound-guided nerve block includes proper positioning of the patient and ultrasound machine with a linear array probe.[38,39] It is recommended that the patient be placed on a cardiac monitor and have intravenous access.[35] Consent must be obtained and a time out completed. The ultrasound machine should be placed on the opposite side of where the procedure is being performed. Materials include a sterile probe cover, short beveled spinal needle (to reduce the risk of unintentional intravascular infiltration), standard infiltration materials to include a control syringe, and added room if performing a two-provider approach. The control syringe provides more precise targeting of the nerve. The two-provider technique is simpler to perform as it allows for better control of the needle during placement but requires additional staff, which can be difficult with limited resources. If administrating large volumes of anesthetic, the two-provider technique is preferred.[35] **Fig. 3**

The 2 most common medications used for nerve blocks are lidocaine and bupivacaine. It is recommended to utilize a weight-based dosing chart and confirm the dose with a colleague prior to beginning.[35] Clinical documentation should include a pre and postneurological exam, type and location of block performed, time of

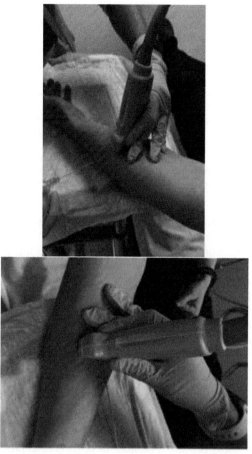

Fig. 3. In-plane and out-of-plane approach. (*Courtesy of* Jason Ausmus, MS, PA-C Weill Cornell Medicine, New York, NY.)

completion, and type/amount/concentration of analgesic used. The extremity should be placed in a neutral positioned and padded from injury. Any consult services and department staff should be made aware of the procedure.

While discussion of specific nerve blocks is beyond the scope of this article, peripheral nerves are best visualized in the short axis view and run adjacent to vascular structures and facial planes.[39] Peripheral nerves appear as hyperechoic structures (dark stripe surrounded by a white line) in either round, oval, or triangular shapes.[39,40] Localization of the nerve requires knowledge of anatomic structures. Fanning of the probe or the use of color Doppler will aid in identification adjacent structures.[35] It is also important to note that nerves do not collapse when pressure is applied.[40] The 2 common approaches to needle insertion during ultrasound-guided nerve blocks are in-plane and out-of-plane. With the in-plane view of the nerve, the probe is held in the provider's nondominant hand, resting the palm on the skin and the needle is parallel to the long axis of the probe.[26,38–40] The needle is inserted by the provider's dominant hand under the ultrasound probe with the entire length of the needle visualized along its trajectory.[36,38–40] With the out-of-plane technique, the needle is inserted along perpendicular to the probe midline to the long axis.[36,38–40] During the out-of-plane technique, the needle will be only visualized as a dot as it passes under the probe.[36,38–40] With either technique, the angle of approach will depend on the depth of the nerve and length of the needle. Placement of a small amount of analgesia in your target area can aid in the visualization of your target.[35,39]

Approach	Advantage	Disadvantage
In-plane	Most direct visualization	Some unimaged needle path occurs, but typically less than the out-of-plane approach. Longer needle paths.
Out-of-plane	Shorter needle path	Unimaged needle path

Although the overall complications of performing a peripheral nerve block are rare, they can include vascular injury, hematoma, and infection.[35–40] More adverse events include a persistent sensory or motor deficit specifically to the phrenic or recurrent laryngeal nerve while performing an interscalene block or pneumothorax during a supraclavicular block.[2,36] Local anesthetic systemic toxicity (LAST) occurs when an anesthetic enters the intravascular system. Minor reactions include lightheadedness, nausea, tinnitus, visual disturbances, oral tingling, metallic taste and nausea.[35,39] Severe reactions to lidocaine toxicity include seizures, respiratory depression, cardiac arrhythmias, bradycardia, and cardiac arrest.[35,39] Patients who experience severe symptoms should be treated with lipid emulsion therapy.[35,41] Benzodiazepines are the treatment of choice for patients who experience seizures associated with LAST.[35]

SUMMARY

Emergency medicine providers should have a number of pain management resources at their disposal. Although the idea of no pain may be desired endpoint, emergency medicine providers could provide a number of options to improve a patient's level of comfort to tolerable. While the utilization of pain scales may be the standard approach to management, there are limitations in interpretation as they are subjective in their data. The traditional treatment options of oral and parenteral analgesia provided in the emergency department may be above the therapeutic limits and provided in intervals that may not have an additional effect. In addition to traditional approaches with oral or parenteral analgesia, regional and ultrasound-guided nerve blocks may be an option for those requiring incremental doses of analgesia or with extended length of stays. Through a patient-centered, balanced approach to pain management directed at the initial cause of pain, emergency medicine providers could provide analgesia in a safe and effective manner.

CLINICS CARE POINTS

- Most analgesics provided in the emergency department are dosed above the therapeutic level. Caution should be used with those analgesics that are central nervous system depressants.
- Patients who develop seizures during lidocaine injections should be treated with Benzodiazepines. Patients who develop other reactions should be treated with lipid emulsion therapy.

- When performing ultrasound-guided nerve blocks, note any previous neurological deficits and inform consult services of when the block was performed.

DISCLOSURES

The author has nothing to disclose.

REFERENCES

1. Centers for disease control national hospital ambulatory care survey: 2018 emergency department summary tables. 2021. Available at: https://www.cdc.gov/nchs/ahcd/web_tables.htm. Accessed January 3, 2022.
2. Cisewski DH, Motov SM. Essential pharmacologic options for acute pain management in the emergency setting. Turk J Emerg Med 2018;19(1):1–11.
3. Cisewski D, Motov S. Pain recognition and assessment. In: Cisewski D, editor. Emergency medicine resident association pain management guide. 1. Irving, TX: Emergency Medicine Resident Association; 2020. Available at: https://www.emra.org/books/pain-management/pain-recognition-assessment/. Accessed January 20, 2022.
4. Motov SM, Nelson LS. Advanced concepts and controversies in emergency department pain management. Anesthesiol Clin 2016;34(2):271–85.
5. Green SM, Krauss BS. The numeric scoring of pain: this practice rates a zero out of ten. Ann Emerg Med 2016;67(5):573–5.
6. Pollack CV Jr, Viscusi ER. Improving acute pain management in emergency medicine. Hosp Pract (1995) 2015;43(1):36–45.
7. Cohen V, Motov S, Rockoff B, et al. Development of an opioid reduction protocol in an emergency department. Am J Health Syst Pharm 2015;72(23):2080–6.
8. Motov S, Strayer R, Hayes BD, et al. The treatment of acute pain in the emergency department: a white paper position statement prepared for the american academy of emergency medicine. J Emerg Med 2018;54(5):731–6.
9. Optimizing the treatment of acute pain in the emergency department. Ann Emerg Med 2017;70(3):446–8. https://doi.org/10.1016/j.annemergmed.2017.06.043.
10. Almehlisi A, Tainter C. Emergency department pain management: beyond opioids. Emerg Med Pract 2019;21(11):1–24.
11. Voepel-Lewis T, Zanotti J, Dammeyer JA, et al. Reliability and validity of the face, legs, activity, cry, consolability behavioral tool in assessing acute pain in critically ill patients. Am J Crit Care 2010;19(1):55–62.
12. Gaglani A, Gross T. Pediatric pain management. Emerg Med Clin North Am 2018; 36(2):323–34.
13. Voepel-Lewis T, Malviya S, Tait AR, et al. A comparison of the clinical utility of pain assessment tools for children with cognitive impairment. Anesth Analg 2008; 106(1). https://doi.org/10.1213/01.ane.0000287680.21212.d0.
14. Rijkenberg S, van der Voort PH. Can the critical-care pain observation tool (CPOT) be used to assess pain in delirious ICU patients? J Thorac Dis 2016; 8(5):E285–7.
15. Koehl J. Pharmacology of pain. In: Cisewski D, editor. Emergency medicine resident association pain management guide. 1. Irving, TX: Emergency Medicine Resident Association; 2020. Available at: https://www.emra.org/books/pain-management/pain-recognition-assessment/. Accessed January 20, 2022.

16. Barkin RL. Topical nonsteroidal anti-inflammatory drugs: the importance of drug, delivery, and therapeutic outcome. Am J Ther 2015;22(5):388–407.

17. da Silva J, Gingras A. Usage analysis of ketorolac in the emergency department. Am J Emerg Med 2021;45:541–2.

18. Furyk J, Levas D, Close B, et al. Intravenous versus oral paracetamol for acute pain in adults in the emergency department setting: a prospective, double-blind, double-dummy, randomised controlled trial. Emerg Med J 2018;35(3): 179–84.

19. Ahern TL, Herring AA, Miller S, et al. Low-dose ketamine infusion for emergency department patients with severe pain. Pain Med 2015;16(7):1402–9.

20. Welch JL, Cooper DD. Should I use lidocaine with epinephrine in digital nerve blocks? Ann Emerg Med 2016;68(6):756–7.

21. Clement P, Doomen L, van Hooft M, et al. Regional anaesthesia on the finger: traditional dorsal digital nerve block versus subcutaneous volar nerve block, a randomized controlled trial. Injury 2021;52(4):883–8.

22. Kelly J, Younga J. Regional anesthesia of the thorax and extremities. In: Roberts and hedges procedures in emergency medicine and acute care. 7th ed. Philadelphia, PA: Elesvier; 2018. Available at: https://www-clinicalkey-com.ezproxy.med. cornell.edu/#!/content/book/3-s2.0-B9780323354783000762. Accessed July 20, 2022.

23. Ilicki J. Safety of epinephrine in digital nerve blocks: a literature review. J Emerg Med 2015;49(5):799–809.

24. Cummings AJ, Tisol WB, Meyer LE. Modified transthecal digital block versus traditional digital block for anesthesia of the finger. J Hand Surg Am 2004; 29(1):44–8.

25. Waterbrook AL, Germann CA, Southall JC. Is epinephrine harmful when used with anesthetics for digital nerve blocks? Ann Emerg Med 2007;50(4):472–5.

26. Reed KL, Malamed SF, Fonner AM. Local anesthesia part 2: technical considerations. Anesth Prog 2012;59(3):127–37.

27. Tomaszewska IM, Zwinczewska H, Gładysz T, et al. Anatomy and clinical significance of the maxillary nerve: a literature review. Folia Morphol (Warsz) 2015; 74(2):150–6.

28. Wang YH, Wang DR, Liu JY, et al. Local anesthesia in oral and maxillofacial surgery: a review of current opinion. J Dent Sci 2021;16(4):1055–65.

29. Lee CR, Yang HJ. Alternative techniques for failure of conventional inferior alveolar nerve block. J Dent Anesth Pain Med 2019;19(3):125–34.

30. Dougall A, Apperley O, Smith G, et al. Safety of buccal infiltration local anaesthesia for dental procedures. Haemophilia 2019;25(2):270–5.

31. Kim C, Hwang KG, Park CJ. Local anesthesia for mandibular third molar extraction. J Dent Anesth Pain Med 2018;18(5):287–94.

32. Decloux D, Ouanounou A. Local anaesthesia in dentistry: a review. Int Dent J 2020;71(2):87–95, published online ahead of print, 2020 Sep 17.

33. Acham S, Truschnegg A, Rugani P, et al. Needle fracture as a complication of dental local anesthesia: recommendations for prevention and a comprehensive treatment algorithm based on literature from the past four decades. Clin Oral Investig 2019;23(3):1109–19.

34. American College of Emergency Physicians. Ultrasound-guided nerve blocks. 2021. Available at: https://www.acep.org/patient-care/policy-statements/ ultrasound-guided-nerve-blocks/. Accessed January 22, 2022.

35. Nagdev A, Becherer-Bailey G, Farrow RA II, et al. Ultrasound guided nerve blocks. In: Cisewski D, editor. Medicine resident association pain management

guide. 1. Irving, TX: Emergency Medicine Resident Association; 2020. Available at: https://www.emra.org/books/pain-management/pain-recognition-assessment/. Accessed January 21, 2022.
36. Cogan CJ, Kandemir U. Role of peripheral nerve block in pain control for the management of acute traumatic orthopaedic injuries in the emergency department: diagnosis-based treatment guidelines. Injury 2020;51(7):1422–5.
37. Strakowski JA. Ultrasound-guided peripheral nerve procedures. Phys Med Rehabil Clin N Am 2016;27(3):687–715.
38. Steinfeldt T, Volk T, Kessler P, et al. Peripheral nerve blocks on the upper extremity: technique of landmark-based and ultrasound-guided approaches. Anaesthesist 2015;64(11):846–54.
39. Capek A, MBChB FRCA, Dolan J, et al. Ultrasound-guided peripheral nerve blocks of the upper limb. BJA Education 2015;15(3):160–5.
40. Gray AT. Ultrasound-guided regional anesthesia: current state of the art. Anesthesiology 2006;104(2):368-5A.
41. Ok SH, Hong JM, Lee SH, et al. Lipid emulsion for treating local anesthetic systemic toxicity. Int J Med Sci 2018;15(7):713–22.

Behavioral Health Emergencies

Karla Juvonen, MPAS, PA-C

KEYWORDS

- Psychosis • Anxiety • Agitation • Suicidal • Intoxication • Withdrawal • Panic
- Mania

KEY POINTS

- The angry/aggressive/agitated patient.
- The anxious patient (including acute panic).
- The disorganized/psychotic patient.
- The acutely depressed/actively suicidal patient.
- Medical emergencies of the psychiatric patient (serotonin syndrome, tardive dyskinesia, neuroleptic malignant syndrome).
- The chemically dependent, intoxicated, or withdrawing patient.

INTRODUCTION

One in five adults experience mental illness annually, according to the National Institutes of Health.[1] The rates are even higher among the drug or alcohol dependent, homeless, and those incarcerated or in detention centers. With a current shortage of easily accessible mental health care, especially after hours and on weekends, the emergency department (ED) is frequently where patients experiencing a behavioral health crisis land. A single chapter on such emergencies follows, limited by length to only the most serious situations and the immediate management of those situations. This section does not provide recommendations for ongoing psychiatric management other than recommendations for referrals nor does it include mental illnesses outside of the realm of emergent.

Department of Psychiatry and Addiction Medicine, 711 Nereid Avenue, Bronx, NY 10466, USA
E-mail address: karlarae123@gmail.com

Physician Assist Clin 8 (2023) 167–192
https://doi.org/10.1016/j.cpha.2022.09.003
2405-7991/23/© 2022 Elsevier Inc. All rights reserved.

THE ANGRY, AGGRESSIVE, OR AGITATED PATIENT

In all patient care settings, but particularly in the ED, encountering violent or agitated patients is common. Prolonged waiting times and confusion frequently seen is busy EDs, along with serious illness, can exacerbate agitation and violent tendencies among patients and their families. Alcohol, drugs, and weapon accessibility further amplify the problem.

The first step in assessing any patient who seems agitated or violent is to ensure the safety of staff, patient, and surrounding bystanders.

Agitated or violent patients should be assessed for weapons and disarmed if necessary and seen in a semiprivate, but not isolated, area that is free of heavy or dangerous objects (syringes, scissors, scalpels, electrical cords).[2,3] Leaving the door open with security personnel standing nearby and situating the clinician closest to the door provides additional safety. Before entering the room, the clinician should remove anything that could be used to harm them such as neckties, non-breakaway lanyards, earrings, and necklaces. If an accompanying visitor seems to be escalating the situation, ask them to wait elsewhere.

It is very difficult to perform any type of evaluation while a patient is acutely agitated or violent. In this case, evaluation and management may occur simultaneously or in a somewhat disorganized fashion, as some means of management may be required before further evaluation can take place.

Management

Verbal deescalation techniques

If at all possible, using verbal techniques as the first line is standard. The clinician will rapidly detect, while using such tactics, if the patient will be cooperative or not. The mental status of the patient can also be observed during this time. The clinician should attempt to assess patient orientation, signs of hallucinations or delusions, speech pattern and language skills, mood, affect, suicidal/homicidal statements, body posture, and any obvious physical abnormalities.

Using a calm voice, and avoiding prolonged eye contact, the clinician should stand at least 2 arms' length away from the patient.[2,4] The patient should be asked about violence directly. "Do you feel like hurting yourself?" "Do you feel like hurting someone else?" "Do you carry a knife or a gun?"

Most importantly, take all threats of violence seriously. If verbal techniques are unsuccessful, the clinician should discreetly request help (panic button/code word) or leave the room to assemble a team to move on to the next phase of managing the violent or agitated/aggressive.

Physical restraints may be required in situations where verbal techniques are unsuccessful. In such a case, the clinician and staff should follow guidelines set forth within their specific institution to achieve physical restraint.

Chemical restraint

Ultimately, chemical restraint may be necessary for the safety of the patient and staff. Many EDs have their own protocol for chemical restraint, but in the absence of institutional guidelines, the following algorithm may be used.

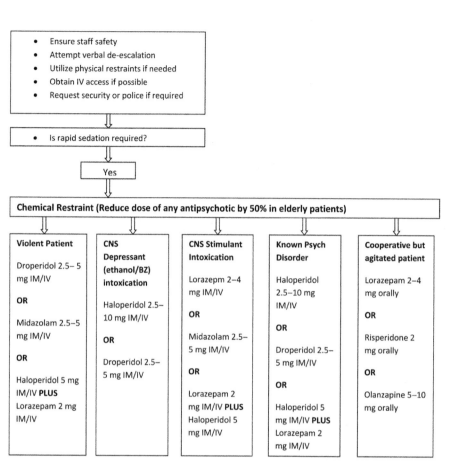

- Ensure staff safety
- Attempt verbal de-escalation
- Utilize physical restraints if needed
- Obtain IV access if possible
- Request security or police if required

⟱

- Is rapid sedation required?

⟱

Yes

⟱

Chemical Restraint (Reduce dose of any antipsychotic by 50% in elderly patients)

Violent Patient	CNS Depressant (ethanol/BZ) intoxication	CNS Stimulant Intoxication	Known Psych Disorder	Cooperative but agitated patient
Droperidol 2.5– 5 mg IM/IV **OR** Midazolam 2.5–5 mg IM/IV **OR** Haloperidol 5 mg IM/IV **PLUS** Lorazepam 2 mg IM/IV	Haloperidol 2.5–10 mg IM/IV **OR** Droperidol 2.5–5 mg IM/IV	Lorazepm 2–4 mg IM/IV **OR** Midazolam 2.5–5 mg IM/IV **OR** Lorazepam 2 mg IM/IV **PLUS** Haloperidol 5 mg IM/IV	Haloperidol 2.5–10 mg IM/IV **OR** Droperidol 2.5–5 mg IM/IV **OR** Haloperidol 5 mg IM/IV **PLUS** Lorazepam 2 mg IM/IV	Lorazepam 2–4 mg orally **OR** Risperidone 2 mg orally **OR** Olanzapine 5–10 mg orally

Fig. 1. Chemical Restraint Algorithm.[5–25]

As quickly as possible, once safety is assured, assessment for organic causes of agitation should be initiated.

Box. 1
Differential diagnosis for psychosis/aggression[21–41]

General Medical Conditions
- Infections (UTI, COVID-19, HIV/AIDS, malaria, leprosy)
- Hypo-/hyperthyroidism
- Shock (all causes)
- Systemic lupus erythematosis
- Hypo-/hyperglycemia, DKA
- Vitamin deficiency (including Wernicke encephalopathy)
- Tumor/brain metastasis
- Sarcoidosis

Medications
- Systemic steroids
- Anticholinergic medications (diphenhydramine, scopolamine)
- Antibiotics
- Anticonvulsants
- Some chemotherapy agents

Illicit Drugs (chronic use, intoxication, or withdrawal)
- LSD
- PCP
- Cocaine
- GHB
- Alcohol (alcoholic hallucinations, delirium tremens)
- Antihistamines
- Marijuana
- Synthetic marijuana (K2), not often detected on standard toxicology panel
- Methamphetamines
- Kratom, not often detected on standard toxicology panel
- Bath salts, not often detected on standard toxicology panel
- Opioids (fentanyl, "pressed Percocet," heroin, oral opioids)

Psychiatric
- Primary psychotic disorder (schizophrenia, major depression, brief psychotic disorder, delusional disorder, schizoaffective disorder, schizophreniform disorder)
- Mood disorder (major depression with psychotic features, bipolar disorder, mania)
- Trauma disorders (complex PTSD)
- Personality disorders (borderline, paranoia, schizoid, schizotypal)
- Other (peripartum psychosis, autism spectrum disorder with acute decompensation)

Neurodegenerative Disease
- Alzheimer disease
- Lewy body dementia
- Parkinson disease (and associated dementia)
- Vascular dementia

Other neurologic diseases
- Huntington disease
- CVA
- Epilepsy (ictal, postictal, interictal psychosis)
- Multiple sclerosis
- Primary brain tumor
- Encephalitis (infectious, autoimmune)
- TBI

Workup

Initially, obtain a comprehensive metabolic panel, complete blood count, urine toxicology, urinalysis, thyroid stimulating hormone (TSH), and chest radiograph (CXR) as well as frequent vital sign and pulse oximetry checks.

If initial workup is unrevealing, follow-up with vitamin B12, folate, thiamine, cortisol, human immunodeficiency virus (HIV), rapid plasma reagin (RPR), COVID-19 polymerase chain reaction (PCR), erythrocyte sedimentation rate (ESR)/C-reactive protein (CRP), and serum antinuclear antibody (ANA).

If agitation and/or psychosis rapidly progresses, move forward to electroencephalogram (EEG) and lumbar puncture (LP) for cerebrospinal fluid (CSF) counts and glucose.

Head computed tomography (CT) scan is appropriate for agitation and delirium (to rule out intracranial abnormality) but is rarely useful for isolated psychosis.

Treatment

The treatment will depend greatly on the cause. If chemical sedation was required, the patient's symptoms may have already improved.

If rapid chemical restraint was not required, workup is unremarkable, yet symptoms of agitation persist, a trial of an atypical antipsychotic is appropriate. Oral administration is preferred, if possible.

Table 1
Commonly used atypical antipsychotics for aggression and/or agitation (consider lower doses in elderly)[41–43]

Antipsychotic	Form	Typical ER Dosage	Caution
Risperidone (Risperdal)	Tablet/liquid/IM	1–2 mg (max 8 mg/d)	Dystonia
Olanzapine (Zyprexa)	Tablet/oral/IM	5–10 mg (max 30 mg/d)	Possible cardiorespiratory suppression if given along with lorazepam
Ziprasidone (Geodon)	Tablet/IM	20 mg PO/10–20 mg IM (max 40 mg/d)	QTc interval prolongation
Aripiprazole (Abilify)	Tablet/liquid/IM	10–15 mg PO/9.75 mg IM (max 30 mg/d)	Akathisia, nausea
Quetiapine (Seroquel)	Oral	25–50 mg	Sedation

Abbreviations: ER, extended release; IM, intramuscular.

Disposition/Referral

Prognosis varies according to cause. If general medical causes are ruled out, psychiatric consultation (face to face or telemedicine) should be obtained for definitive treatment and discharge planning and to ensure prompt and appropriate follow-up and ongoing medication management. The agitated patient who is reporting suicidal or homicidal ideation or intent should be admitted. In addition, those patients who have been found to be agitated due to significant substance use disorder with toxicity or withdrawal (particularly alcohol and/or benzodiazepines) should be admitted to a detoxification floor or center for ongoing, medically monitored management.

THE ANXIOUS PATIENT (INCLUDING PANIC)

Anxiety and related disorders account for a staggering number of ED visits annually. Panic attacks are the most frequent of the anxiety disorder that result in ED presentation. Current literature estimates the prevalence of at least one lifetime panic attack is approximately 20% among adults in the United States.[44,45] Because of the severe and frightening symptoms of a panic attack, many patients experiencing them will seek care in the ED.

Definition

According to the Diagnostic and Statistical Manual of Mental Disorders, Fifth Edition (DSM-V), a panic attack is a sudden, unexpected, intense fear response during which anxiety rapidly escalates within minutes (**Boxes 2 and 3**).[46]

Box 2
Common somatic manifestations of anxiety[44,45,47–52]

Cardio/Pulmonary
• Chest pain
• Palpitations
• Shortness of breath/sensation of being smothered

Gastrointestinal

- Nausea, sometimes with vomiting or dry heaving
- Diarrhea
- Sensation of choking
- Abdominal bloating or pain
- Dyspepsia

Genitourinary
- Urinary frequency
- Urinary urgency

Neurologic/Autonomic
- Diaphoresis
- Dizziness or presyncope
- Hot flashes/chills
- Tremor
- Headache

Box 3
Differential diagnosis for anxiety[44,45,47–52]

Cardio/Pulmonary
- Arrhythmias
- Myocardial infarction
- COPD
- Asthma
- Mitral valve prolapsed
- Pulmonary embolism

Endocrine
- Hyperthyroidism
- Hyperparathyroidism
- Pheochromocytoma
- Cancerous tumor

Metabolic
- Electrolyte imbalances
- Hypoglycemia
- Porphyria

Seizure disorders

Psychiatric disorders
- Obsessive-compulsive disorder
- Posttraumatic stress disorder
- Generalized anxiety disorder
- Specific phobia/social phobia

Therapeutic drugs
- Theophylline
- Oral/IM/IV steroids

Recreational drugs
- Amphetamines/methamphetamines
- Cocaine
- Caffeine
- Diet/weight loss pills

Withdrawal
- Alcohol
- Cannabis
- Benzodiazepines
- Barbiturates

Abbreviations: COPD, chronic obstructive pulmonary disease; IM, intramuscular; IV, intravenous.

Workup

Although a panic attack is not a diagnosis of exclusion, underlying causes must be ruled out. The workup should be tailored to the presenting symptoms and may include the following:

- Electrocardiogram (EKG), electrolytes plus calcium, toxicology screen, thyroid profile, and in some cases, telemetry and serial cardiac enzyme monitoring may be warranted
- Obtain CXR, arterial blood gas (ABG's), or pulmonary function testing (PFT) if respiratory compromise is suspected
- Brain CT or MRI or an EEG may be reasonable to obtain depending on presenting symptoms
- Holter monitor

Treatment

In the ED, once concomitant medical or substance-related conditions are ruled out, the mainstay of treatment of a persistent panic attack is benzodiazepines. Used in the acute setting, these are highly effective. Given the addictive nature, however, these should not be prescribed for ongoing use through the ED but rather used only while the patient is being treated within the facility.

Generally, short-acting benzodiazepines are recommended in this setting due to the rapid onset and shorter duration of action.[53] A single dose of lorazepam, 1 mg PO, or alprazolam, 0.5 mg PO, is frequently sufficient. The dosage may be repeated in 1 hour if needed. Poor response to treatment indicates that further workup is needed, which may include psychiatry consultation.

Disposition/Referral

Patients should be referred back to their PCP within a week of their ED visit for ongoing management and, if warranted, referral on to psychiatry and/or counseling services.

THE DISORGANIZED/PSYCHOTIC PATIENT

Psychosis is a state in which reality is distorted due to delusions and/or hallucinations. It is a key finding in many primary psychiatric illnesses including schizophrenia. It can be a component of a severe mood disorder (major depressive disorder with psychotic features, a manic episode of bipolar disorder), as a result of withdrawal or active intoxication from a substance or as a sign of an underlying medical or neurologic problem. Medical, neurologic, and substance-related causes of psychosis must be given consideration and ruled out as quickly as possible.

Assessment

As with the agitated patient, first and foremost, ensure safety of the patient, staff, and bystanders. The assessment and management may become intertwined and follow a disorganized pattern, depending on the level of patient impairment. Refer to **Fig. 1** if immediate chemical restraint is warranted.

When observing the patient, assess for the following:

- Altered or bizarre thought pattern
- Suicidal or homicidal ideation/intent
- Disorganized or abnormal speech (word salad, pressured, ruminative)
- Abnormal motor skills (ie, catatonia, Parkinsonism, cogwheeling, pill-rolling)
- Memory impairment

- Attentional difficulties
- Lack of insight or judgment
- Cognitive delay, limited intellect
- Evidence of response to internal stimuli

Differential Diagnosis

Workup

Initially, obtain a comprehensive metabolic panel, complete blood count, urine toxicology, urinalysis (UA), TSH, and CXR as well as frequent vital signs with pulse oximetry Refer to **Box 1**.

If initial workup is unrevealing, follow-up with vitamin B12, folate, thiamine, cortisol, HIV, RPR, COVID-19 PCR, ESR/CRP, and serum ANA.

If agitation and/or psychosis rapidly progresses, move forward to EEG and LP for CSF counts and glucose.

Head CT is appropriate for agitation and delirium (to rule out intracranial abnormality) but is rarely useful for isolated psychosis.

Treatment

The goal of treatment of psychosis in the ED is to identify the root cause of the psychotic break and treat accordingly. If medical and substance-related causes are ruled out, and a primary psychiatric condition is likely, next steps are partially determined by the resources available within the ED. If psychiatric consultation services are available, use them.

In situations where such services are not readily available, manage the patient's symptoms with an antipsychotic. Selection of agent varies based on availability of agents, allergies, potential side effects, comorbidities, and clinician comfort/familiarity.

In all but the most severe cases, second-generation antipsychotics are recommended due to their more favorable side-effect profile (fewer extrapyramidal symptoms, in particular).[54–67] The route of administration will vary depending on agent formulations as well as the patient's willingness to cooperate. Use the least invasive means of administration when possible (See **Table 1**).

For the psychotic patient with agitation, haloperidol, 2–10 mg, orally or intramuscularly (IM), along with benztropine or diphenhydramine to reduce extrapyramidal symptoms (EPS)/dystonic reactions is recommended.

For the *severely* psychotic patient with agitation where safety is a concern, the addition of a benzodiazepine is suggested. The combination of Haldol, 5 mg IM; lorazepam, 2 mg IM; and benztropine, 2 mg IM, is often effective in managing the acute psychosis, calming agitation, and preventing EPS.

Disposition/referral

Referral depends on the cause. In the absence of any underlying medical or substance-related cause, the acutely psychotic patient requires immediate psychiatric consultation and/or transfer to an inpatient psychiatric unit for monitoring and stabilization.

THE ACUTELY DEPRESSED/SUICIDAL PATIENT

Each year, approximately 45,000 people die by suicide in the United States alone, with an estimated 800,000 annual suicides worldwide.[68] These numbers are likely underestimated. The death may have been misclassified as unintentional, especially if there was uncertainty about the intent. Social sensitivity regarding suicide and stigma can also be a factor, and in some areas of the world, suicide is considered illegal **Box 4**.[69]

Assessment

If the patient has been brought to the ED following a serious attempt, the initial course of treatment will clearly be acute stabilization.

If there has been no attempt that requires immediate medical management, start by determining the presence of suicidal ideation to determine if the thoughts are active or passive. Follow-up questions should include the following:[70,71]

- Is there a specific plan? A method, place, and time?
- What does the patient hope suicide would accomplish? (Escape, punishing others)
- How easily could the patient execute their suicide plan? (The patient has guns and knows how to use them versus wants to but has no access to firearms or does not know how to use them)
- What is the lethality of the plan?
- Is rescue likely within the plan?
- What preparations for the plan have been made?
- Is there associated substance use/abuse that may increase impulsivity?
- Past suicidal ideation, attempts, self-injurious behavior
- Current or past psychiatric diagnoses and medications
- Family history of completed suicide
- Current stressors (relationship breakdown, job loss, financial struggle)

Box 4
Factors increasing suicide risk[68–74]

- Prior suicide attempt with highly fatal method (hanging, firearm)

- Disappointment that prior suicide attempt was not successful

- Steps to avoid detection were included in prior suicide attempt

- Unwillingness or inability to discuss safety planning

- Inability to openly and honestly discuss ideations, intent, plan, or precipitating factors

- Psychiatric disorders
  1. Anxiety disorder
  2. Bipolar disorder
  3. Personality disorder
  4. Posttraumatic stress disorder
  5. Psychotic disorder
  6. Substance use disorder
  7. Mood disorder

- Poor social support/isolation

- Current state of agitation

- History of childhood trauma

- History of military active combat or trauma/veteran status

- Ease of access to weapons or other lethal measures

- White (non-Hispanic) men older than 70 years

- History of or current incarceration

- Sexual minority status

- Prior death by suicide of a family member

- Chronic pain
- History of traumatic brain injury
- History of or current impulsivity
- Lack of hope for the future

Workup

The self-inflicted gunshot wound victim will likely require trauma services first, before any psychiatric intervention. Similarly, a patient presenting with an intentional overdose, will initiatlly require management in accordance to Poison Control (1-800-222-1222) before a psychiatric evaluation.

At minimum, obtain the following:

- Complete set of vital signs
- Urine or blood toxicology
- Thyroid profile
- Electrolytes

Treatment

The treatment of the suicidal patient will depend on circumstances specific to their presentation.

Disposition/Referral

Consultation with psychiatry or a mental health crisis team, face-to-face or telemedicine, should be obtained for ALL suicidal patients. If unavailable within the facility, the patient should be transferred to a site with such services to provide definitive care and manage follow-up.

MEDICAL EMERGENCIES OF THE PSYCHIATRIC PATIENT
Serotonin Syndrome

Definition

Serotonin syndrome is a drug-induced disorder, with the classic characterizations of mental status changes, autonomic dysfunction, and neuromuscular hyperactivity. It is potentially life-threatening Box 5.[75]

Assessment

Serotonin syndrome is a clinical diagnosis, with no laboratory test for confirmation. The Hunter criteria for serotonin syndrome are widely used for diagnosis,[76] which confirm if the patient has taken a serotonergic agent (usually in the context of a dosage increase or addition of second agent) and has one or more of the following:

- Inducible clonus AND agitation or diaphoresis
- Spontaneous clonus
- Tremor AND hyperreflexia
- Hypertonia
- Temperature greater than 38°C AND ocular clonus or inducible clonus
- Ocular clonus AND agitation or diaphoresis

Box 5
Examples of drug agents that can precipitate serotonin syndrome[75-82]

- SSRIs (fluoxetine, sertraline, citalopram, escitalopram, paroxetine, fluvoxamine)
- SNRIs (desvenlafaxine, duloxetine, venlafaxine, milnacipran)
- Monoamine oxidase inhibitors (selegiline, isocarboxazid, phenelzine, tranylcypromine)
- Atypical antispsychotics (risperidone, aripiprazole, quetiapine, olanzapine)
- Trazodone
- Bupropion
- Tricyclic antidepressants (amitriptyline, clomipramine, nortriptyline, trimipramine)
- St. John's wort (hypericum perforatum)
- Psychostimulants (methylphenidate, dextroamphetamine, phentermine)
- Buspirone
- Mirtazapine
- Antiemetics (ondansetron, granisetron)
- Cyclobenzaprine
- Lithium
- Analgesics (meperidine, tramadol, fentanyl)
- Triptans (almotriptan, eletriptan, frovatriptan, naratriptan, rizatriptan, sumatriptan, zolmitriptan)
- Cough suppressants (dextromethorphan)
- Illicit drugs (methamphetamine, MDMA, cocaine, LSD)

Abbreviations: LSD, lysergic acid diethylamide; MDMA, 3,4-methylenedioxymethamphetamine.

Workup

Although the history and physical examination alone are diagnostic,[77] additional tests may be warranted to narrow the differential and rule out other life-threatening conditions. Consider the following:

- CBC); electrolytes; blood, urea, nitrogen (BUN)/creatinine
- CK), liver profile, coagulation studies
- UA, urine culture (UC), blood cultures
- EKG/telemetry
- CXR
- Head CT
- Lumbar puncture
- Urine or blood toxicology
- Thyroid panel

Differential diagnosis

- Anticholinergic crisis/toxicity
- Malignant hyperthermia
- Meningitis/encephalitis
- Sympathomimetic toxicity
- Neuroleptic malignant syndrome (typically presents in a more gradual manner over days to weeks, where serotonin syndrome develops rapidly over 24 hours)
- Drug toxicity (amphetamines, cocaine, LSD, PCP, lithium, salicylates)

Treatment (**Fig. 2**) (**Box 6**)

Box 6
Management of Serotonin Syndrome[77–82]

- Discontinue use of ALL potential precipitating drugs
- Control symptoms (agitation, clonus, tremor, palpitations, HTN) with benzodiazepines. Recommend lorazepam, 1 to 2 mg, IV Q 30 minutes, titrating the dosage as necessary for desired effect. Diazepam, 5 to 10 mg, IV is an alternative.
- Provide oxygen to maintain saturations greater than 94%
- Monitor patient with continuous telemetry
- Hypotensive patients may require both IV fluids and vasopressor therapy
- Hypertensive patients should be treated with short-acting agents (eg, esmolol or nitroprusside)
- If benzodiazepines fail to improve symptoms, trial cyproheptadine, 12 mg, orally (adult dosage) every 2 hours up to 32 mg/d[79,80]
- For significant hyperthermia (greater than 41.1°C), patient should undergo rapid sequence intubation and be transferred to ICU for ongoing management and standard hyperthermia measures. AVOID antipyretics such as acetaminophen.

Abbreviations: HTN, hypertension; ICU, intensive care unit; IV, intravenous.

Disposition/referral
Disposition will depend on severity of symptoms and response to treatment. Some patients will require transfer to the ICU. Those with mild symptoms, who seem appropriate for discharge, should first undergo face-to-face or telemedicine psychiatry consult for aftercare planning.

Tardive Dyskinesia

Definition
Tardive dyskinesia (TD) is a neurologic disorder of involuntary movements associated with the long-term use of antipsychotic medication, particularly first-generation antipsychotics. Patients exhibit rapid, repetitive, stereotypic movements that mostly involve the oral, lingual, trunk, and limb areas. Although most cases of TD are managed outside of the ED/hospital setting, many patients experiencing TD will present to the ED as their first point of contact for these particular symptoms.

Assessment
TD is a diagnosis of exclusion. A thorough neuropsychiatric and medication history and a complete physical examination are generally the extent of that which is required to formulate a TD diagnosis. The Abnormal Involuntary Movement Scale can be used to evaluate and monitor the severity of TD.[87]

- TD typically appears with the withdrawal or reduction of an antipsychotic medication
- Lip smacking and puckering, tongue protrusion and twisting, and facial grimacing are the classic symptoms, but in some cases there may be truncal or limb involvement
- Oral symptoms associated with TD may be suppressed by voluntary actions such as eating, drinking, or talking

Workup
Although the history and physical examination alone are diagnostic, additional tests may be warranted to narrow the differential and rule out other life-threatening conditions. Consider the following:

- CBC, electrolytes, BUN/Creatinine
- CK, liver profile, coagulation studies
- UA, UC, blood cultures
- EKG/telemetry
- CXR
- Head CT
- Lumbar puncture
- Urine or blood toxicology
- Thyroid panel

Differential diagnosis

- Acute EPS such as short-term withdrawal dyskinesias, akathisia, or Parkinsonism
- Basal ganglia disorders (Tourette syndrome, levodopa-induced dyskinesia in Parkinson disease, Wilson disease, Huntington chorea)
- Hyperthyroidism-induced choreoathetosis
- Dyskinesias related to improperly fitted dentures (edentulous dyskinesia)
- Autoimmune diseases such as multiple sclerosis
- Neurologic damage (mercury or lead toxicity, neurosyphilis, prior head injury, brain damage secondary to illicit substances)

Treatment

Disposition/referral

Patients should follow-up with their psychiatrist or mental health prescriber as soon as possible on discharge from the ER. If TD is refractory, consider referral to multidisciplinary movement disorder center.

Neuroleptic Malignant Syndrome

Definition

Neuroleptic malignant syndrome (NMS), a life-threatening emergency, is associated with the use of antipsychotic agents. Mental status change, fever, rigidity, and dysautonomia are distinct characteristics of the syndrome.[95–97]

Although most frequently seen in relation to high-potency first-generation antipsychotic agents (Haldol, fluphenazine), every class of antipsychotic drug has been implicated, including the low-potency (chlorpromazine) and second-generation antipsychotic drugs (Clozaril, olanzapine, risperidone) as well as antiemetic drugs (promethazine, metoclopramide).

Assessment

Typically, NMS symptoms evolve over 1 to 3 days and include the following tetrad of symptoms:

- Mental status change (agitated delirium with confusion rather than psychosis; catatonia with mutism)
- Muscular rigidity, which is generalized and often extreme
- Hyperthermia
- Autonomic instability (hypertension, tachycardia, tachypnea, profuse diaphoresis)

Workup

The diagnosis of NMS is made in a patient who develops the typical clinical syndrome in the context of taking an associated causative medication. There is no diagnostic

Is ongoing treatment with dopamine receptor-blocking agent (DRBA) necessary?

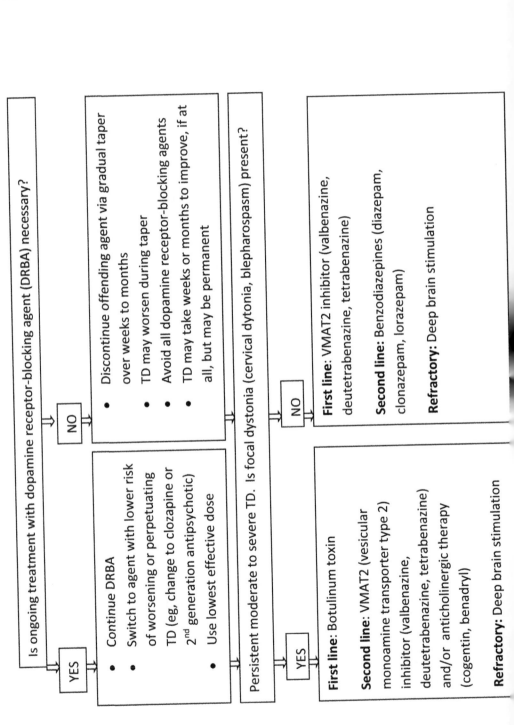

YES

- Continue DRBA
- Switch to agent with lower risk of worsening or perpetuating TD (eg, change to clozapine or 2ⁿᵈ generation antipsychotic)
- Use lowest effective dose

NO

- Discontinue offending agent via gradual taper over weeks to months
- TD may worsen during taper
- Avoid all dopamine receptor-blocking agents
- TD may take weeks or months to improve, if at all, but may be permanent

Persistent moderate to severe TD. Is focal dystonia (cervical dytonia, blepharospasm) present?

YES

First line: Botulinum toxin

Second line: VMAT2 (vesicular monoamine transporter type 2) inhibitor (valbenazine, deutetrabenazine, tetrabenazine) and/or anticholinergic therapy (cogentin, benadryl)

Refractory: Deep brain stimulation

NO

First line: VMAT2 inhibitor (valbenazine, deutetrabenazine, tetrabenazine)

Second line: Benzodiazepines (diazepam, clonazepam, lorazepam)

Refractory: Deep brain stimulation

test for NMS, but laboratory abnormalities can aid in the confirmation of the clinical diagnosis and ruling out other conditions.

- CK is typically greater than 1000 IU/L and can be seen as high as 100,000/IU/L. CK may be normal during the earlier stages of the syndrome
- Leukocytosis is generally present (WBC 10,000–40,000)
- Mild elevations of liver function testing (alkaline phosphatase/ALT/AST/LDH) commonly seen
- Electrolyte abnormalities common (hypomagnesemia, hyponatremia, hypernatremia, hypocalcemia, hyperkalemia) along with metabolic acidosis
- Acute renal failure may be present secondary to rhabdomyolysis
- Low serum iron concentration frequently present

Brain imaging studies and lumbar puncture are necessary to exclude brain disease (structural and/or infectious).

- Brain MRI/CT are typically normal in NMS
- CSF analysis is typically normal in NMS
- EEG, to rule out nonconvulsive status epilepticus, will frequently show generalized slow wave activity

Differential diagnosis

- Anticholinergic crisis/toxicity
- Malignant hyperthermia
- Meningitis/encephalitis
- Sympathomimetic toxicity
- Neuroleptic malignant syndrome (typically presents in a more gradual manner over days to weeks, where serotonin syndrome develops rapidly over 24 hours)
- Drug toxicity or withdrawal (amphetamines, cocaine, LSD, PCP, lithium, salicylates)
- Serotonin syndrome
- Malignant hyperthermia
- Malignant catatonia
- Central nervous system (CNS) infection (encephalitis, meningitis)
- Systemic infections (sepsis, pneumonia, urinary tract infection)
- Tetanus
- Thyrotoxicosis
- Seizure disorder
- Acute dystonia
- Heat stroke (impaired thermoregulation secondary to antipsychotic use)
- Pheochromocytoma
- Acute Porphyria

Treatment
Stop causative agent
- Removal of the causative agent is the single most important treatment in NMS. Other potential contributing psychotropic agents (anticholinergic medications, serotonergic medications, lithium) should also be stopped if possible. When the precipitant is discontinuation of dopaminergic therapy, resuming the agent is recommended.

Supportive therapy
- Maintain cardiorespiratory stability

- Maintain euvolemic state using intravenous fluids
- Lower fever using cooling blankets. More aggressive physical measures may be required: ice water gastric lavage and ice packs in the axilla.
- Lower blood pressure if markedly elevated. Both clonidine and nitroprusside are effective in NMS, although if patient is hyperthermic, nitroprusside may have advantages by also facilitating cooling through cutaneous vasodilation.[92]
- Prescribe heparin or low-molecular-weight heparin for prevention of deep venous thrombosis.
- For agitation, use benzodiazepines (lorazepam, 0.5–1 mg)

Disposition/referral. The intensive nature of the required monitoring and supportive treatment is such that admission to the ICU is required.

ACUTE SUBSTANCE INTOXICATION AND/OR WITHDRAWAL

For the purpose of this brief overview, only acute intoxication and acute withdrawal with life-threatening potential will be covered, in the format of reference tables. Referral to psychiatry, addiction medicine, and/or placement of patient in a detoxification or rehabilitation facility may be warranted **Boxes 7–11**.

Box 7
Opioids (central nervous system depressant)[98–100]

Classic Presentation of Toxicity
- Pinpoint pupils
- Hypoventilation
- Reduced consciousness/unconsciousness
- Diminished or absent bowel sounds

Workup
- Urine or blood toxicology (awaiting laboratory confirmation does NOT preclude naloxone)
- Assess for track marks
- Rapid bedside serum glucose
- CK if suspect lengthy immobilization
- Acetaminophen/salicylate levels
- Pregnancy test in women (positive test does NOT preclude naloxone)

Emergency Management of Toxicity (beyond ABC/ACLS management)
- Naloxone (Narcan) administration as soon as possible (IV, IM, SQ, nasal spray)
- Partial response indicates need for repeat dosage
- Concern for potential precipitated opioid withdrawal is not a contraindication to naloxone administration (toxicity can be fatal, withdrawal does not kill)
- Observation and symptomatic management for withdrawal
- Consultation with addiction medicine/psychiatry or substance abuse team if possible
- Patient medically stable for transfer to detox (preferable) or discharge when ventilation and mental status are stabilized for more than 1 hour following last naloxone dosage

Classic Presentation of Withdrawal
- Nausea and vomiting
- Insomnia
- Diarrhea
- Rhinorrhea/lacrimation
- Muscle aches, pains, or cramps
- Anxiety

- Diaphoresis
- Hot and cold flashes

Workup
- Use COWS assessment scale (Clinical Opiate Withdrawal Scale) or similar[99]
- Pregnancy test in women

Emergency Management of Withdrawal (beyond ABC/ACLS management)
- Manage nausea and vomiting with promethazine or ondansetron
- Manage diarrhea with loperamide
- Manage severe anxiety or muscle cramps with diazepam
- If naloxone-induced withdrawal, do not use methadone or buprenorphine
- If naturally occurring withdrawal, clinician may use methadone (10 mg IM or 20 mg orally) or buprenorphine, 4 to 8 mg, sublingual (SL) (do NOT initiate until COWS score 8 or greater)

Referral/Disposition
- Consultation with addiction medicine/psychiatry or substance abuse team if possible
- If buprenorphine or methadone have been initiated, patient must have appropriate follow-up arranged to ensure ongoing management

---

Box 8
Amphetamines (central nervous system stimulant)[98,101–108]

Classic Presentation of Toxicity
- Tachycardia
- CNS stimulation (delirium, agitation, psychosis)
- Diaphoresis
- Dilated pupils
- Hypertension
- Hyperthermia may occur

Workup
- EKG
- Glucose
- Acetaminophen/salicylate levels
- Pregnancy test in women
- BUN and creatinine
- Electrolytes
- Urine toxicology testing

Emergency Management of Toxicity (beyond ABC/ACLS)
- Manage agitation with aggressive sedation (lorazepam, diazepam, midazolam) (see **Fig. 1**)
- Manage psychosis if necessary (**Table 1**)
- Manage hypertension with benzodiazepines; if ineffective use nitroprusside or phentolamine
- For significant hyperthermia (greater than 41.1°C), patient should undergo rapid sequence intubation and be transferred to ICU for ongoing management and standard hyperthermia measures. AVOID antipyretics such as acetaminophen.

Referral/Disposition
- Consultation with addiction medicine/psychiatry or substance abuse team if possible

---

Box 9
Cocaine (central nervous system stimulant)[98,109–116]

Classic Presentation of Toxicity
- Tachycardia
- CNS stimulation (delirium, agitation, psychosis)
- Diaphoresis

- Dilated pupils
- Hypertension
- Hyperthermia may occur

Workup
- EKG
- Glucose
- Acetaminophen/salicylate levels
- Pregnancy test in women
- BUN and creatinine
- Electrolytes
- Urine toxicology testing (confirms use in last few days but does NOT confirm acute toxicity)
- Further tests as indicated based on presentation (such as cardiac biomarkers or chest CT)

Emergency Management of Toxicity (Beyond ABC/ACLS)
- Manage agitation with aggressive sedation (lorazepam, diazepam, midazolam) (see **Fig. 1**)
- Manage psychosis if necessary (see **Table 1**)
- Manage hypertension with benzodiazepines; if ineffective use nitroprusside or phentolamine
- Avoid β-blockers, which are contraindicated in acute cocaine toxicity
- For significant hyperthermia (greater than 41.1°C), patient should undergo rapid sequence intubation and be transferred to ICU for ongoing management and standard hyperthermia measures. AVOID antipyretics such as acetaminophen
- For cocaine-associated myocardial ischemia administer aspirin, 325 mg, orally (unless aortic dissection is suspected), nitroglycerin, 0.4 mg SL, and supplemental O2
- For QRS widening suggesting profound toxicity, administer sodium bicarbonate 1 to 2 mEq/kg IV push

Referral/Disposition
- Consultation with addiction medicine/psychiatry or substance abuse team if possible
- Observe uncomplicated cocaine toxicity until symptom resolution
- Monitor patients with cocaine-associated chest pain with serial cardiac biomarkers and EKG; if normal after 12 hours, may discharge
- Admit patients with evidence of end-organ toxicity

Box 10
Benzodiazepines (central nervous system depressant)[117–122]

Classic Presentation of Toxicity
- Ataxia
- Amnesia
- Stupor or somnolence
- Altered consciousness/unconscious
- Typically, normal vital signs
- Additive effects with alcohol

Workup
- Urine or blood toxicology
- Rapid bedside serum glucose
- Acetaminophen/salicylate levels
- Pregnancy test in women

Emergency Management of Toxicity (Beyond ABC/ACLS Management)
- Although flumazenil is available as an antagonist, it can precipitate seizures in those who depend on benzodiazepines and should be used with extreme caution, if at all
- Most of the patients require only observation and airway monitoring/support while "sleeping it off"

Classic Presentation of Withdrawal
- Seizures (life-threatening)

- Tremor
- Insomnia
- Anxiety
- Perceptual disturbance

Workup
- Urine or blood toxicology
- Rapid bedside serum glucose
- Acetaminophen/salicylate levels
- Pregnancy test in women

Emergency Management of Withdrawal (Beyond ABC/ACLS Management)
- Benzodiazepines—generally diazepam or lorazepam, titrated to eliminate withdrawal symptoms without causing respiratory depression or altered mental state

Referral/Disposition
- Consultation with addiction medicine/psychiatry or substance abuse team if possible
- Patient must have appropriate follow-up arranged to ensure ongoing management of a monitored benzodiazepine taper

---

Box 11
Alcohol (central nervous system depressant)[123–129]

Classic Presentation of Toxicity
- Ataxia/incoordination
- Memory impairment
- Stupor or somnolence
- Slurred speech
- Disinhibited behavior
- Altered consciousness/unconscious
- Hypotension and tachycardia may be present secondary to volume loss
- Additive effects with benzodiazepines

Workup
- BAC (blood alcohol concentration)
- Urine or blood toxicology
- Rapid bedside serum glucose
- Acetaminophen/salicylate levels
- Pregnancy test in women

Emergency Management of Toxicity (Beyond ABC/ACLS Management)
- patients require only observation and airway monitoring/support while "sleeping it off"
- Fluid replacement, with dextrose if hypoglycemic
- Thiamine, 100 mg

Classic Presentation of Withdrawal
- Seizures (life-threatening)
- Tremor (limbs, tongue)
- Insomnia
- GI upset (nausea, vomiting, anorexia)
- Anxiety
- Tachycardia
- Hypertension
- Perceptual disturbance
- Delirium Tremens

Workup
- BAC (in the chronic alcoholic, withdrawal may be present despite high BAC)
- Urine or blood toxicology to assess for additional substances
- Rapid bedside serum glucose

- Acetaminophen/salicylate levels
- Liver function testing
- BUN with creatinine
- Electrolytes
- Pregnancy test in women

Emergency Management of Withdrawal (Beyond ABC/ACLS Management)
- Use CIWA scoring (Clinical Institute Withdrawal Assessment for Alcohol) or similar[124]
- Generally, scores of 10 or greater require management with benzodiazepines[124]
- Benzodiazepines—generally IV or PO diazepam, lorazepam, or chlordiazepoxide, titrated to eliminate withdrawal symptoms without causing respiratory depression or altered mental state
- Manage psychosis per **Fig. 1.** Obtain EKG before administering antipsychotic due to potential for QT prolongation with many antipsychotic agents
- Fluid replacement, with dextrose if hypoglycemic
- Thiamine, 100 mg, IV or PO

Referral/Disposition
- Transfer to medically monitored detoxification unit

DISCLOSURE

The author has nothing to disclose.

REFERENCES

1. https://pubmed.ncbi.nlm.nih.gov/29261480/. [Accessed 20 December 2021].
2. Rice MM, Moore GP. Management of the violent patient. Therapeutic and legal considerations. Emerg Med Clin North Am 1991;9:13.
3. Kuhn W. Violence in the emergency department. Managing aggressive patients in a high-stress environment. Postgrad Med 1999;105:143.
4. Richmond JS, Berlin JS, Fishkind AB, et al. Verbal De-escalation of the Agitated Patient: Consensus Statement of the American Association for Emergency Psychiatry Project BETA De-escalation Workgroup. West J Emerg Med 2012;13:17.
5. Yildiz A, Sachs GS, Turgay A. Pharmacological management of agitation in emergency settings. Emerg Med J 2003;20:339.
6. Battaglia J. Pharmacological management of acute agitation. Drugs 2005;65:1207.
7. Mendoza R, Djenderedjian AH, Adams J, et al. Midazolam in acute psychotic patients with hyperarousal. J Clin Psychiatry 1987;48:291.
8. Battaglia J, Moss S, Rush J, et al. Haloperidol, lorazepam, or both for psychotic agitation? A multicenter, prospective, double-blind, emergency department study. Am J Emerg Med 1997;15:335.
9. Knott JC, Taylor DM, Castle DJ. Randomized clinical trial comparing intravenous midazolam and droperidol for sedation of the acutely agitated patient in the emergency department. Ann Emerg Med 2006;47:61.
10. Martel M, Sterzinger A, Miner J, et al. Management of acute undifferentiated agitation in the emergency department: a randomized double-blind trial of droperidol, ziprasidone, and midazolam. Acad Emerg Med 2005;12:1167.
11. Nobay F, Simon BC, Levitt MA, et al. A prospective, double-blind, randomized trial of midazolam versus haloperidol versus lorazepam in the chemical restraint of violent and severely agitated patients. Acad Emerg Med 2004;11:744.

12. Klein LR, Driver BE, Miner JR, et al. Intramuscular Midazolam, Olanzapine, Ziprasidone, or Haloperidol for Treating Acute Agitation in the Emergency Department. Ann Emerg Med 2018;72:374.
13. Thomas H Jr, Schwartz E, Petrilli R. Droperidol versus haloperidol for chemical restraint of agitated and combative patients. Ann Emerg Med 1992;21:407.
14. Richards JR, Derlet RW, Duncan DR. Chemical restraint for the agitated patient in the emergency department: lorazepam versus droperidol. J Emerg Med 1998;16:567.
15. Isbister GK, Calver LA, Page CB, et al. Randomized controlled trial of intramuscular droperidol versus midazolam for violence and acute behavioral disturbance: the DORM study. Ann Emerg Med 2010;56:392.
16. Martel ML, Driver BE, Miner JR, et al. Randomized Double-blind Trial of Intramuscular Droperidol, Ziprasidone, and Lorazepam for Acute Undifferentiated Agitation in the Emergency Department. Acad Emerg Med 2021;28:421.
17. Kao LW, Kirk MA, Evers SJ, et al. Droperidol, QT prolongation, and sudden death: what is the evidence? Ann Emerg Med 2003;41:546.
18. Shale JH, Shale CM, Mastin WD. A review of the safety and efficacy of droperidol for the rapid sedation of severely agitated and violent patients. J Clin Psychiatry 2003;64:500.
19. Gaw CM, Cabrera D, Bellolio F, et al. Effectiveness and safety of droperidol in a United States emergency department. Am J Emerg Med 2020;38:1310.
20. Marco CA, Vaughan J. Emergency management of agitation in schizophrenia. Am J Emerg Med 2005;23:767.
21. Bergman H, Soares-Weiser K. Anticholinergic medication for antipsychotic-induced tardive dyskinesia. Cochrane Database Syst Rev 2018;1:CD000204.
22. Carbon M, Kane JM, Leucht S, et al. Tardive dyskinesia risk with first- and second-generation antipsychotics in comparative randomized controlled trials: a meta-analysis. World Psychiatry 2018;17(3):330–40.
23. Chakraborti D, Tampi DJ, Tampi RR, et al. Melatonin and melatonin agonist for delirium in the elderly patients. Am J Alzheimers Dis Other Demen 2015; 30(2):119–29.
24. Cipriani A, Barbui C, Salanti G, et al. Comparative efficacy and acceptability of antimanic drugs in acute mania: a multiple-treatments meta-analysis. Lancet 2011;378(9799):1306–15.
25. Freudenreich O. In: Rosenbaum J, editor. Psychotic disorders: a practical guide. Cham, Switzerland: Springer International; 2020. p. 127–36.
26. Glasner-Edwards S, Mooney LJ. Methamphetamine psychosis: epidemiology and management. CNS Drugs 2014;28(12):1115–26.
27. González-Rodríguez A, Catalán R, Penadés R, et al. Antipsychotic response in delusional disorder and schizophrenia: a prospective cohort study. Actas Esp Psiquiatr 2016;44(4):125–35.
28. Huhn M, Nikolakopoulou A, Schneider-Thoma J, et al. Comparative efficacy and tolerability of 32 oral antipsychotics for the acute treatment of adults with multiepisode schizophrenia: a systematic review and network meta-analysis. Lancet 2019;394(10202):939–51.
29. Leentjens AFG, Rundell J, Rummans T, et al. Delirium: an evidence-based medicine (EBM) monograph for psychosomatic medicine practice, commissioned by the Academy of Psychosomatic Medicine (APM) and the European Association of Consultation Liaison Psychiatry and Psychosomatics (EACLPP). J Psychosom Res 2012;73:149–52.

30. Leucht S, Crippa A, Siafis S, et al. Dose-response meta-analysis of antipsychotic drugs for acute schizophrenia. Am J Psychiatry 2020;177(4):342–53.
31. Moreno C, Nuevo R, Chatterji S, et al. Psychotic symptoms are associated with physical health problems independently of a mental disorder diagnosis: results from the WHO World Health Survey. World Psychiatry 2013;12(3):251–7.
32. Moreno-Küstner B, Martin C, Pastor L, et al. Prevalence of psychotic disorders and its association with methodological issues. A systematic review and meta-analyses. PLoS One 2018;13(4).
33. Sit D, Rothschild AJ, Wisner K, et al. A review of postpartum psychosis. J Womens Health (Larchmt) 2006;15(4):352–68.
34. Tiihonen J, Lönnqvist J, Wahlbeck K, et al. 11-year follow-up of mortality in patients with schizophrenia: a population-based cohort study (FIN11 study). Lancet 2009;374(9690):620–7.
35. Vinogradov S, Fisher M, Warm H, et al. The cognitive cost of anticholinergic burden: decreased response to cognitive training in schizophrenia. Am J Psychiatry 2009;166(9):1055–62.
36. . https://www.poison.org. [Accessed 3 January 2022].
37. Klein LR, Driver BE, Horton G, et al. Rescue Sedation When Treating Acute Agitation in the Emergency Department With Intramuscular Antipsychotics. J Emerg Med 2019;56:484.
38. Cole JB, Stang JL, DeVries PA, et al. A Prospective Study of Intramuscular Droperidol or Olanzapine for Acute Agitation in the Emergency Department: A Natural Experiment Owing to Drug Shortages. Ann Emerg Med 2021;78:274.
39. Schneider A, Mullinax S, Hall N, et al. Intramuscular medication for treatment of agitation in the emergency department: A systematic review of controlled trials. Am J Emerg Med 2021;46:193.
40. Rund DA, Ewing JD, Mitzel K, et al. The use of intramuscular benzodiazepines and antipsychotic agents in the treatment of acute agitation or violence in the emergency department. J Emerg Med 2006;31:317.
41. Glassman AH, Bigger JT Jr. Antipsychotic drugs: prolonged QTc interval, torsade de pointes, and sudden death. Am J Psychiatry 2001;158:1774.
42. Seitz DP, Gill SS, van Zyl LT. Antipsychotics in the treatment of delirium: a systematic review. J Clin Psychiatry 2007;68:11.
43. Fitzgerald P. Long-acting antipsychotic medication, restraint and treatment in the management of acute psychosis. Aust N Z J Psychiatry 1999;33:660.
44. de Jonge P, et al. Cross-national epidemiology of panic disorder and panic attacks in the world mental health surveys. Depress Anxiety 2016;33(12):1155–77.
45. Kessler RC, Petukhova M, Sampson N A,, et al. Twelve-month and lifetime prevalence and lifetime morbid risk of anxiety and mood disorders in the United States. Int J Methods Psychiatr Res 2012;21(3):169–84.
46. American Psychiatric Association. Diagnostic and Statistical Manual of Mental Disorders. Fifth Edition. Arlington, VA: American Psychiatric Association; 2013.
47. Barlow DH, Farchione TJ, Bullis JR, et al. The unified protocol for transdiagnostic treatment of emotional disorders compared with diagnosis-specific protocols for anxiety disorders. JAMA Psychiatry 2017;74(9):875–84.
48. Boettcher J, Aström V, Påhlsson D, et al. Internet-based mindfulness treatment for anxiety disorders: a randomized controlled trial. Behav Ther 2014;45(2):241–53.
49. Foldes-Busque G, Denis I, Poitras J, et al. A closer look at the relationships between panic attacks, emergency department visits and non-cardiac chest pain. J Health Psychol 2019;24(6):717–25.

50. Hettema JM, Neale MC, Kendler KS, et al. A review and meta-analysis of the genetic epidemiology of anxiety disorders. Am J Psychiatry 2001;158(10): 1568–78.
51. Hettema JM, Prescott CA, Myers JM, et al. The structure of genetic and environmental risk factors for anxiety disorders in men and women. Arch Gen Psychiatry 2005;62(2):182–9.
52. Hofmann SG, Sawyer AT, Witt AA, et al. The effect of mindfulness-based therapy on anxiety and depression: a meta-analytic review. J Consult Clin Psychol 2010; 78(2):169–83.
53. Stein M, Goin M, Pollack M, et al. Practice Guideline for the treatment of patients with panic disorder: Second edition. Am J Psychiatry 2009;166(2):1.
54. Sikich L, Frazier JA, McClellan J, et al. Double-blind comparison of first- and second-generation antipsychotics in early-onset schizophrenia and schizo-affective disorder: findings from the treatment of early-onset schizophrenia spectrum disorders (TEOSS) study. Am J Psychiatry 2008;165:1420.
55. Buchanan RW, Kreyenbuhl J, Kelly DL, et al. The 2009 schizophrenia PORT psychopharmacological treatment recommendations and summary statements. Schizophr Bull 2010;36:71.
56. Reus VI, Fochtmann LJ, Eyler AE, et al. The American Psychiatric Association Practice Guideline on the Use of Antipsychotics to Treat Agitation or Psychosis in Patients With Dementia. Am J Psychiatry 2016;173:543.
57. Takeuchi H, MacKenzie NE, Samaroo D, et al. Antipsychotic Dose in Acute Schizophrenia: A Meta-analysis. Schizophr Bull 2020;46:1439.
58. Komossa K, Rummel-Kluge C, Schmid F, et al. Aripiprazole versus other atypical antipsychotics for schizophrenia. Cochrane Database Syst Rev 2009;4: CD006569.
59. Leucht S, Corves C, Arbter D, et al. Second-generation versus first-generation antipsychotic drugs for schizophrenia: a meta-analysis. Lancet 2009;373:31.
60. Misdrahi D, Tessier A, Daubigney A, et al. Prevalence of and Risk Factors for Extrapyramidal Side Effects of Antipsychotics: Results From the National FACE-SZ Cohort. J Clin Psychiatry 2019;80.
61. Fusar-Poli P, Papanastasiou E, Stahl D, et al. Treatments of Negative Symptoms in Schizophrenia: Meta-Analysis of 168 Randomized Placebo-Controlled Trials. Schizophr Bull 2015;41:892.
62. Zhang JP, Gallego JA, Robinson DG, et al. Efficacy and safety of individual second-generation vs. first-generation antipsychotics in first-episode psychosis: a systematic review and meta-analysis. Int J Neuropsychopharmacol 2013;16: 1205.
63. Leucht S, Cipriani A, Spineli L, et al. Comparative efficacy and tolerability of 15 antipsychotic drugs in schizophrenia: a multiple-treatments meta-analysis. Lancet 2013;382:951.
64. Huhn M, Nikolakopoulou A, Schneider-Thoma J, et al. Comparative efficacy and tolerability of 32 oral antipsychotics for the acute treatment of adults with multiepisode schizophrenia: a systematic review and network meta-analysis. Lancet 2019;394:939.
65. Yildiz A, Vieta E, Leucht S, et al. Efficacy of antimanic treatments: meta-analysis of randomized, controlled trials. Neuropsychopharmacology 2011;36:375.
66. Wijkstra J, Lijmer J, Burger H, et al. Pharmacological treatment for psychotic depression. Cochrane Database Syst Rev 2013;7:CD004044.
67. Wang HR, Woo YS, Bahk WM. Atypical antipsychotics in the treatment of delirium. Psychiatry Clin Neurosci 2013;67:323.

68. Centers for Disease Control and Prevention. Web-based injury statistics query and reporting system (WISQARS). Leading causes of death reports 1981 - 2016. Atlanta, GA. U.S department of Health and Human Services. Available at: https://www.cdc.gov/injury/wisqars/fatal.html. Accessed April 17, 2018.

69. World Health Organization. Preventing Suicide: A Global Imperative. Geneva, Switerland. 2014. Available at: www.who.int. Accessed April 24, 2018.

70. Practice guideline for the assessment and treatment of patients with suicidal behaviors. Am J Psychiatry 2003;160:1.

71. Silverman JJ, Galanter M, Jackson-Triche M, et al. The American Psychiatric Association Practice Guidelines for the Psychiatric Evaluation of Adults. Am J Psychiatry 2015;172:798.

72. Horowitz L, Snyder D, Ludi E, et al. Ask suicide-screening questions to everyone in medical settings: the asQ'em Quality Improvement Project. Psychosomatics 2013;54(3):239–47.

73. Tsai A, Lucas M, Sania A, et al. Social integration and suicide mortality among men: 24-year cohort study of U.S. health professionals. Ann Intern Med 2014; 161:85–95.

74. Norris D, Clark M. Evaluation and treatment of the suicidal patient. Am Fam Physician 2012;85(6):602–5.

75. Boyer EW, Shannon M. The serotonin syndrome. N Engl J Med 2005;352:1112.

76. Dunkley EJ, Isbister GK, Sibbritt D, et al. The Hunter Serotonin Toxicity Criteria: simple and accurate diagnostic decision rules for serotonin toxicity. QJM 2003; 96:635.

77. Mason PJ, Morris VA, Balcezak TJ. Serotonin syndrome. Presentation of 2 cases and review of the literature. Medicine (Baltimore) 2000;79:201.

78. Mills KC. Serotonin syndrome. A clinical update. Crit Care Clin 1997;13:763.

79. Graudins A, Stearman A, Chan B. Treatment of the serotonin syndrome with cyproheptadine. J Emerg Med 1998;16:615.

80. McDaniel WW. Serotonin syndrome: early management with cyproheptadine. Ann Pharmacother 2001;35:870.

81. Sternbach H. The serotonin syndrome. Am J Psychiatry 1991;148:705.

82. Ables AZ, Nagubilli R. Prevention, recognition, and management of serotonin syndrome. Am Fam Physician 2010;181(9):1139–42.

83. Ricciardi L, Pringsheim T, Barnes TRE, et al. Treatment Recommendations for Tardive Dyskinesia. Can J Psychiatry 2019;64:388.

84. Correll CU. Epidemiology and Prevention of Tardive Dyskinesia. J Clin Psychiatry 2017;78:e1426.

85. Correll CU, Kane JM, Citrome LL. Epidemiology, Prevention, and Assessment of Tardive Dyskinesia and Advances in Treatment. J Clin Psychiatry 2017;78:1136.

86. Lieberman JA, Saltz BL, Johns CA, et al. The effects of clozapine on tardive dyskinesia. Br J Psychiatry 1991;158:503.

87. Stacy M, Sajatovic M, Kane JM, et al. Abnormal involuntary movement scale in tardive dyskinesia: Minimal clinically important difference. Mov Disord 2019;34: 1203.

88. Kazamatsuri H, Chien CP, Cole JO. Long-term treatment of tardive dyskinesia with haloperidol and tetrabenazine. Am J Psychiatry 1973;130:479.

89. Kang UJ, Burke RE, Fahn S. Natural history and treatment of tardive dystonia. Mov Disord 1986;1:193.

90. Lang AE, Marsden CD. Alpha methylparatyrosine and tetrabenazine in movement disorders. Clin Neuropharmacol 1982;5:375.

91. Gregorakos L, Thomaides T, Stratouli S, et al. The use of clonidine in the management of autonomic overactivity in neuroleptic malignant syndrome. Clin Auton Res 2000;10:193.

92. Blue MG, Schneider SM, Noro S, et al. Successful treatment of neuroleptic malignant syndrome with sodium nitroprusside. Ann Intern Med 1986;104:56.

93. Caroff SN, Mann SC, Keck PE Jr. Specific treatment of the neuroleptic malignant syndrome. Biol Psychiatry 1998;44:378.

94. Modi S, Dharaiya D, Schultz L, et al. Neuroleptic Malignant Syndrome: Complications, Outcomes, and Mortality. Neurocrit Care 2016;24:97.

95. Levenson JL. Neuroleptic malignant syndrome. Am J Psychiatry 1985;142:1137.

96. Velamoor VR. Neuroleptic malignant syndrome. Recognition, prevention and management. Drug Saf 1998;19:73.

97. Caroff SN, Mann SC. Neuroleptic malignant syndrome. Med Clin North Am 1993;77:185.

98. The DAWN Report. Highlights of the 2010 drug abuse warning network (DAWN) findings on drug-related emergency department visits [Internet]. [cited 2015 Apr 19]. Available at: http://archive.samhsa.gov/data/2k12/DAWN096/SR096EDHighlights2010.htm. Accessed 2 Feb 2018.

99. Wesson DR, Ling W. The Clinical Opiate Withdrawal Scale (COWS). J Psychoactive Drugs 2003;35:253.

100. Herring AA, Perrone J, Nelson LS. Managing Opioid Withdrawal in the Emergency Department With Buprenorphine. Ann Emerg Med 2019;73:481.

101. Drug policy information clearinghouse fact sheet: methamphetamine. Office of National Drug Control Policy, Rockville, MD, 2003. Available at: www.whitehousedrugpolicy.gov. Accessed June 15, 2007.

102. Hendrickson RG, Cloutier R, McConnell KJ. Methamphetamine-related emergency department utilization and cost. Acad Emerg Med 2008;15:23.

103. Drug fact sheet: methamphetamine. Available at: https://www.dea.gov/druginfo/drug_data_sheets/Methamphetamine.pdf. Accessed November 14, 2016.

104. Gray SD, Fatovich DM, McCoubrie DL, et al. Amphetamine-related presentations to an inner-city tertiary emergency department: a prospective evaluation. Med J Aust 2007;186:336.

105. Derlet RW, Rice P, Horowitz BZ, et al. Amphetamine toxicity: experience with 127 cases. J Emerg Med 1989;7:157.

106. Chan P, Chen JH, Lee MH, et al. Fatal and nonfatal methamphetamine intoxication in the intensive care unit. J Toxicol Clin Toxicol 1994;32:147.

107. Richards JR, Bretz SW, Johnson EB, et al. Methamphetamine abuse and emergency department utilization. West J Med 1999;170:198.

108. Swanson SM, Sise CB, Sise MJ, et al. The scourge of methamphetamine: impact on a level I trauma center. J Trauma 2007;63:531.

109. Weber JE, Shofer FS, Larkin GL, et al. Validation of a brief observation period for patients with cocaine-associated chest pain. N Engl J Med 2003;348:510.

110. Hollander JE. The management of cocaine-associated myocardial ischemia. N Engl J Med 1995;333:1267.

111. Albertson TE, Dawson A, de Latorre F, et al. TOX-ACLS: toxicologic-oriented advanced cardiac life support. Ann Emerg Med 2001;37:S78.

112. Chan GM, Sharma R, Price D, et al. Phentolamine therapy for cocaine-association acute coronary syndrome (CAACS). J Med Toxicol 2006;2:108.

113. Hoffman RS. Cocaine and beta-blockers: should the controversy continue? Ann Emerg Med 2008;51:127.

114. Richards JR, Hollander JE, Ramoska EA, et al. β-Blockers, Cocaine, and the Unopposed α-Stimulation Phenomenon. J Cardiovasc Pharmacol Ther 2017; 22:239.

115. Richards JR, Garber D, Laurin EG, et al. Treatment of cocaine cardiovascular toxicity: a systematic review. Clin Toxicol (Phila) 2016;54:345.

116. Flaque-Coma J. Cocaine and rhabdomyolysis: report of a case and review of the literature. Bol Asoc Med P R 1990;82:423.

117. Drug Abuse Warning Network. The DAWN Report. April 2004. Benzodiazepine in Drug-Abuse Related Emergency Department Visits: 1995-2002. Available at: www.oas.samhsa.gov/2k4benzodiazepinesTrends.pdf. Accessed May 04, 2009.

118. Soyka M. Treatment of Benzodiazepine Dependence. N Engl J Med 2017;376: 1147.

119. Kaufmann CN, Spira AP, Alexander GC, et al. Emergency department visits involving benzodiazepines and non-benzodiazepine receptor agonists. Am J Emerg Med 2017;35:1414.

120. Weinbroum AA, Flaishon R, Sorkine P, et al. A risk-benefit assessment of flumazenil in the management of benzodiazepine overdose. Drug Saf 1997;17:181.

121. Seger DL. Flumazenil–treatment or toxin. J Toxicol Clin Toxicol 2004;42:209.

122. Authier N, Balayssac D, Sautereau M, et al. Benzodiazepine dependence: focus on withdrawal syndrome. Ann Pharm Fr 2009;67:408.

123. Mo Y, Thomas MC, Laskey CS, et al. Current Practice Patterns in the Management Of Alcohol Withdrawal Syndrome. P T 2018;43:158.

124. Sullivan JT, Sykora K, Schneiderman J, et al. Assessment of alcohol withdrawal: the revised clinical institute withdrawal assessment for alcohol scale (CIWA-Ar). Br J Addict 1989;84:1353.

125. Mayo-Smith MF. Pharmacological management of alcohol withdrawal. A meta-analysis and evidence-based practice guideline. American Society of Addiction Medicine Working Group on Pharmacological Management of Alcohol Withdrawal. JAMA 1997;278:144.

126. Amato L, Minozzi S, Vecchi S, et al., Benzodiazepines for alcohol withdrawal, 2010, Cochrane Database Syst Rev, (3), CD005063. https://doi.org/10.1002/14651858.CD005063.pub3.

127. Amato L, Minozzi S, Davoli M. Efficacy and safety of pharmacological interventions for the treatment of the Alcohol Withdrawal Syndrome. Cochrane Database Syst Rev 2011;6:CD008537.

128. Schmidt KJ, Doshi MR, Holzhausen JM, et al. Treatment of Severe Alcohol Withdrawal. Ann Pharmacother 2016;50:389.

129. Kosten TR, O'Connor PG. Management of drug and alcohol withdrawal. N Engl J Med 2003;348:1786.

Emergency Evaluation and Management of Sepsis and Septic Shock

Kasey Dillon, DScPAS, PA-C

KEYWORDS

- Sepsis • Septic shock • Sepsis screening tools • Management of sepsis
- Treatment of sepsis

KEY POINTS

- Sepsis and septic shock are medical emergencies, and the early recognition of both reduces mortality.
- Several screening tools are used to assist in the early recognition of sepsis and septic shock, with varying sensitivities and specificities.
- The Surviving Sepsis Guidelines are regularly updated and provide recommendations in the management of sepsis and septic shock.
- Despite varied evidence, the Surviving Sepsis Guidelines are accepted as the standard of care for emergency medicine and critical care providers.

INTRODUCTION

In 2016, the Sepsis Task Force revised the accepted definition of sepsis as life-threatening organ dysfunction characterized by a dysregulated host response to infection.[1,2] Septic shock, a subset of sepsis, is a form of distributive shock causing inadequate distribution of blood flow, leading to significant circulatory, metabolic, and cellular abnormalities.[3,4] Clinically and as defined by Sepsis-3 criteria, septic shock is sepsis with persistent hypotension requiring vasopressors to maintain an adequate mean arterial pressure (MAP).[5] Historically, sepsis screening tools have been used to assist clinicians in the rapid identification and, therefore, management of sepsis. Clinical variables include the systemic inflammatory response syndrome (SIRS) criteria, the Sequential Organ Failure Score (SOFA), the quick Sequential Organ Failure Score (qSOFA), the National Early Warning Sign Score (NEWS), and the Modified Early Warning Sign Score (MEWS).[1,2]

Sepsis and septic shock carry a large global health burden. Globally, estimates range from 19 to 49 million cases of sepsis annually leading the World Health

1260 Elm Street, Manchester, NH 03110, USA
E-mail address: Kasey.dillon@mcphs.edu

Physician Assist Clin 8 (2023) 193–204
https://doi.org/10.1016/j.cpha.2022.08.007
2405-7991/23/© 2022 Elsevier Inc. All rights reserved.

physicianassistant.theclinics.com

Organization (in 2017) to recognize the prevention and management of sepsis as a global health priority.[2,5] In developed countries, sepsis and septic shock account for 30% to 50% of all in-hospital deaths.[6] The trend of sepsis and septic shock is consistent in the United States as well, with an annual approximate of 1.7 million cases of sepsis and 250,000 deaths.[2] In 2015, the US Centers for Medicare and Medicaid Services (CMS) prioritized and implemented the Severe Sepsis and Septic Shock Early Management Bundle (SEP-1) tying hospital reimbursement to compliance with these established guidelines, further establishing early recognition and treatment of sepsis and septic shock as essential.[7] These estimates do not include the global burden of sepsis, septic shock, and death from COVID-19. Severe infection from COVID-19 does, by definition, meet Sepsis-3 criteria as viral sepsis with potential bacterial or fungal co-infection.[8] Although the overall target goals and management of sepsis and septic shock remain consistent regardless of cause, and including COVID-19, there are nuanced and rapidly changing approaches to the treatment of critically ill patients infected with COVID-19. This article does not address those specifically.

The decision to focus efforts on early recognition of sepsis is directly proportional to the overall mortality rates of septic shock. When defining sepsis by Sepsis-3 criteria, the in-hospital mortality rate is greater than 10%, which increases to greater than 40% when patients meet established criteria for septic shock.[4,9] There are multiple factors that contribute to the high rates of mortality associated with septic shock. Patients with preexisting comorbidities, compromised immunity, and poor access to health care and health care resources have demonstrated higher overall rates of sepsis, septic shock, and death. In addition, age greater than 65 years, female gender, and African American ethnicity predict higher mortality rates in patients with septic shock.[10,11] As clinicians, these risks factors are imperative to consider when evaluating patients for suspected sepsis or septic shock and must contribute to the decision-making process in the management of these same patients.

CLINICAL PRESENTATION

The clinical presentation of patients with sepsis is varied, making the diagnosis often difficult to efficiently determine. Patients who are experiencing symptoms of shock are easier to identify, based on clinical features. The cause of sepsis and septic shock is often not immediately recognizable. Because of this, sepsis screening tools and sepsis and septic shock treatment bundles and clinical guidelines have been established. Although these tools have a wide range of diagnostic accuracy and associated poor predictive values, the Surviving Sepsis Campaign of international guidelines for the diagnosis and management of sepsis and septic shock in 2021 make a strong recommendation that a screening tool be used by hospitals and health systems for all acutely ill and high-risk patients.[1,2] Because these screening tools have been shown to drive higher compliance with achieving sepsis bundle recommendations, overall mortality is decreased.[1]

SIRS Criteria Screening Tool

Although the SIRS criteria are still widely used as a screening tool in Emergency Medicine clinical practice, it has been criticized for its lack of sensitivity and specificity (as shown in **Table 1**).[6,12] In 2016, SEPSIS-3 was accepted as a more accurate definition of sepsis and septic shock. This redefined description of sepsis included life-threatening organ dysfunction, which is not detected by using SIRS criteria as a screening tool; this led to the creation of SOFA.

Table 1	
Systemic inflammatory response syndrome (SIRS) screening tool.	
Body Temperature	>38C or <36C
Heart Rate	<90
Respiratory Rate	>20
White blood cell count	>12,000 or <4,000 or the presense of <10% neutrophils

SOFA Criteria Screening Tool

Using the scale, SOFA criteria evaluate level of consciousness, respiratory function, hemodynamic stability, coagulation parameters, and liver and renal function. Laboratory test results are needed to accurately use this screening tool (as Shown in **Table 2**); this can be cumbersome and may limit the clinician's ability to initiate treatment bundles in a timely manner in the emergency department.[2,6] The SEPSIS-3 working group attempted to accelerate assessment using the SOFA screening tool by creating the q-SOFA (quickSOFA score).[1,2,6]

qSOFA Screening Tool

qSOFA as a screening tool uses 3 variables, instead of 5, to determine potential sepsis. These variables include the Glasgow Coma Scale, respiratory rate and systolic blood pressure (as shown in **Table 3**). Although qSOFA has been shown to be an accurate predictor of mortality and prolonged intensive care unit (ICU) stay, experts agree that it has not been shown to be an effective screening tool for sepsis and septic shock.[1,2,6,12]

NEWS Screening Tool

A large retrospective study of emergency department patients showed that the NEWS screening tool demonstrated greatest accuracy for predicting sepsis endpoints (as shown in **Table 4**, **Figs. 1** and **2**).[13] It was shown to be more specific than SIRS with similar sensitivity. It does not require laboratory testing for calculation, thus is expedient, and however may require automated computation for improved adherence.[13] Clinical risk is based on aggregate score (>7 indicates high risk for sepsis).

MEWS Screening Tool

The MEWS screening tool is similar to the NEWS screening tool; however, it adds an additional category and point for the "nurse being worried." It is frequently used in long-term monitoring and care of patients with sepsis and septic shock, and there are slight variations to the parameters associated with each point value.

In summary, the Surviving Sepsis Campaign revised 2021 guidelines do recommend the use of at least one of the aforementioned single sepsis screening tools. These guidelines state a strong recommendation *against* using the qSOFA screening tool compared with SIRS, NEWS, or MEWS, given the lack of quality evidence in its efficacy to predict sepsis and septic shock.[1,2] To be effective, a screening tool score must discriminate sepsis from other competing diagnoses in the emergency setting and be capable of predicting the development of sepsis in infected patients.[14] A gold standard for the diagnosis of sepsis and septic shock does not exist and likely will not, given the heterogeneity of symptoms and cause.[6] Several high-quality studies show consistent data, demonstrating the NEWS screening tool as most sensitive and specific, when compared with SIRS, SOFA, qSOFA, and MEWS, in predicting

Table 2
Sequential Organ Failure Assessment (SOFA) scale.

Points	1	2	3	4
Respiration (PaO2/FiO2)	<400	<300	<200	<100
Coagulation (Platelet count)	<150	<100	<50	<25
Liver function Bilirubin (mg/dL)	1.2-1.9	2.0-5.9	6.0-11.9	>12.0
Cardiovascular Hypotension	MAP<70	Dopamine <or=5 or dobutamine (any dose)	Dopamine >5 or epi <or=0.1 or norepi < or= 0.1	Dopamine >15 or epi >0.1 or norepi > 0.1
Neurologic (GCS)	13-14	10-12	6-9	<6
Renal (Crt) or urine output (UOP)	1.2-1.9	2.0-3.4	3.5-4.9 or UOP <500 mL/day	>5.0 or UOP <200 mL/day

mortality.[13–16] Although screening tools are recommended for use, they are not meant to replace clinician decision-making and experience in the overall assessment of patients.

EVALUATION AND MANAGEMENT

The Surviving Sepsis Campaign released updated international guidelines for the management of sepsis and septic shock in 2021. There are 93 recommendations, and each guideline recommendation is described as strong or weak based on available evidence and the quality of that evidence that exists. There are best practice statements included in these guidelines as well.[2] This article attempts to summarize those recommendations based on relevance to emergency medicine. As emergency medicine clinicians, much time is dedicated to the rapid and early detection of disease states and to the stabilization of patients. Given the overall surge in use of the emergency department in addition to the complexity of COVID-19 hospitalizations since March of 2019, emergency departments are experiencing overcrowding and prolonged patient boarding. This, in turn, is requiring emergency medicine providers to have a more complete understanding of sepsis and septic shock management guidelines, moving beyond identification and immediate treatment alone.[17]

Screening and Early Treatment—Blood Lactate Level

Recommendation—measure blood lactate if suspected sepsis (weak/low-quality evidence).[1]

Blood lactate levels are used to biochemically assess tissue perfusion, often in the setting of infection or ischemia. Lactate is typically used in combination with the clinical evaluation of blood pressure and heart rate measurement in addition to skin mottling indicators and capillary refill time.[18] Many experts agree that blood lactate levels are also reflective of cellular dysfunction and, in the setting of sepsis and septic shock, is a predictive marker of illness severity and mortality.[4,18] Most emergency settings have rapid access to laboratory testing and can have a blood lactate level resulted within a brief time period, although not immediately on initial assessment,

Table 3	
Quick sequential organ failure assessment (qSOFA).	
Respiratory Rate	< or = 22
Systolic blood pressure	< or = 100
Glasgow Coma Scale	< or = 13

making the use of several screening tools disadvantageous. Point-of-care blood lactate level testing shows variable diagnostic accuracy when compared with venous blood and some arterial blood sampling, limiting its use in prehospital settings.[18] In 2016, a task force, composed of the Society of Critical Care Medicine and the European Society of Intensive Care Medicine determined that although commonly available, serum lactate levels are not universally accessible. Therefore, clinical criteria including both hypotension and hyperlactatemia, for septic shock, were accepted.[4] Although blood lactate levels are prognostic, limited evidence exists that serial lactate measurements or lactate measurements alone improve outcomes when compared with clinical evaluation.[7]

Initial Resuscitation—Fluid Resuscitation

Best practice statement—immediate treatment and resuscitation is recommended with sepsis and septic shock and both should be considered medical emergencies.[1]

Recommendation—in adults with sepsis or septic shock, intravenous (IV) crystalloids are recommended as first-line fluids for fluid resuscitation (strong/moderate-quality evidence)[1]

Recommendation—in adult patients, IV crystalloid fluid should be given at 30 mL/kg within the first 3 hours of resuscitation if evidence of hypoperfusion or if septic shock is diagnosed/suspected (weak/low-quality evidence).[1]

Immediate fluid resuscitation is currently viewed as the mainstay for treatment of sepsis and septic shock; however, there lacks sufficient, high-quality data to support this practice.[1,19,20] The 2018 Surviving Sepsis Campaign recommends 30 mL/kg of IV crystalloid fluid be given within the first 3 hours of resuscitation if a patient is hypotensive or produces a serum lactate level of greater than or equal to 4 mmol/L. There is concern that high-volume fluid resuscitation may increase 28-day mortality. Effective fluid resuscitation depends on cardiac output and vascular responsiveness to maintain tissue perfusion. Sepsis causes increased inflammation and endothelial dysfunction, leading to subsequent third space loss of volume, pulmonary edema, and ischemic organ dysfunction.[19,20] There are high-quality data to support fluid resuscitation in decreasing 28-day mortality in patients with septic shock; however, the volume and speed with which this is done is debated still.[19–21]

Initial Resuscitation—Antimicrobial Use

Best practice statement—continuous reevaluation of cause of infection is recommended until source is confirmed and empirical antimicrobial therapy should be discontinued if an alternative cause of illness is strongly suspected.[1]

Best practice statement—prompt removal of intravascular access devices that are the possible source of infection is recommended.[1]

Recommendation—in adult patients with evidence of septic shock, antimicrobials should be administered immediately and within 1 hour of recognition (strong/low-quality evidence).[1]

Table 4
National Early Warning System (NEWS).

	3	2	1	0	1	2	3
Respiration rate	< or =8		9-11	12-20		21-24	> or= 25
SpO2 Scale 1	<or= 91	92-93	94-95	>or= 96			
SpO2 Scale 2	<or= 83	84-85	86-87	88-92 >or= 93RA	93-94 on O2	95-96 on O2	>or= 97 on O2
Air or O2?		O2		Air			
Systolic blood pressure	<or= 90	91-100	101-110	121-219			>or=220
Pulse	<or=40		41-50	51-90	91-110	111-130	>or=131
Consciousness				Alert			CVPU
Temperature	<or=35.0		35.1-36.0	36.1-38.0	38.1-39.0	>or=39.1	

CVPU, confusion, voice, pain, unresponsiveness.

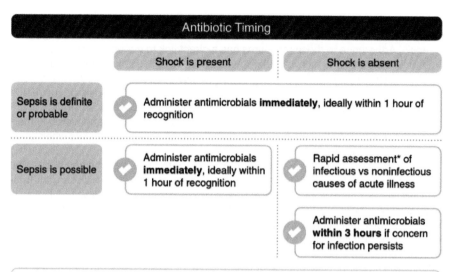

Fig. 1. Antibiotic timing in sepsis management.[1]

Recommendation—in adult patients with evidence of sepsis without shock, antimicrobials should be administered immediately and within 1 hour of recognition (strong/very low-quality evidence).[1]

High-quality evidence exists proving the effectiveness of early, broad-spectrum, and empirical antimicrobial use in decreasing mortality in sepsis and septic shock.[22,23]

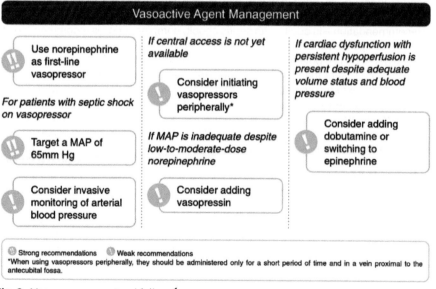

Fig. 2. Vasopressor agent guidelines.[1]

Early antimicrobial use, in addition to blood lactate levels and fluid resuscitation, are timed core measures established by the CMS in the recognition and management of sepsis. Adherence to these measures has a direct link to hospital reimbursement.[24] Time to first dose of antimicrobial therapy has been linked to improved mortality rates in patients with septic shock; however, there are weak associations between time to first dose of antimicrobial therapy and mortality of patients with sepsis or suspected sepsis.[7] Mortality reduction has been most closely linked to rapid administration of antimicrobials in patients with septic shock. The guidance to provide antimicrobial therapy quickly must be balanced with the potential harm imposed on patients when given antimicrobials unnecessarily.[1]

Data from several high-quality, large cohort, retrospective studies show that approximately 1 in 5 individuals with sepsis or septic shock receive discordant first-dose empirical antimicrobial therapy, leading to increased mortality.[22,23] Delay in blood culture laboratory results, confirming the causative agent, is a limiting factor in antimicrobial selection and poses a challenge for the clinician. The timing of second-dose antimicrobial therapy is critical to decreasing mortality and reducing the requirement of mechanical ventilation. Factors associated with delayed timing of second-dose therapy include selection of antimicrobials requiring more frequent dosing and increased emergency department boarding time. Many empirical antimicrobial regimes require more frequent dosing.[17]

Best practice statement—in adults with sepsis or septic shock at high-risk of methicillin-resistant *Staphylococcus aureus* (MRSA) infection, the use of empirical antimicrobials with MRSA coverage is recommended.[1]

Recommendation—in adults with sepsis or septic shock and high risk for multidrug-resistant organisms, the use of 2 antimicrobials with gram-negative coverage over one agent with gram-negative coverage is recommended for empirical treatment (weak/very low-quality evidence)[1]

Hemodynamic Management—Vasopressor Use

Recommendation—in adult patients with septic shock requiring vasopressors, an initial target MAP of 65 mm Hg is recommended (strong/moderate-quality evidence).[1]

Recommendation—in adults with septic shock, norepinephrine is recommended as the first-line agent over other vasopressors (strong).[1]

Norepinephrine is a potent vasoconstrictor although it has negligible effect on heart rate. It is more potent than dopamine and carries a reduced risk of arrhythmias, with lower mortality, when compared with dopamine. Epinephrine, too, carries with it a risk of arrhythmias as well as splanchnic circulatory impairment. Epinephrine may increase aerobic lactate production rendering serum lactate levels inaccurate when being used to guide resuscitation. Unlike other vasopressors, vasopressin is dosed at a fixed rate and does not allow for titration to response. Increased doses of vasopressin have been linked to cardiac, distal, and splanchnic ischemia. These findings led the Surviving Sepsis Campaign experts to recommend the use of norepinephrine as first-line treatment in the management of hypotension instead of dopamine, vasopressin, or epinephrine.[1]

The Surviving Sepsis Guidelines do make several recommendations regarding ventilation and resuscitation in the setting of hypoxemia and acute respiratory distress syndrome (ARDS). These recommendations are not discussed in this article and can be considered consistent with guidelines in the setting of hypoxemia and ARDS not associated with sepsis or septic shock and in accordance with advanced cardiac life support protocols.[1]

DISCUSSION

The early recognition and appropriate and effective management of sepsis and septic shock continue to present challenges to the emergency medicine provider. Alhough several screening tools have been implemented in an attempt to increase early recognition, sepsis and septic shock are complex diagnoses without consistent defining clinical criteria across any given patient population. The Surviving Sepsis Campaign updated guidelines, and the National Severe Sepsis and Septic Shock Early Management Bundle Sepsis Quality Measures have been established in an attempt to further standardize care and decrease mortality rates of patients with sepsis and septic shock. There are limitations, however, to the effectiveness of these measures, as gaps exist in available high-quality data from which these standards and guidelines are based.

As emergency medicine providers, it is critical to use screening tools consistently when attempting to diagnosis a patient with sepsis or septic shock. However, these tools must never replace our clinical decision-making. Instead, screening tools should be used in conjunction with clinical reasoning and reliance on professional expertise and experience. Recent data have shown that the NEWS screening tool is more specific than the SIRS or qSOFA screening tools and has similar sensitivity to SIRS. The SOFA screening tool is not efficient for use in the early identification of sepsis or septic shock in the emergency department when compared with the other screening tools due to the requirement of blood lactate levels for calculation.

Guidelines have been established in the management of patients with sepsis and septic shock. Although varied evidence exists supporting the quality of data from which these guidelines are created, they are considered the standard of care. In addition, financial reimbursement is linked to adherence to several of these guidelines. As an emergency department provider, early recognition of sepsis and septic shock is essential, and this requires attention to vital signs, laboratory testing, and imaging studies. Recognition of the source of infection and cause of sepsis is critical in determining appropriate treatment and mortality reduction. Appropriate selection of empirical antimicrobial therapy is crucial. Consultation with pharmacists trained in emergency and critical care as well as understanding of established guidelines when selecting treatment of individual patients will increase accuracy and should limit discordance in therapy and outcomes.

The Surviving Sepsis Campaign guidelines recommend that patients with sepsis or septic shock be admitted to the ICU within 6 hours of arrival in the emergency department. There are low-quality data to support this recommendation; nonetheless, it remains the goal of most hospitals. The data that do exist show improved mortality rates when patients receive more immediate care in the ICU.[1] Overcrowding in emergency departments, understaffing, and at- or over-capacity hospital admissions contribute to the increased length of time a patient spends in the emergency department; this is not predicted to change, which will force emergency medicine clinicians and staff to provide care longer for admitted patients; this will require emergency providers to become familiar with the guidelines and recommendations set for septic and septic shock patients after initial recognition, resuscitation, and stabilization occurs. This article does not address the long-term management of sepsis and septic shock.

There are 2 further areas regarding the management of sepsis and septic shock that bare consideration for continued future research. The 2016 Surviving Sepsis guidelines made a weak recommendation for the use of IV hydrocortisone in a patient with sepsis or septic shock refractory to fluid resuscitation and vasopressor therapy. The current data continue to present mixed results regarding decreased 28-day mortality in patients with sepsis and/or septic shock receiving corticosteroid therapy. In fact, 2 systematic reviews were published between 2019 and 2021. The study findings of one review suggested that the use of IV corticosteroids was associated with a reduced 28-day mortality, and the other study found that use of corticosteroids had no significant effect on mortality.[24–26] In addition, the benefit of early use of IV vitamin C on overall mortality is being researched. One small study evaluating the effect of high-dose vitamin C in patients with sepsis and septic shock revealed promising results, warranting further consideration.[27]

SUMMARY

Patients meeting clear criteria for septic shock are often easily recognizable to the emergency medicine provider. Adhering to set recommendations established by The Surviving Sepsis Campaign and the National SEP-1 bundle can appear straightforward and effective in appropriate patient care. The Infectious Disease Society of America (IDSA) released a position paper in 2021 applauding CMS for its attention to sepsis and septic shock as emergencies in medicine. The IDSA did, however, state several concerns with the CMS bundle. Because of the focus on timed intervention, providers often feel rushed in their decision-making, leading to the overdiagnosis and treatment of sepsis. Unnecessary antimicrobial use carries its own risks including patient allergy, the development of clostridium difficile, and the overall global increase in antimicrobial resistance.[7] Emergency medicine providers must consider these factors when the diagnosis of sepsis, in particular, is unclear and when the sepsis screening tools are imprecise.

As has been stated, several guidelines exist that are based on low-quality data. Further research and attention must be given in order to further decrease the mortality rates of septic shock and to minimize the complications associated with inappropriate empirical treatment or misdiagnosis. Although screening tools are indicated, emergency medicine providers must have the power to make clinical decisions based on individualized patient history, risk, and presentation. And although the SEP-1 bundle has been shown to improve time to first dose of antimicrobial administration, further high-quality research must be pursued in order to provide the most appropriate guidance in sepsis and septic shock care.

CLINICS CARE POINTS

- Sepsis and septic shock are medical emergencies, and delayed recognition leads to increased mortality.
- There are several screening tools used for the early detection of sepsis and septic shock. All have limitations in specificity and sensitivity. The NEWS tool has the highest specificity when compared with the other screening tools and equivalent sensitivity to the (SIRS) screening tool.
- The CMS has established sepsis and septic shock as a national priority. Because of this, the SEP-1 measure has been established linking financial reimbursement to compliance with these measures.
- The Surviving Sepsis Campaign was established in 2002 and is a joint initiative between the Society of Critical Care Medicine, the European Society of Intensive Medicine, and the International Sepsis Forum. Guidelines are updated regularly and most recently in 2021. The mission of the global initiative is to reduce mortality from sepsis. These guidelines are considered the standard of care for emergency medicine providers in the management of sepsis and septic shock.

- Blood lactate levels should be included in the initial evaluation of patients with suspected sepsis or septic shock.
- IV crystalloid fluids should be initiated immediately at 30 mL/kg over 3 hours if there is evidence of septic shock.
- Empirical, broad-based, antimicrobial therapy should be initiated within 1 hour of arrival to the emergency department in patients with evidence of sepsis or septic shock.
- Norepinephrine is the first-line therapy for the management of hypotension associated with septic shock. Target MAP is 65 mm Hg.
- It is recommended that patients diagnosed with sepsis or septic shock be transferred to the ICU within 6 hours of admission to the emergency department.

DISCLOSURE

This author declares that she has no conflict of interest. This author declares that she has no competing monetary interests or personal relationships that could have influenced the work reported here.

REFERENCES

1. Evans L, Rhodes A, Alhazzani W, et al. Surviving Sepsis Campaign: international guidelines for management of sepsis and septic shock. Intensive Care Med 2021;47:1181–247.
2. Font MD, Braghadhesswar T, Khanna AK. Sepsis and septic shock-Basics of diagnosis, pathophysiology and clinical decision making. Med Clin North Am 2020;104:573–85.
3. Backer DD, Ricottilli F, Ospina-Tascon GA. Septic shock: a microcirculation disease. Curr Opin Anesthesiol 2021;34:85–91.
4. Singer M, Deutschman CS, Seymour CW, et al. The Third International Consensus Definitions for Septic and Septic Shock (Sepsis-3). JAMA 2016;315(8):801–10.
5. Chiu C, Legrand M. Epidemiology of sepsis and septic shock. Curr Opin Anesthesiol 2021;34:71–6.
6. Horak J, Martinkova V, Radej J, et al. Back to Basics: Recognition of sepsis with new definition. J Clin Med 2019;8:1838.
7. Rhee C, Chiotos K, Cosgrove SE, et al. Infectious Disease Society of American Position Paper: Recommended revisions to the National Severe Sepsis and Septic Shock Early Management Bundle (SEP-1) Sepsis Quality Measure. Clin Infect Dis 2021;72(4):541–52.
8. Ramos FJ, Rezende de Freitas FG, Machado FR. Sepsis in patients hospitalized with coronavirus 2019: how often and how severe? Curr Opin Crit Care 2021;27: 474–9.
9. Asner SA, Desgranges F, Schrijver IT, et al. Impact of the timeliness of antibiotic therapy on the outcome of patients with sepsis and septic shock. J Infect 2021; 82:125–34.
10. Hidalgo DC, Tapaskar N, Rao S, et al. lower socioeconomic factors are associated with higher mortality in patients with septic shock. Heart Lung 2021;50: 477–80.
11. Cerceo E, Rachoin J, Gaughan J, et al. Association of gender, age, and race on renal outcomes and mortality in patients with severe sepsis and septic shock. J Crit Care 2021;61:52–6.

12. Sinha S, Ray B. Sepsis-3: How useful is the new definition? J Anaesthesiol Clin Pharmacol 2018;34(4):542–3.
13. Usman OA, Usman AA, Ward MA. Comparison of SIRS, qSOFA, and NEWS for the early identification of sepsis in the Emergency Department. Am J Emerg Med 2019;37(8):1490–7.
14. Melhammar L, Linder A, Tverring J, et al. NEWS2 is superior to qSOFA in detecting sepsis with organ dysfunction in the Emergency Department. J Clin Med 2019;8(8):1128.
15. McGrath SP, Perreard I, Mackenzie T, et al. Improvement of sepsis identification through multi-year comparison of sepsis and early warning scores. Am J Emerg Med 2022;51:239–47.
16. Liu VX, Lu Y, Carey KA, et al. Systems for hospitalized patients with and without infection at risk for in-hospital mortality and transfer to intensive care unit. JAMA Netw Open 2020;3(5).
17. Lykins JD, Kuttab HI, Rourke EM, et al. The effects of delays in second-dose antibiotics on patients with severe sepsis and septic shock. Am J Emerg Med 2021; 47:80–5.
18. Jouffroy R, Leguillier T, Gilbert JP, et al. Prehospital lactate clearance is associated with reduced mortality in patients with severe shock. Am J Emerg Med 2021;46:367–73.
19. Wang H, Shao J, Liu W, et al. Initial fluid resuscitation (30 ml/Kg) in patients with septic shock: more or less? Am J Emerg Med 2021;50:309–15.
20. Jiang S, Wu M, Lu X, et al. Is restrictive fluid resuscitation beneficial not only for hemorrhagic shock but also for septic shock? A meta-analysis. Medicine 2020; 100(12).
21. Rowan KM, Angus DC, Bailey M, et al. Early, goal-directed therapy for septic shock – a patient-level meta-analysis. N Engl J Med 2017;376:2223–34.
22. Kadri SS, Lai YL, Warner S, et al. Inappropriate empirical antibiotic therapy for bloodstream infections based on discordant in-vitro susceptibilities: a retrospective cohort analysis of prevalence, predictors, and mortality risk in US hospitals. Lancet Infect Dis 2021;21:241–51.
23. Taylor SP, Shah M, Kowalkowski MA, et al. First-to-second antibiotic delay and hospital mortality among emergency department patients with suspected sepsis. Am J Emerg Med 2021;46:20–2.
24. Liang H, Song H, Zhai R, et al. Corticosteroids for treating sepsis in adult patients: A systematic review and meta-analysis. Front Immunol 2021;12.
25. Fang F, Zhang JT, Tang J, et al. Association of corticosteroid treatment with outcomes in adult patients with sepsis: A systematic review and meta-analysis. JAMA Intern Med 2019;179(2):213–23.
26. Prescott HC, Sussman JB. Smarter use of corticosteroids in treating patients with septic shock. JAMA Netw Open 2020;3(12).
27. Lv S, Zhang G, Xia J, et al. Early use of high-dose vitamin C is beneficial in treatment of sepsis. J Med Sci 2021;190:1183–8.

"Can't Miss" Orthopedic Diagnoses

Michael Smith, MS, PA-C[a],*, James A. Johanning, MPAS, PA-C[b]

KEYWORDS

- Orthopedic trauma • Compartment syndrome • Cauda equina • Septic joint
- Septic arthritis • Bone tumor • Osteosarcoma • Flexor tenosynovitis

KEY POINTS

- Focused recognition and approach to workup of compartment syndrome.
- Focused recognition and approach to workup of cauda equina syndrome.
- Focused recognition and approach to and workup of septic arthritis.
- Focused recognition and approach to workup of sarcoma.
- Special mention section regarding recognition and workup of flexor tenosynovitis.

"CANNOT MISS" ORTHOPEDIC DIAGNOSES

Physician Assistants, and other medical providers who see patients with musculoskeletal complaints, find that the vast majority of these are nonemergent and can usually be managed with stabilization and referral to an orthopedic surgeon. In fact, limb-threatening, much less life-threatening, emergencies in orthopedics are very uncommon. Those orthopedic injuries serious enough to warrant hospital admission and emergent surgical intervention are usually evident from the history and clinical presentation. However, patients occasionally present with subtle or unclear musculoskeletal complaints that do in fact pose a limb-threatening or life-threatening condition. The astute clinician must be able to recognize these conditions on presentation without delay.

The goal of this article is to present certain critically important orthopedic syndromes where failure to diagnose and treat correctly could have disastrous sequelae. Discussion of definitive surgical treatment techniques of these syndromes is beyond the focus of this article but the signs, symptoms, clinical presentation, and diagnostic findings will be presented so that medical providers will be better prepared to accurately diagnosis and treat them.

[a] Boston University School of Medicine, 72 East Concord Street, Boston, MA 02118, USA; [b] St. Catherine University, Henrietta Schmoll School of Health, 2009 Randolph Avenue, Saint. Paul, MN 55105, USA
* Corresponding author.
E-mail address: Msmith64@bu.edu

Physician Assist Clin 8 (2023) 205–224
https://doi.org/10.1016/j.cpha.2022.09.004
2405-7991/23/© 2022 Elsevier Inc. All rights reserved.
physicianassistant.theclinics.com

Certainly, patients do not present to the Emergency Department with a chief complaint of, say, compartment syndrome. Rather they arrive with a complaint of pain that is out of proportion to the apparent injury or history. There may even be a suspicion on the part of the provider that the patient is coming to the ED for secondary gain, perhaps work restrictions or to be prescribed narcotic medications. If the treating provider is misdirected or distracted by an extraneous issue such as department workload, or even personal bias, the correct diagnosis may be missed. It is important to keep in mind that sick people get sick too and the likelihood of an actual compartment syndrome in a malingering patient is the same as in the general population. Secondary gain should only enter into the scenario once ominous pathology is definitively ruled out.

In the case of a patient who falls onto an outstretched hand (FOOSH) and has wrist pain, a scaphoid fracture may not be identified on the initial X-ray. If the treating provider does not suspect scaphoid fracture after obtaining the history, physical examination and imaging, the diagnosis may simply be "wrist sprain." In that case, treatment will be suboptimal with inadequate immobilization and lack of follow-up.

Occasionally, a patient may present with a complaint that can be explained by another diagnosis. This is a potential trap for medical providers. A patient with symptoms consistent with urinary retention or an uncomplicated UTI may in fact have cauda equina syndrome. Alternatively, what appears as superficial cellulitis of the skin may in reality be a joint infection.

Multitrauma patients in particular are at risk of having injuries missed if there is an inadequate secondary and tertiary survey, decrease in mental status, or the patient is obtunded. That patient will not be able to describe pain out of proportion or numbness and tingling in a specific region. It is incumbent on the treating provider to have a high index of suspicion of other injuries or sequelae from such an event.[1]

Fortunately, the widespread use of in-hospital medical interpreters, or "language line" via telephone, has reduced language barriers between patient and provider. Yet, items in the history of present illness or even clinical signs may be under appreciated and cause delayed or missed diagnosis. Cultural differences also can contribute to a provider not appreciating the level of pain or disability the patient presents with.

An appropriate musculoskeletal evaluation demands a directed yet detailed history and physical examination as well as the ordering and correct interpretation of appropriate imaging studies. The authors strongly recommend that providers maintain a low threshold for obtaining imaging studies for a patient presenting with a musculoskeletal complaint. There is no surer way to miss diagnosing a fracture or osseous lesion than by not ordering the initial X-ray.

This article will discuss the evaluation and appropriate treatment of patients who present with one of the following syndromes:

- Acute compartment syndrome
- Septic arthritis (SA)
- Sarcoma
- Scaphoid fracture
- Flexor tenosynovitis–honorable mention

ACUTE COMPARTMENT SYNDROME

Acute compartment syndrome (ACS) is an extremely painful condition, which occurs when tissue pressure within a fascial compartment increases to such a level that impedes arterial blood flow and causes ischemia of the tissues contained within. Any condition that decreases the volume capacity of a compartment, or the fluid within it, will increase intracompartmental pressure and place the patient at risk for ACS.

Epidemiology/Cause

ACS usually develops after significant trauma, particularly to an extremity. There are instances, however, when compartment syndrome can develop secondary to other sequelae and the risk of a missed diagnosis resultantly increases. A comminuted tibia and fibula fracture is often correctly recognized by most practitioners as a high-risk injury. However, compartment syndrome in the patient with a minimally displaced distal radius fracture immobilized by a tightly fitting cast may not be as readily apparent because the fracture seems stable and the initial treatment thought to be appropriate.

Additionally, compartment syndrome resulting from various nonfracture injuries is more difficult to recognize without a high index of suspicion for ACS. These include the following:[1]

- Muscle injury due to
  - Blunt trauma
  - Crush
- Prolonged immobilization
- Severe burns
- Tightly fitting splints/casts

Clinical Presentation

A detailed history and physical examination in a patient with a chief complaint of severe pain should alone suffice in raising clinical suspicion of ACS. During training, medical providers are taught mnemonic devices such as "the 5 P's" to recall the signs and symptoms of compartment syndrome. As useful as these mnemonics may be, it is critical for providers to understand that the hallmark sign of compartment syndrome is pain.

The pain will appear to be "out of proportion" and thus the clinician may suspect the patient has a low tolerance for discomfort or is seeking secondary gain. These assumptions must be avoided until ACS is ruled out. Of note, the "P" of pulselessness is inherently unreliable as arterial blood flow continues early in the process of developing ACS. Diastolic pressures at this point will have been overcome, and therefore, no effective blood flow and oxygen delivery is present despite still having a pulse.

The "5 P's" of Acute Compartment Syndrome[1]
• Pain
• Pallor
• Pulselessness
• Paresthesia
• Paralysis

The anterior compartment of the lower leg containing the anterior tibialis muscle and the dorsal compartment of the forearm containing the extensor muscles are the most commonly affected compartments. However, during the evaluation, the provider must measure pressure in all compartments of the affected extremity.

If there were a sixth "P" in the list presented above, it would be pain on passive motion. Aggravation of pain by passive or active stretching of muscles in the compartment in question occurs early, and is the most sensitive clinical finding in ACS.

Intracompartmental pressure increases as the muscle is stretched, and the patient's pain level responds in kind. If there were a seventh "P" in the list presented above, it would be pain on palpation. Early in the development of ACS, palpation of the affected extremity will reliably reveal a tense and exquisitely tender muscle compartment. Compression of the affected compartment will exacerbate pain as well.[2] In the authors' opinion, these 2 additional P's would be the second and third in importance and priority to pain in the presentation of ACS.

As the compartment pressure continues to increase, the patient will develop diffuse, nondermatomal dysesthesia in the sensory nerves and weakness of the muscles in the affected compartment.[2] Again, it must be emphasized that pain out of proportion alone should prompt the medical provider to suspect ACS and measure compartment pressures accordingly. Paresthesia is a late finding and the provider must not wait for it to develop before initiating prompt surgical consult. A high index of suspicion with a patient presenting with pain out of proportion must be the mindset of the provider rather than waiting for dysesthesia or paresthesia to develop.

It is generally recognized that an absolute compartmental pressure of 30 to 45 mm Hg puts the patient at risk of developing ACS and that surgical consultation is required. However, absolute numbers must be approached with caution as a hypotensive patient may still be at risk even with compartment pressures less than 30 mm Hg.[2]

The provider should also keep in mind that compartment pressures within 10 to 30 mm Hg of the patient's diastolic blood pressure can cause tissue ischemia because the intercompartment pressure begins to match arterial pressure. The astute provider relies on history and physical examination findings and then proceeds with appropriate evaluation in order to rule out compartment syndrome.[2]

Diagnostic/Imaging Studies

The diagnosis of ACS is made from clinical findings with support from compartment pressure measurement readings. Neither laboratory values nor imaging studies should be used in order for the diagnosis to be made. In fact, if ACS is suspected, surgical consultation must not be delayed in order to obtain a laboratory result or X-ray, or, if delayed, even to measure compartment pressures themselves.

A common instrument to measure intracompartmental pressure is the Stryker Intra-Compartmental Pressure Monitor. Measuring compartment pressures with this hand-held manometer is the most common and effective way to accurately measure the compartment pressure[3] (**Fig. 1**).

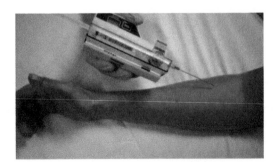

Fig. 1. The Stryker Intra-compartmental Pressure Monitor being utilized to measure compartment pressure in the proximal volar forearm. Courtesy of: Tintinalli, J.E. et al, Tintinalli's Emergency Medicine: A Comprehensive Study Guide, 9th Edition.

Whichever instrument or method is used to measure compartment pressure, it is critical that the catheter or device tip be placed in close enough proximity to the site of injury to accurately measure the true pressure. Optimally, this should be no more than 5 cm away from the fracture/injury site. Accuracy decreases the further away the measurement is taken from the fracture or injury site.[3]

The provider should keep in mind that a single measurement performed within 5 cm of the fracture or injury site will not by itself suffice in ruling out ACS. Continuous measurements in an at-risk patient are necessary when clinical suspicion is high but again the serial measuring of compartment pressures should not delay surgical consult. In addition, it is critical to document the date and time of the measurement to provide for an accurate assessment of trends. In a patient with hypotension, an absolute compartment pressure of 30 mm Hg may not be attained. However, a trend revealing increasing intercompartmental pressure in the presence of decreasing diastolic pressure can alert the clinician to developing ACS.[4]

Interpretation of measurements—The normal pressure of a tissue compartment falls between 0 and 8 mm Hg. Clinical findings associated with ACS generally correlate with the degree to which tissue pressure within the affected compartment approaches systolic blood pressure:

- Capillary blood flow becomes compromised when tissue pressure increases to within 25 to 30 mm Hg of mean arterial pressure.
- Pain may develop as tissue pressures reach between 20 and 30 mm Hg.
- Ischemia occurs when tissue pressures approach diastolic pressure.

Prognosis

The prognosis for the patient is good with early detection and treatment. Even a simple cast removal can be definitive treatment in the early stage of a developing compartment syndrome (**Figs. 4** and **5**). However, delayed diagnosis can result in muscle necrosis, sensory deficits, paralysis, infection, and limb amputation. Muscle necrosis can lead to rhabdomyolysis, which can then result in myoglobinuria and acute kidney injury. Serious adverse sequelae can be avoided with early recognition.

Treatment

Definitive surgical treatment entails open fasciotomy of all involved compartments to fully decompress the tissues (**Figs. 2** and **3**). Immediate steps that can be taken before this include removing all possible extrinsic causes of pressure. Casts or splints must be removed and the affected area closely examined. Jewelry, watches, or even constrictive clothing must also be removed. The affected limb should then be placed at patient's heart level to allow for return of blood flow. It is critical that the limb not hang dependent.[4]

Other measures depend on the clinical situation. For example, if the patient is hypotensive, fluid resuscitation is in order as is maximizing oxygenation of the tissues (See Pearls and Pitfalls of Trauma Management Chapter).

The successful treatment of ACS requires at first a high degree of clinical suspicion that the condition exists or is imminent. Then a detailed physical examination and accurate compartment measurement will confirm the diagnosis. Surgical consultation must not be delayed waiting for a physical examination sign or absolute number in the compartment pressure measurement.

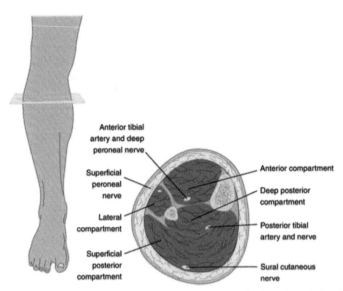

Fig. 2. The four compartments of the lower extremity. Note the location of the deep posterior compartment illustrating how difficult it can be to access. Courtesy of: Tintinalli, J.E. et al, Tinitinalli's Emergency Medicine: A Comprehensive Study Guide, 9th Edition.

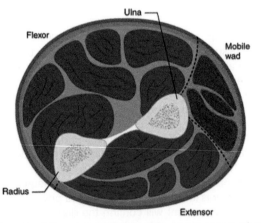

Fig. 3. The compartments of the upper extremity forearm. Courtesy of: Tintinalli, J.E. et al, Tinitinalli's Emergency Medicine: A Comprehensive Study Guide, 9th Edition.

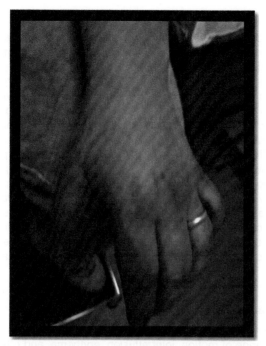

Fig. 4. Impending compartment syndrome in a 26-year-old woman complaining of severe, increasing pain in left hand and thumb. Numbness and tingling had begun to develop, which prompted patient visit to the Walk-In Clinic. Patient had been placed in a thumb spica cast less than 24 hours after sustaining a "Bennet" type thumb fracture. Pictures taken after cast removal. Note the swollen fingers and the wedding ring, which was not removed before casting. (*Source*: Michael Smith, PA-C, author.)

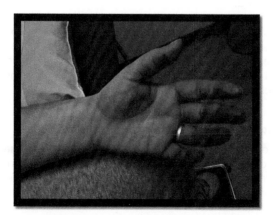

Fig. 5. Impending compartment syndrome in a 26-year-old woman complaining of severe, increasing pain in left hand and thumb. Numbness and tingling had begun to develop which prompted patient visit to Walk-In Clinic. Patient had been placed in a thumb spica cast less than 24 hours after sustaining a "Bennet" type thumb fracture. Pictures taken after cast removal. Note the swollen fingers and the wedding ring, which was not removed before casting. (*Source*: Michael Smith, PA-C, author.)

SEPTIC ARTHRITIS

SA is a potentially destructive arthropathy caused by an intra-articular infection, which has been seeded from an outside source.[5] Although thankfully uncommon in an otherwise healthy patient with no previous trauma, SA of a joint can have potentially devastating sequalae if not diagnosed and properly treated at the time of initial presentation. The incidence of musculoskeletal infection is increasing coincident with an increase in the elderly demographic and higher rates of diabetes and obesity in the general population. The most critical aspect to timely and accurate diagnosis and treatment of SA is a high index of suspicion of its presence.

In this section, the authors will specifically exclude discussion of patients who present with painful, swollen joints in the perioperative or postoperative period from a joint arthroplasty or who have sustained trauma to the affected area. Any patient presenting with joint pain, fever or effusion in the setting of previous arthroplasty, or a trauma should prompt the ED provider to quickly consult with orthopedics. Joint infections in the setting of total arthroplasty are referred to as periprosthetic joint infections. Further, a suspected joint infection in the setting of open fracture will also not be examined here because any patient with such an injury must also have an immediate ortho consult.

Epidemiology/Cause

The classic presentation of a patient with SA is an insidious onset of severe joint pain, decreased range of motion, joint effusion, erythema, and often fever. Overall, it is uncommon in an otherwise healthy patient. Providers should be suspicious of the presence of SA in any patient who reports joint pain without improvement or worsening of previous symptoms despite appropriate conservative treatment. In immunocompromised patients, SA may present without fever, so this clinical sign cannot be relied on as sufficient in itself to rule out SA. Diabetics and paraplegics often have sensory deficits and may not appreciate pain from infection or even skin breakdown. The first indication of the presence of infection may be erythema or even a draining wound.[5]

SA in a nonimmunocompromised patient is most commonly due to bacterial organisms with *Neisseria gonorrhea*, *Staphylococcus aureus*, and group A streptococcus being the most common. In addition, a swollen, warm, and erythematous joint may indeed have Lyme or a crystalline arthropathy as the source. Notably, immunocompromised patients are at risk for not only the preceding organisms but also fungal and atypical mycobacteria.[6]

Clinical Presentation

The atraumatic, otherwise healthy patient who presents with severe joint pain, decreased range of motion, and swelling with or without fever can be confounding to the ED provider. In a patient with no history of trauma, the differential diagnosis of a painful, swollen joint includes the following:

- Infection
- Gout
- Lyme disease
- Arthritic effusion
- Effusion secondary to anticoagulation
- Prepatellar bursitis

It is important for the ED provider to understand that, in an atraumatic patient, the inability or refusal of the patient to perform either active or passive range of motion is almost pathognomonic for SA. The increased pain caused by range of motion will cause patients to avoid movement of more than 10° in either direction. This must be differentiated from pain that a patient has at the extremes of flexion and extension that a knee effusion will often cause. In that case, the comfortable plane of motion is usually much greater than 10°.

In addition, a thorough skin examination is critical as even an innocuous skin penetration in the crevices between toes or elsewhere can be the source of infection.

Diagnostic/Imaging Studies

Once suspected, laboratory and diagnostic evaluation of the patient should be done without delay. The ubiquity of ultrasound (US) in the ED setting allows the provider to quickly assess for the presence of a joint effusion. In addition, US is effective in visual guidance during joint aspiration. Standard X-rays of the affected joint should be done on any patient suspected of having SA. If there is no associated osteomyelitis, the X-rays will likely only show an effusion, which is also suggestive of SA.[5]

The gold standard laboratory diagnostic tool is needle aspiration of an affected joint. Again, US can assist in the collection of joint aspirate, and the reduction in size of the effusion can itself be therapeutic for the patient simply through pain relief. Fluid aspirated should be visually assessed for clarity and the presence of particles. A joint aspirate that appears turbid and has a WBC greater than 75,000 should be considered to be positive for infection while awaiting the laboratory determination.

Laboratory studies should include the following:

- WBC with a differential
  - WBC >50,000
- Gram stain
- Cell count
- Fluid culture—aerobic and anaerobic
- Inflammatory markers: ESR/CRP
- Crystals
- Lyme titer

Most common pathogens are as follows:[6]

- S aureus
- Neisseria
- Group A beta strep

Treatment

Treatment of a patient with SA is multidisciplinary and requires the close coordination of the surgical and medical teams in order to optimize patient outcome and minimize adverse sequelae. Once fluid has been aspirated in the ED and is being analyzed by the laboratory, empiric IV antibiotics, often vancomycin 15 mg/kg, should be initiated until Gram stain analysis identifies the causative organism.[6]

Referral to orthopedics should quickly follow with emergent irrigation and drainage of the affected joint. This likely will be performed in the operating room setting through either an open or arthroscopic "washout" of the joint. An orthopedic maxim is that "the solution to pollution is dilution" which means that irrigation of an infected joint with a large volume of normal saline and drain placement is the appropriate treatment of SA. By debulking the joint of pus, the increased perfusion gradient allows for more successful antibiotic treatment.

Prognosis

Orthopedic infections are frequently subtle, and without a high level of suspicion, the diagnosis will be missed and definitive treatment delayed. Even with an astute clinician rapidly diagnosing and treating SA, the patient is at risk for complications. Specifically, the articular cartilage of the joint is at risk of breakdown in the setting of infection, thus the nomenclature "Septic Arthritis." Incidence of postjoint infection arthritis is proportional to patient comorbidities and the duration of infection.

The prognosis for the patient is dependent on early diagnosis and treatment. Even if treatment is not overly delayed, potential sequelae include the following:[5]

- Articular cartilage degradation (**Figs. 6 and 7**)
- Tissue loss
- Amputation
- Loss of mobility
  - Decreased social status
  - Decreased income
- Death

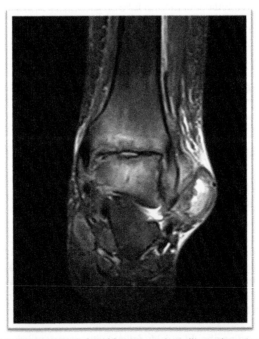

Fig. 6. A 25-year-old woman with left ankle pain and swelling: There is erosion of the articular cartilage of the talar dome and distal tibia. Note the abscess by the medial malleolus. Copyright 2022. Dr Naqibullah Foladi Image courtesy of Dr Naqibullah Foladi and Radiopaedia.org. Used under licence.

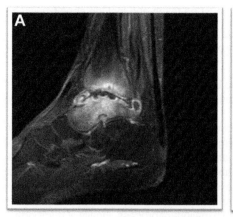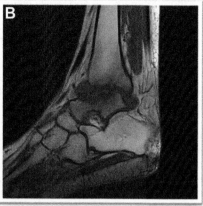

Fig. 7. 25 y/o female with left ankle pain and swelling: The erosion of the articular cartilage in the talar dome is evident in this lateral view. Copyright 2022. Dr Naqibullah Foladi Image courtesy of Dr Naqibullah Foladi and Radiopaedia.org. Used under licence.

Sarcoma

The incidence of osteo or soft-tissue sarcoma and other malignant lesions is relatively rare and thus increases the risk of missed diagnosis in a patient presenting with an atraumatic complaint of pain. In addition, guidelines developed for reducing the frequency of ordering X-rays in Emergency Departments and the primary care setting can lead to delay in discovering such lesions and ultimately reduce the 5-year survivability of the patient.[7]

Epidemiology

Sarcomas are a heterogeneous group of tumors that originate from mesenchymal or connective tissue. It was estimated that in 2018, soft-tissue sarcomas represented 0.8% of all cancers in the United States and were among the top 5 causes of cancer deaths for people aged younger than 20 years. It is currently estimated that approximately 13,000 to 16,000 new cases and up to 6,000 deaths can be attributed to sarcomas in the United States annually.[8]

Clinical Presentation

When assessing any patient with a complaint of indolent pain, which cannot be attributed to trauma, it is critically important to get a complete history, including a full Review of Systems and a complete family history. It will not be readily apparent to the patient or clinician that there is a potential osseous or soft-tissue lesion. Pain, resultant weakness, and reduced joint movement should alert the provider to the possibility of malignancy because benign lesions are very often painless.

The history of present illness must include the following:[7]

- Patient age
- Duration of complaint. Acute (<4 weeks) vs chronic (>4 weeks)
- Onset: trauma related or not
- Worsening or improving symptoms: worsening symptoms can indicated growth of a lesion
- Location of pain
- Alleviating or aggravating factors

A thorough personal and family history must be taken and include specifically:[7]

- Does the patient have a history of cancer?
- Does a primary relative have a history of lung, breast, prostate, or renal disease or cancer?

A complete review of systems must also be documented. In particular unintentional weight loss, night pain, night sweats, fatigue, or a change in appetite should be investigated.

Once the HPI and ROS have been documented, a thorough physical examination must be performed, including current weight, which should be compared with prior visits if available. The skin overlying the area of pain should be carefully assessed. The provider should check both active and passive range of motion of the joint(s) involved and palpate the area of tenderness, noting any swelling, firmness, or bogginess. Regional lymph nodes in the area of pain should be assessed as well. A firm mass greater than 5 cm can be indicative of a malignant process. Finally, it is important to perform and document a through neurovascular examination and document any disability at the time of presentation.

Diagnostics/Imaging Studies

X-rays are the initial diagnostic imaging study of choice in detecting osteo or soft-tissue sarcoma and other lesions. Should an osseous lesion be found on imaging, the entire bone must be included in the X-ray. In the case of osteosarcoma, "skip lesions" may be found at a higher level in the femur in addition to the more commonly located lesions in the distal femur and proximal tibia. Such a lesion is associated with a lower probability of survival.[7]

The initial radiographic images must be scrutinized carefully by the provider and a radiologist familiar with the evaluation of osseous lesions. For long bone lesions, the location within the bone (diaphysis, metaphysis) can aid in the initial diagnosis because primary sarcomas of bone are usually metaphyseal.

If an osseous lesion is found, computed tomographic (CT) scan is then the next appropriate imaging study to assess the extent of bone involvement. Should a soft-tissue lesion be detected, MRI is the imaging study of choice not only to delineate the extent of soft-tissue involvement but also to assess for the presence of occult bone marrow extension (**Figs. 8** and **9**).

Unless the patient's underlying medical condition necessitates further investigation, laboratory studies are not required at the initial visit. For instance, a patient with renal disease would need creatinine clearance assessed before administration of contrast medium. In most cases however, the patient is otherwise healthy and specific laboratory studies should be ordered by the treating oncologist.[7]

Prognosis

Before the use of adjuvant chemotherapy, treatment of sarcoma was basically amputation with wide resection of the tumor. The rate of mortality from this was exceedingly high with only 20% of patients having a 5-year survival after diagnosis. Today, sarcomas remain ominous but with early detection and the combination of chemotherapy and surgical treatment, the prognosis for 5-year survival approaches 70%.[8]

Treatment

For most stable patients, the treatment depends on chief complaint. If a fracture occurred through a lesion, then appropriate immobilization is indicated as with any other fracture. It cannot be overstated that the most important element in assuring the best

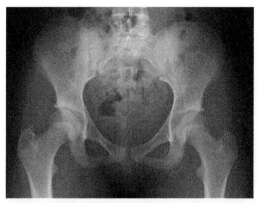

Fig. 8. AP Pelvis X-ray of 12-year-old girl complaining of 5-week history of atraumatic onset left anterior hip pain with reduced range of motion. Physical examination revealed reduced passive range of motion and tenderness to palpation in left groin but no mass. Note the approx. 3.5 cm × 5 cm, dense, calcified mass in the soft tissue around the hip joint, anterior to the inferior pubic rami. (*Source*: Michael Smith, PA-C, author.)

outcome for the patient is early diagnosis. Failure to obtain radiographs due to overdependence on exclusion criteria can have adverse, even fatal, implications for the patient and should have no place when evaluating musculoskeletal complaints.

SCAPHOID FRACTURE
Epidemiology

The scaphoid is the most commonly injured carpal bone and accounts for approximately 10% of all hand fractures. Acute scaphoid fractures account for approximately 3% of all fractures in patients aged older than 18 years. The male/female ratio is approximately 2.5/1.0, respectively, and men are often younger at the time of injury. Approximately 65% of fractures occur at the scaphoid waist.[9]

Cause

The most common mechanism of injury is a FOOSH with the wrist frequently in extension on impact. Older women with scaphoid fracture are more likely to have sustained

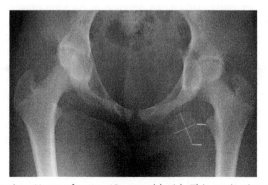

Fig. 9. Pelvic inlet view X-ray of same 12-year-old girl. This projection helped make the initial diagnosis of soft-tissue mass rather than osseous. Further evaluation by MRI showed the lesion to be a soft-tissue sarcoma. (*Source*: Michael Smith, PA-C, author.)

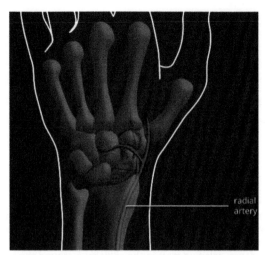

Fig. 10. The blood supply to the scaphoid. Note that the blood flow to the proximal pole is retrograde. Copyright 2022. Dr Maciej Debowski Image courtesy of Dr Maciej Debowski and Radiopaedia.org. Used under licence.

a fall from standing height, whereas younger men are more likely to sustain a high-energy injury during sports or due to a motor vehicle collision. In all ages, football, basketball, cycling, skateboarding, or physical assault have been associated with an increased risk of scaphoid fracture.[9]

An important reason why scaphoid fractures can be so debilitating is that the bone has a tenuous blood supply whereby it receives approximately 80% its blood *via retrograde* flow from the dorsal carpal branch of radial artery (**Fig. 10**). Fractures through the scaphoid disrupt this blood flow, thus proper immobilization or early surgical intervention is key to preserve this blood supply, promote healing, and avoid avascular necrosis.

BLOOD SUPPLY
Clinical Presentation

The most common chief complaint is radial sided wrist pain, which often develops immediately after the inciting event. The pain is worse with movement, extension of the wrist, or overall use of the hand. In addition, the patient will usually report associated weakness due to pain; particularly when gripping or carrying objects in the hand. The patient may report an initial period of swelling but depending on when they present for evaluation, this swelling may have resolved and not be noticeable to the examiner.

A careful physical examination will reveal pain on focal palpation in the anatomic snuffbox of the wrist. This is the region on the radial side of wrist just distal the radial styloid and at the base of the first metacarpal. It can be best palpated with ulnar deviation of the wrist and extension and abduction of the thumb. Additionally, an axial load applied to the first metacarpal through grasping the thumb and pushing down has been found to be 90% sensitive and 40% specific in detecting a scaphoid fracture. Another common physical finding is decreased strength with the wrist in extension secondary to pain.[9]

Imaging Studies

In a patient presenting with a wrist injury and similar physical examination as described above, the treating provider should order a 3-view X-ray of the wrist, with one being a specific "scaphoid view." It is not uncommon for the initial X-rays to be "negative" with no fracture being visualized. Approximately 30% to 40% of scaphoid fractures are not initially identified through the combination of clinical assessment and plain X-rays. Unfortunately, other imaging modalities, which could be utilized by the Emergency Department provider either are not readily available (MRI) or are less than optimal in detecting scaphoid fractures (US).[10]

If initial X-rays do not detect a scaphoid fracture, MRI is the next appropriate imaging study. It is excellent in detecting cancellous bone edema and is able to show subtle disruptions in the cortical integrity of the bone. However, MRI is expensive, not always readily available in nontertiary care centers, and often requires insurance preauthorization.[10]

A CT scan would then be the next choice but its use entails higher radiation exposure than plain x-ray and is not recommend by the authors for early use as the results of CT scan will not change the recommended initial treatment plan.[11]

Prognosis

Failure to diagnose a scaphoid fracture at initial presentation will result in inadequate immobilization and can subsequently contribute to a nonunion of the fracture. In order to avoid avascular necrosis of the proximal pole of the scaphoid, surgical intervention in necessary. Simply put, delayed diagnosis turns an otherwise nonsurgical condition into a condition that requires surgery. Surgical repair of the nonunion uses a vascular

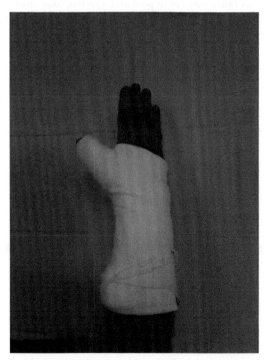

Fig. 11. Example of a proper thumb spica splint. Webril is placed prior to the Orthoglass splint application so as to protect the skin from breakdown. *Courtesy* of the author Michael Smith, PA-C.[12]

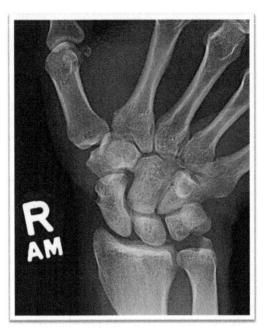

Fig. 12. Scaphoid view of Right wrist of 45 y/o male complaining of radial sided wrist pain 5 days after falling on his outstretched right hand while skiing at a high rate of speed. Patient had immediate onset of radial sided wrist pain and now has "dull" pain rated at 5/10 which is worsened with movement or trying to grasp/hold objects. Initially had swelling in wrist, but resolved after 2 days. (*Source*: Michael Smith, PA-C, author.)

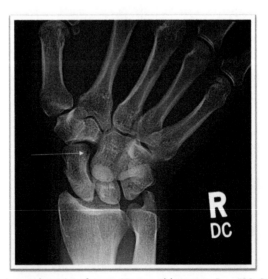

Fig. 13. Scaphoid view right wrist of same 45-year-old man on Day #30. Still complaining of pain on palpation once cast removed. Note the now apparent distal apparent distal pole scaphoid fracture. (*Source*: Michael Smith, PA-C, author.)

graft harvested from the patient's distal radius and compression screw placement. Immobilization of the wrist is then necessary for 6 to 12 weeks. Each delay in treatment, whether conservative or surgical, increases the incidence of avascular necrosis of the scaphoid, radial sided wrist pain, limited range of motion, osteoarthritis of the wrist, and long-term functional deficits.

Treatment

Any patient with radial sided wrist pain, particularly with anatomic snuffbox pain, should be considered to have a scaphoid fracture. It cannot be overstated that the absence of a fracture on X-ray does not definitively rule out the presence of a scaphoid fracture. Similar to all other fractures, even in the setting of negative X-rays, if the patient is symptomatic, the clinician must treat the injury as if a fracture does indeed exist and apply the appropriate splint.

The patient then should be referred for orthopedic follow-up to be seen optimally within 7 days. A thumb spica splint along the radial border of the forearm should be applied and come to at least the interphalangeal (IP) joint of the thumb so as to limit both wrist and thumb motion (**Fig. 11**).

The patient should remain in a thumb spica splint for 3 to 5 days until the swelling resolves and then follow-up with orthopedics. At the initial visit, the splint will be removed and repeat X-rays taken. If no fracture is visualized, the patient will be transitioned into a thumb spica cast for 14 days and instructed to return to clinic for cast removal and repeat X-rays (**Figs. 12 and 13**).

At that second visit, if the patient is asymptomatic, has a benign physical examination, including resolution of anatomic snuff box tenderness, and no fracture is seen, there is low probability of scaphoid fracture. The patient can safely be transitioned into a removable thumb spica splint and return to normal activity as tolerated. However, if the patient is still symptomatic with continued physical findings, but no fracture is seen on X-ray, he/she will then be recasted and referred for MRI.[13]

If the MRI reveals a nondisplaced scaphoid fracture, the patient will remain in a thumb spica cast for 6-weeks followed by serial short thumb-spica casting until clinical and radiographic signs of union are seen. This can be frustrating for the patient as immobilization is commonly indicated for 6 to 10 weeks and sometimes necessary for 4 to 6 months with cast changes every 14 days for the first 6 weeks.

It has been stated repeatedly that a negative X-ray does not rule out a scaphoid, or any other type of fracture. The authors stress that if a patient has radial sided wrist pain after trauma, especially with concurrent anatomic snuff box tenderness, a scaphoid fracture must be considered and the patient appropriately immobilized in a thumb spica splint and referred to orthopedics.

Flexor Tenosynovitis

An article on "Can't miss" orthopedic emergencies would not be complete without an honorable mention to flexor tenosynovitis. Hand infections may not be readily apparent and can be notoriously difficult to treat. Flexor tenosynovitis is a specific hand infection in which bacteria invade the flexor tendon sheath (FDS or FDP or both of any finger) and spread through the tenosynovium (**Figs. 14 and 15**).

Due to the minimal blood supply within the flexor tendon sheath and its dark, warm, walled off and moist environment, it is an ideal medium for bacterial replication. In addition, perfusion is further compromised during this condition and leads to rapid progression of flexor tenosynovitis. Early recognition is key in order to minimize potential residual functional deficits and decrease the need for amputation.

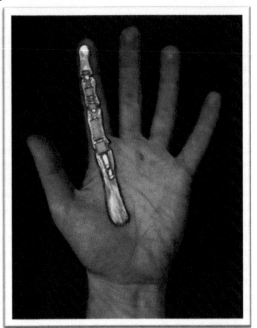

Fig. 14. The location of the flexor tendon sheath on the volar aspect of hand and finger. Courtesy of: Emily Chan, Bernard F Robertson and Simon M Johnson British Journal of General Practice 2019; 69 (683): 315-316. DOI: https://doi.org/10.3399/bjgp19X704081

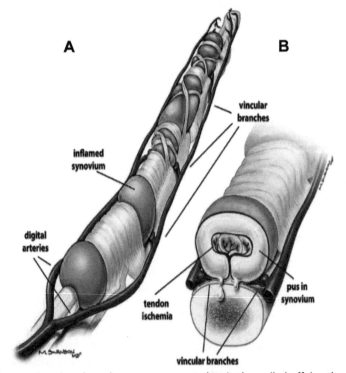

Fig. 15. Cross section view shows how pus can accumulate in the walled-off sheath and lead to rapid compression of the tendon. This illustrates why active/passive motion is so painful in this condition. Courtesy of: Patel A, Ascha M, Punjabi A, et al. (May 14, 2020) Pyogenic Flexor Tenosynovitis Caused by Shewanella putrefaciens. Cureus 12(5): e8113. doi:10.7759/cureus.8113

Table 1	
Kanavel signs/additional information	
Finger Held in Slight Flexion	*Patients Preferred Position of the Digit on Inspection*
Fusiform swelling of the affected digit	*Circumferential swelling entire digit*
Tenderness along the flexor tendon sheath	*Tender palmar surface of the affected digit*
Pain with passive extension of the digit	*Single most reliable sign. Gentle passive extension often leading to patient retraction*

In 1912, Dr A.B. Kanavel described key recognition findings in flexor tenosynovitis, which are still in use today and commonly referred to as Kanavel's signs.[14] (**Table 1**). It is important for physician assistants who see and evaluate hand conditions in any setting to be able to quickly recognize Kanavel's signs without requiring reference. Although there are some exceptions to the need for emergent surgical intervention, all patients who have a suspected flexor tenosynovitis require an urgent / same day / as soon as reasonably possible hand surgery consultation.

SUMMARY

During the course of a career, an Emergency Medicine provider will see at least hundreds of patients with musculoskeletal complaints. Most of these patients will have routine strains, sprains, and fractures, which will be properly assed, stabilized, and referred to orthopedics. This can give the ED provider a false sense of security, or an artificially high comfort level, when evaluating a patient with musculoskeletal complaints and can lead to missed diagnosis. In addition, numerous factors may cause stress or distraction to the provider leading to a missed diagnosis. Among these are clinic workload, staffing shortages, language barriers, cultural differences, and difficult patients.

The emergency medicine physician assistant must always be vigilant and maintain a high index of suspicion that a serious disease or injury state is present before them. Knowledge of the classic features of ominous orthopedic pathologic condition without reference is of utmost importance. Overreliance on radiologic exclusionary criteria can lead to appropriate imaging studies not being ordered. Patient volume and a language barrier or altered mental status can lead to a complaint of severe pain not being appreciated in a case of compartment syndrome. Finally, a "negative" finding on the initial X-ray can give the false impression that no fracture is present. It is the job of every medical provider to always maintain the highest level of awareness of orthopedic syndromes that can cause limb-threatening or life-threatening consequences.

CLINICS CARE POINTS

- The critical element in diagnosing and managing orthopedic syndromes that present in a subtle manner but have potentially disastrous sequelae is a high index of suspicion.
- Overdependence on diagnostic exclusion criteria, such as the Ottawa Ankle Rules, can lead to delayed or missed diagnosis and have no place when evaluating musculoskeletal complaints.
- Patients with a scaphoid fracture, or any fracture, can have physical signs and symptoms but "negative": X-ray findings. It is the standard of care to treat the injury as a fracture and splint the patient and refer for orthopedic follow-up.

DISCLOSURE

The authors have nothing to disclose.

REFERENCES

1. Hammerberg, E. M. (2022). Acute Compartment Syndrome of the Extremities. UpToDate.com.
2. Shadgan BM. Diagnostic techniques in acute compartment syndrome of the leg. J Orthop Trauma 2008;22(#8).
3. Tintinalli, J.E. et al, Tinitinalli's Emergency Medicine: A Comprehensive Study Guide, 9th Edition.
4. Schmidt AM. Management of acute compartment sydrome, clinical practice guideline. Chicago, IL: American Academy of Orthopaedic Surgeons; 2018.
5. McGough, RL., Current diagnosis & treatment in orthopedics, 6th Ed. Chaper 9: Orthopedic Infections: Basic Principles of Pathogenesis, Diagnosis, and Treatment.
6. Burton, John H., Tintinalli's Emergency Medicine: A Comprehensive Study Guide, 9e Chapter 284: Joints and Bursae.
7. Randall R, Ward R, Hoang BH. Chapter 5. Musculoskeletal oncology. In: Skinner HB, McMahon PJ, editors. Current diagnosis & treatment in orthopedics. 5e. McGraw Hill; 2014. Available at: https://accesssurgery.mhmedical.com/content.aspx?bookid=675&sectionid=45451711.
8. Bernthal NM, Burke ZC, Blumstein GW, et al. Musculoskeletal Oncology. In: McMahon PJ, Skinner HB, editors. Current Diagnosis & Treatment in Orthopedics. Sixth Edition. McGraw Hill; 2021. Available at: https://accessmedicine.mhmedical.com/content.aspx?bookid=3066&sectionid=255723740.
9. Jones BM. Scaphoid fracture of the wrist. Chicago, IL: American Academy of Orthopaedic Surgeons; 2016.
10. Donovan AM. Imaging musculoskeletal trauma: interpretation and reporting. Hoboken, NJ: Wiley-Blackwell; 2012.
11. Daniels AM. Improved detection of scaphoid fractures with high-resolution quantitative CT compared with conventional CT. J Bone Joint Surg 2020;102(24).
12. Kronfol, Rana MD, et al. Splinting of Musculoskeletal Injuries. UpToDate.com. Feb 23, 2016
13. Beutler, Anthony, MD, et al. General Principles of Definitive Fracture Management, UpToDate.com, November 18, 2014.
14. Adams Julie. Tendinopathies of the wrist and hand. J Am Acad Orthop Surg 2015;23(12).

The Evolving Role of Ultrasound in Prehospital and Emergency Medicine

Adam Broughton, MScPA, PA-C[a,b,c,d],*

KEYWORDS

- POCUS • Ultrasound • Prehospital • Emergency medicine • Diagnostic
- Procedural

KEY POINTS

- Point-of-care ultrasound (POCUS) is rapidly expanding in access and utility in emergency medicine for the diagnosis and treatment of a wide range of clinical conditions.
- There are several high-yield applications of POCUS in emergency medicine.
- POCUS has been shown to aid in evaluation and treatment of patients in several emergency scenarios.
- Multiple trials have shown integration of POCUS in prehospital care as feasible.
- The use of POCUS should be done within a specific clinical context to answer specific diagnostic questions. In the prehospital and emergency medicine setting, POCUS can rapidly answer binary questions pertaining to a critically ill or injured patient.

INTRODUCTION

Bedside ultrasound has become an essential tool for emergency medicine (EM) providers for the evaluation and treatment of patients in the emergency department (ED). Recently, studies have looked at the use of ultrasound to aid in prehospital care (PHC) including augmenting resuscitation protocols and early identification of critical disease states. As ultrasound equipment becomes more affordable and portable and more studies show the diagnostic and procedural utility of sonography, it is likely to have a growing number of applications which could make the ultrasound probe as common as the stethoscope.[1,2]

Ultrasound is no longer only used by trained technicians and radiologists to confirm diagnoses and aid in procedures with ultrasonography now being done at the bedside

[a] Physician Assistant Studies (Northeastern University 2007), 336 Huntington Avenue, Boston, MA 02115, USA; [b] Bachelor of Science in Kinesiology (Gordon College 2004), 255 Grapevine Road, Wenham, MA 01984, USA; [c] Northeastern University PA Program (2020-Present), 360 Huntington Avenue, Boston, MA 02115, USA; [d] Lahey Beverly Hospital Emergency Department Physician Assistant (2015-Present), 85 Herrick Street. Beverly, MA 01915, USA
* Corresponding author. 202 Robinson Hall, 360 Huntington Avenue, Boston, MA 02115.
E-mail address: a.broughton@northeastern.edu

Physician Assist Clin 8 (2023) 225–236
https://doi.org/10.1016/j.cpha.2022.08.004
2405-7991/23/© 2022 Elsevier Inc. All rights reserved.
physicianassistant.theclinics.com

Abbreviations	
POCUS	Point-of-care Ultrasound
PHC	Prehospital care
EM	Emergency medicine
ED	Emergency department
ATLS	Advanced trauma life support
CPR	Cardiopulmonar resuscitation
PEA	Pulseless electrical activity

rather than only in radiology suites. The term point-of-care ultrasonography (POCUS) has been defined as "the acquisition, interpretation, and immediate clinical integration of ultrasonographic imaging performed by a treating clinician at the patient's bedside rather than by a radiologist or cardiologist."[3]

The use of POCUS requires successful acquisition of images at the bedside including probe selection, placement, and manual manipulation to obtain useful images which is a skill that requires repetition and practice. In addition, users must understand the basic physics of the ultrasound waves and the numerous ways to adjust, manipulate, and capture images. This is known as "knobology,"[4] referring to the standard knobs and buttons of traditional machines that are rapidly being replaced by touchscreens.

Experience is also needed obtaining as well as interpreting sonographic images in real time at the bedside. Like other radiographic studies, knowledge of normal anatomic structures and pathologic states are needed to successfully interpret the images obtained. This requires further training beyond the technical and manual skills needed to clearly visualize subcutaneous structures. Thus, the implementation of POCUS into clinical care requires education and training on the use of the ultrasound machine and manual manipulation of the ultrasound probe to obtain images while simultaneously interpreting those images and applying it to the clinical scenario at hand.

HISTORY

Before the routine use of ultrasound in the ED at the bedside, sonography had and continues to be used as a diagnostic test with images obtained by trained technicians and interpreted by experts, including radiologists and cardiologists. Trained interventional radiologists also use ultrasound in therapeutic procedures. Today, many EM providers are integrating POCUS into clinical care for immediate diagnostic purposes as well as visualization prior or during common procedures.[3]

The role of POCUS in the ED continues to evolve[5] as technology advances and more literature on the subject is published. Research has shown the value of POCUS at the bedside in a variety of settings in the hospital,[3] which has expanded to the field including the use of POCUS in the evaluation and management of patients in the field and during transport by emergency medical services (EMS) in the prehospital setting.[6]

POINT-OF-CARE ULTRASOUND IN PATIENT ASSESSMENT

POCUS has been shown to significantly change diagnosis and treatment,[7] although it should always be done within the training, experience, and scope of practice of the practitioner. There are limitations in its use including patient factors such as bowel gas or body habitus that can obscure useful images as well as findings that must be carefully considered when making diagnostic or therapeutic decisions.

POCUS can be thought of as an adjunct to the physical examination, like ausculta-tion with a stethoscope, or it can be used as a bedside test to provide more data about a potential diagnosis, such as obtaining a bedside glucose reading in the assessment of altered mental status. In either approach, it is important to know the meaning and significance of POCUS findings and the limitations of its use. For example, just as a heart murmur is rarely diagnostic alone, a singular POCUS finding is rarely pathogno-monic. Similarly, when interpreting POCUS as a test, the sensitivity and specificity must be considered when formulating the most likely diagnosis. POCUS must always be used in conjunction with the clinical picture and probability of the diagnosis in question.

HIGH-YIELD POINT-OF-CARE ULTRASOUND

The use of POCUS to reliably detect a finding that results in a change in the diagnosis or treatment of a patient can be considered high yield. This includes both *emergent* applications in the critically ill patient, such as finding and treating a reversible cause for cardiac arrest, and *urgent* applications of POCUS in non-life-threatening condi-tions like identifying an abscess in a soft tissue infection and can change the course of treatment of a patient. In addition, a potential reduction of radiation exposure and/or reduction in time to diagnosis or disposition[5] could also be considered high yield. **Table 1** is a list of high yeild uses of POCUS in diagnostics and therapeutics that can readily inform and be performed by EMS and EM providers (**Table 1**).

CLINICAL SCENARIOS AIDED BY POINT-OF-CARE ULTRASOUND

When looking at the use of POCUS within clinical scenarios, the following applications of POCUS potentially have high-yield findings in clinical management:

- In *trauma*, the eFAST (extended Focused Assessment with Sonography in Trauma) as a diagnostic aid for potentially immediate life threats: tension pneu-mothorax, pericardial effusion with tamponade, and thoracic and intra-abdominal hemorrhage.[8] The full application and interpretation of results are taught in Advanced Trauma Life Support (ATLS) and will not be reiterated here.
- In *respiratory failure or distress and intubation*, POCUS can be used to evaluate for a misplaced esophageal tube[9] and potential iatrogenic or pathologic pneu-mothorax.[10] More nuanced findings of interstitial edema, consolidation, small pleural effusions, and pulmonary embolism might not be considered high yield because they can be difficult to interpret.
- In *cardiac arrest*, there are several reversible causes within advanced cardiac life support (ACLS) algorithms where POCUS[11–14] can aid identification and need for treatment including tension pneumothorax, pericardial tamponade, presence or absence of pulse, true pulseless electrical activity (PEA), ventricular fibrillation, and cardiac standstill. All will need to be supported by electrocardiogram and other findings.
- In *undifferentiated hypotension*, like the trauma patient with unstable vital signs, the presence of a pericardial effusion can inform decision-making. The rapid ul-trasound in shock (RUSH) examination[15] has been proposed and shows high ac-curacy[16] for further evaluation of cardiogenic, hypovolemic, distributive, or obstructive shock. This examination requires training in obtaining and interpret-ing cardiac and central vascular findings.
- In *abdominal pain and hypotension*, the principles of the FAST (focused assess-ment with sonography for trauma) examination can be applied to look for free

Table 1
Summary of uses of point-of-care ultrasound

Examination	Probe	Easily Identified Findings	Potential Clinical Scenarios
Arterial Doppler	High-frequency linear probe with color Doppler at carotid, femoral, and radial artery	Confirm the presence of absence of pulses	CPR—confirm PEA or asystole Hypotension—identify cardiac activity without palpable pulse Ischemic limb—initiate early treatment or imaging
Lung Pleura	High-frequency linear probe with or without M-mode	Identify lung sliding and A-lines	Respiratory failure including CPR—rule out pneumothorax
Thorax	Low-frequency curvilinear or phased-array probe	Identify fluid in the pleural space	Blunt or penetrating trauma with unstable vital signs—indication for thoracostomy or thoracotomy tube for presumed intrathoracic bleeding
Cardiac	Low-frequency phased-array or curvilinear probe	Identify large pericardial effusion, confirm organized cardiac motion vs standstill vs ventricular fibrillation, distinguish between hyperdynamic vs poor ejection fraction	CPR—to identify a reversible cause of cardiac arrest or confirm cardiac standstill in PEA or asystole. Profound hypotension—help distinguish hypovolemia from other potential causes of heart failure
Abdomen	Low-frequency curvilinear or phased-array probe	Identify intraperitoneal free fluid (assumed to be blood in unstable patient)	Blunt or penetrating trauma with unstable vital signs—for prompt operative treatment intraperitoneal bleeding Unstable patient with possible ruptured ectopic, AAA, or abdominal aortic dissection
Pelvis	Low-frequency curvilinear or phased-array probe	Identify intraperitoneal free fluid, confirmation of urinary retention, and identification of IUP	Blunt or penetrating trauma with unstable vital signs—for prompt operative treatment intraperitoneal bleeding Unstable patient with possible ruptured ectopic, AAA, or abdominal aortic dissection

Abbreviations: CPR, cardiopulmonary resuscitation; PEA, pulseless electrical activity; AAA abdominal aortic aneurysm; IUP, intrauterine pregnancy

fluid that could represent intraperitoneal hemorrhage and necessitate emergent surgery and large-volume transfusion. Interpreting images of the abdominal aorta and uterus, if visualized, can help diagnoses aortic aneurysm or dissection and the presence or absence of an intrauterine pregnancy. These can readily be learned by the novice when good technique is used.

PREHOSPITAL APPLICATION OF POINT-OF-CARE ULTRASOUND

Several POCUS protocols have been proposed and are used by physician sonographers in the ED,[13,15,17,18] but the prehospital setting has unique challenges in an ever changing, noisy, and chaotic environment. One advantage of ultrasound is that it can provide visual information that can be seen and captured in a cost-effective manner outside the hospital. If applied in the appropriate circumstances with the right patient, by an adequately trained professional, ultrasonography can aid in diagnosis and treatment in the prehospital setting. The studies referenced and summarized in **Table 2** have proposed algorithms for the use of ultrasound in the prehospital setting.

Limitations of Prehospital Sonography

With the price of ultrasound units decreasing substantially as well as the availability of hand-held units, price and portability has become less limiting for EMS to purchase and use POCUS. While much more affordable, upkeep, maintenance, and trouble-shooting need to be considered as recurring cost. Another cost to consider is staffing trained professionals and/or training prehospital providers in the appropriate use of ultrasound. Studies[12,13,21] have shown that training paramedics and implementing prehospital ultrasound protocols are feasible.

One potential disadvantage to introducing ultrasound to the prehospital setting is the possible inappropriate use of ultrasound that delays critical interventions. This was seen in studies showing in-hospital delays during pulse checks longer than 10 seconds during cardiopulmonary resuscitation (CPR).[22] Any delay in critical treatment for unnecessary diagnostic testing, including ultrasound verification of an obvious diagnosis, can be detrimental and should be avoided.

In addition, some findings such as massive intraperitoneal hemorrhage may not be able to be addressed outside of the hospital. A clinician caring for a critically ill patient must not "lose the forest for the tree" and become hyper-focused on a finding that may not warrant action at that time. Thus, clinicians must learn to incorporate POCUS into their evaluation and management of patients at the level of their training and in circumstances where ultrasound findings could change diagnosis or management of the patient.

APPLYING POINT-OF-CARE ULTRASOUND TO PRACTICE WITH PERTINENT CLINICAL QUESTIONS

A simplified and helpful approach to the use of ultrasound to make critical decisions and diagnoses is to use POCUS to answer binary (yes/no) pertinent clinical questions. These binary questions are well-suited for the PHC of patients. When posed as a yes or no question, it is plausible that less time would be spent "looking around" for other diagnoses that could delay care and may distract or confuse EMS providers.

Are Pulses Present?

Background: Recognition of the presence of pulses by palpation during CPR has been shown to be time-consuming and inaccurate in CPR trained providers.[23,24] POCUS used to detect pulses has been shown to be rapid,[23] more accurate,[25,26] and helpful in nonexpert sonographers to detect femoral pulses integrated into ACLS.[27]

Table 2
Summary of prehospital protocols integrating point-of-care ultrasound

Protocol	Study	Application	Pertinent Findings
FEEL[13]	Focused Echocardiographic Evaluation in Life support	Identify reversible causes[a] during CPR in cardiac arrest	Pericardial effusion, right heart strain, LV dysfunction, collapsing IVC, fine VF
US-CAB[12]	Ultrasound protocol for Circulation-Airway-Breathing	Sequential evaluation of circulation (heart and IVC), airway (trachea), and breathing (lungs)	Pericardial tamponade, collapsing IVC, esophageal intubation, lack of lung slide
CASA[19]	Cardiac Arrest Sonographic Assessment (CASA) examination: A standardized approach to the use of ultrasound in PEA	Three, < 10 s POCUS examinations that occur at pulse checks during CPR to identify reversible causes[a] of PEA	Cardiac tamponade, right heart strain, cardiac activity
PAUSE[20]	Prehospital Assessment with UltraSound for Emergencies (PAUSE) protocol	Pleura examination followed by focused TTE (subxiphoid, parasternal long views)	Assessment for pericardial effusion, pneumothorax, and the presence/absence of cardiac activity

[a] Reversible causes = pericardial tamponade, tension pneumothorax, pulmonary embolism, hypovolemia. CPR = cardiopulmonary resuscitation, LV = left ventricle, IVC = inferior vena cava, VF = ventricular fibrillation, PEA = pulseless electrical activity, TTE = transthoracic echocardiogram.

Pearls: A rapid assessment of carotid, femoral, or radial pulses can be performed during the pulse checks of CPR or in patients with undetectable BP.

Pitfalls: POCUS is highly accurate for the detection of pulses; therefore, false positives or false negatives would most likely be due to user error in obtaining and interpreting images. Users will need to understand how to operate their specific ultrasound machine with color Doppler and the fact that motion artifact can be confused for presence of a pulse.

Is There Organized Cardiac Motion?

Background: Similar to the use of POCUS for the detection of pulses during resuscitation within the Advanced Cardiac Life Support (ACLS) algorithm, POCUS has been proposed to be used to distinguish "true" Pulseless Electrical Activity (PEA) rhythm on electrocardiogram (ECG) with no cardiac activity from "false" PEA where organized heart motion may not result in palpable BP or adequate end-organ perfusion. Organized heart contractility can be easily recognized by the novice provider if adequate windows are obtained.

Pearls: This is another excellent adjunct to the physical examination during ACLS-guided resuscitation even with nonexpert sonographers.[27] PEA has an established treatment protocol, whereas profound hypotension with organized cardiac activity could be detected and treated appropriately.

Pitfalls: Echocardiography during CPR has been associated with prolonged delays during pulse checks.[22] Unfortunately, there was not good inter-rater reliability of physician interpretation of cardiac standstill,[28] and this finding alone is not an accepted indication for termination of resuscitation. Prehospital workers should not consider a lack of organized cardiac movement as the sole reason to discontinue resuscitative efforts. A systematic review showed little evidence to support the use of a single decision rule in adult or pediatric patients to reliably predict mortality or survival with unfavorable neurologic outcome after in-hospital cardiac arrest.[14] Cardiac motion alone is not sufficient to terminate resuscitation.

Is There a Pericardial Effusion?

Background: One of the aims of the eFAST in ATLS is to identify immediate life threats that include pericardial effusion with tamponade. The absence of a pericardial effusion is valuable information in eliminating cardiac tamponade as an explanation for hypotension or shock. Prehospital providers may not be able to perform pericardiocentesis in the field, but the early identification might improve patient care once in the ED.

Pearls: In the context of hypotension, the absence of pericardial fluid essentially rules out cardiac tamponade as the cause and clinicians should look elsewhere. A large effusion found on POCUS, in the correct clinical context, can help inform the need for intervention with much better accuracy than auscultation and physical examination findings such as Beck's triad with greater speed than CT (computed tomography) imaging.

Pitfalls: It can be difficult to distinguish a pleural effusion from a pericardial effusion as well as a pericardial fat pad. In addition, large chronic effusions may not cause tamponade; thus, the user must understand and distinguish tamponade pathology in real time.

Is a Pneumothorax Potentially Present?

Background: Another aspect of the eFAST in ATLS is examining for the presence of pleural sliding at the apex of the chest where air is most likely to collect in a large, non-loculated pneumothorax. A tension pneumothorax is an immediate life threat in thoracic trauma. The presence of lung sliding bilaterally has a high probability of ruling out tension pneumothorax as an immediate life threat.[29] The absence of lung sliding does not mean that a tension pneumothorax is present, although in the unstable trauma patient with high enough suspicion, the benefits of prompt needle decompression might outweigh the potential risks. Outside of trauma, examination for pleural lung sliding can be applied in other circumstances such as suspicion of iatrogenic pneumothorax from mechanical ventilation or main stem bronchi intubation.

Pearls: Any provider with access to POCUS can learn to identify pleura sliding. Lung POCUS is faster than x-ray or CT imaging and has been shown to be more accurate than auscultation alone.[30] The sonographic setting M-mode can show a "seashore sign" pattern in normal pleural movement and "barcode sign" in pneumothorax.[31] The additional presence of A-lines improves accuracy.[10]

Pitfalls: False positives (lack of lung sliding) can be seen in patients who have had prior pleurodesis, and a large lung bleb also may not show reverberating A-lines. Both should be considered in clinical context and are relatively rare. User error by not selecting the appropriate depth or misinterpreting rib shadowing could also contribute to errors. Main stem bronchi intubation can lead to a lack of lung movement that could be misinterpreted as well.

Is the Endotracheal Tube in the Esophagus?

Background: During intubation, POCUS can be used to assess for successful intubation with accuracy similar to waveform capnography[32] and can be observed sooner than the few breaths it takes to obtain accurate capnography.

Pearls: This is an additional way to help detect a dislodged or inappropriately placed airway. POCUS performed well as a secondary measure to confirm endotracheal (ET) tube placement in pediatric patients as well.[33]

Pitfalls: The correct placement of an airway in the trachea seems essentially the same as a normal patient without an airway. Users are not "seeing" the tube in the trachea. Only tubes placed in the esophagus will be seen. Waveform and color capnography should continue to be used as the gold standard.

Is There Intrathoracic Hemorrhage?

Background: Because fluid is an optimal medium for sonographic detection, pleural effusions or hemorrhage should be easy to see so long as the user has experience with the appearance of normal lungs on ultrasound. In a breathing or ventilated patient, lung parenchyma may be visualized floating around within the surrounding fluid making pleural fluid easy to identify.

Pearls: In the trauma patient, a large collection of fluid could indicate intrathoracic hemorrhage that may prompt intervention such as a thoracostomy tube or open thoracostomy evacuation and examination for source.

Pitfalls: Identification of pleural fluid must be taken within the clinical context. Providers should understand if the finding has clinical significance to need immediate intervention or if an effusion is not likely to cause hemodynamic instability or respiratory failure.

Is There Intra-abdominal Hemorrhage?

Background: The FAST examination was designed to look for free fluid in the abdomen as an indicator of intra-abdominal hemorrhage, and in the unstable patient with no other obvious source of hemodynamic instability, prompt immediate surgical exploration without the delay of CT confirmation. It has, however, performed very poorly in ruling out intra-abdominal injury and cannot detect retroperitoneal hemorrhage, bowel injury, or diaphragmatic injury. Thus, it should always be used to aid in decision-making to proceed to the operating room when positive. Outside of trauma, the same technique can be used looking for free fluid as a sign of intra-abdominal hemorrhage in cases with suspicion of ruptured ectopic pregnancy or vascular catastrophe like a rupture abdominal aortic aneurysm (AAA). The overarching principle of not delaying surgical intervention if free fluid is found, while understanding that intra-abdominal injury or hemorrhage is not ruled out by a negative abdominal POCUS examination, is paramount.

Pearls: The FAST examination includes trauma in the name, but this protocol can be applied in cases with suspicion for nontraumatic intraperitoneal bleeding. This should be in the skillset of any clinician expected to care for trauma patients, thus its inclusion in ATLS, but is valuable beyond trauma in the hemodynamically unstable patient with possible intra-abdominal hemorrhage, thus should be learned by all EM providers.

Pitfalls: The FAST is not sensitive at ruling out intra-abdominal pathology and thus should never be reassuring when negative except to say the patient does not meet criteria for immediate operative management. In the hemodynamically unstable patient without obvious source, intraperitoneal bleeding should remain on the differential diagnosis even with a negative FAST.

SUMMARY

The use of ultrasound in the emergency room and prehospital setting can offer many ways to improve diagnosis and treatment of critically ill patients when used to answer specific clinical questions with easily identified POCUS findings that are pertinent to immediate patient care.

CLINICS CARE POINTS

- Point of care ultrasound (POCUS) can be a very useful tool for immediate diagnosis of life-threatening disease in the hospital and prehospital setting.
- It has been shown that with proper training physicians and physician extenders can learn to identify sonographic findings that can change diagnosis and treatment.
- POCUS has also been shown to delay critical interventions, such as high-quality chest compression, thus should be used judiciously and within proper clinical context.
- Small studies have shown some success in implementation of prehospital sonography protocols.
- Currently, the best application of POCUS in the critically ill patient is the previously well-established incorporation into Advanced Trauma Life Support (ATLS) and the use of POCUS to answer binary (yes/no) questions that may change the diagnosis and immediate treatment of patients. These include more accurate identification of the presence of pulses, pericardial effusion, organized cardiac motion, pneumothorax, endotracheal tube in the esophagus, and intra-thoracic and intra-abdominal free fluid.

DISCLOSURE

Nothing to disclose.

REFERENCES

1. Bledsoe A, Zimmerman J. Ultrasound: The new stethoscope (point-of-care ultrasound). Anesthesiology Clin 2021;39(3):537–53. Available at: https://www.sciencedirect.com/science/article/pii/S1932227521000306. Accessed April 14, 2022.
2. Yn W, Ap L, F F, et al. Beyond auscultation: Acoustic cardiography in clinical practice. Int J Cardiol 2014;172(3). https://doi.org/10.1016/j.ijcard.2013.12.298. Available at: https://pubmed-ncbi-nlm-nih-gov.ezproxy.neu.edu/24529949/. Accessed April 7, 2022.
3. Díaz-Gómez JL, Mayo PH, Koenig SJ. Point-of-care ultrasonography. N Engl J Med 2021;385(17):1593–602. Available at: https://doi.org/10.1056/NEJMra1916062. Accessed April 4, 2022.
4. Enriquez JL, Wu TS. An introduction to ultrasound equipment and knobology. Crit Care Clin 2014;30(1):25–45. Available at: https://www.clinicalkey.es/playcontent/1-s2.0-S0749070413000894.
5. Galdamez LA. The evolving role of ultrasound in emergency medicine. In: Alsheikh AS, editor. Essentials of accident and emergency medicine. London, United Kingdom: IntechOpen [Online]; 2018. Available at: https://www.intechopen.com/chapters/61274. Accessed February 28, 2022.
6. Ketelaars R, Reijnders G, van Geffen G, et al. ABCDE of prehospital ultrasonography: A narrative review. Crit Ultrasound J 2018;10(1):17. Accessed April 14, 2022.
7. Baker DE, Nolting L, Brown HA. Impact of point-of-care ultrasound on the diagnosis and treatment of patients in rural uganda. Trop Doct 2021;51(3):291–6. Accessed April 14, 2022.

8. Montoya J, Stawicki SP, Evans DC, et al. From FAST to E-FAST: An overview of the evolution of ultrasound-based traumatic injury assessment. Eur J Trauma Emerg Surg 2015;42(2):119–26. Available at: https://link.springer.com/article/10.1007/s00068-015-0512-1.

9. Lema PC, O'Brien M, Wilson J, et al. Avoid the goose! paramedic identification of esophageal intubation by ultrasound. Prehosp Disaster Med 2018;33(4):406–10. Available at: https://www.cambridge.org/core/journals/prehospital-and-disaster-medicine/article/abs/avoid-the-goose-paramedic-identification-of-esophageal-intubation-by-ultrasound/92DCBD1EEE703E11AB02A3F74E0D38F1. Accessed February 13, 2022.

10. Khosla R. Bedside lung ultrasound in emergency (BLUE) protocol: A suggestion to modify. Chest 2010;137(6):1487.

11. Hernandez C, Shuler K, Hannan H, et al. Cardiac arrest ultra-sound exam—A better approach to managing patients in primary non-arrhythmogenic cardiac arrest. Resuscitation 2008;76(2):198–206. Available at: https://www.sciencedirect.com/science/article/pii/S0300957207004200. Accessed April 3, 2022.

12. Lien W, Hsu S, Chong K, et al. US-CAB protocol for ultrasonographic evaluation during cardiopulmonary resuscitation: Validation and potential impact. Resuscitation 2018;127:125–31. Available at: https://www.sciencedirect.com/science/article/pii/S0300957218300613. Accessed April 2, 2022.

13. Breitkreutz R, Price S, Steiger HV, et al. Focused echocardiographic evaluation in life support and peri-resuscitation of emergency patients: A prospective trial. Resuscitation 2010;81(11):1527–33. Available at: https://www.sciencedirect.com/science/article/pii/S0300957210004168. Accessed April 2, 2022.

14. Lauridsen KG, Baldi E, Smyth M, et al. Clinical decision rules for termination of resuscitation during in-hospital cardiac arrest: A systematic review of diagnostic test accuracy studies. Resuscitation 2021;158:23–9. Available at: https://www.resuscitationjournal.com/article/S0300-9572(20)30545-1/abstract. Accessed February 25, 2022.

15. Perera P, Mailhot T, Riley D, et al. The RUSH exam: Rapid ultrasound in SHock in the evaluation of the critically Ill. Emerg Med Clin North Am 2010;28(1):29–56. Available at: https://www.sciencedirect.com/science/article/pii/S0733862709001175. Accessed April 4, 2022.

16. Elbaih AH, Housseini AM, Khalifa MEM. Accuracy and outcome of rapid ultrasound in shock and hypotension (RUSH) in Egyptian polytrauma patients. Chin J Traumatol 2018;21(3):156–62. Available at: https://www.sciencedirect.com/science/article/pii/S1008127517301037. Accessed April 4, 2022.

17. Lanctôt J, Valois M, Beaulieu Y. EGLS: Echo-guided life support. Crit Ultrasound J 2011;3(3):123–9. Available at: https://link.springer.com/article/10.1007/s13089-011-0083-2.

18. Seyedhosseini J, Fadavi A, Vahidi E, et al. Impact of point-of-care ultrasound on disposition time of patients presenting with lower extremity deep vein thrombosis, done by emergency physicians. Turkish J Emerg Med 2018;18(1):20–4. Available at: https://www.sciencedirect.com/science/article/pii/S245224731730153X. Accessed April 14, 2022.

19. Gardner KF, Clattenburg EJ, Wroe P, et al. The cardiac arrest sonographic assessment (CASA) exam – A standardized approach to the use of ultrasound in PEA. Am J Emerg Med 2018;36(4):729–31. Available at: https://www.sciencedirect.com/science/article/pii/S0735675717307015. Accessed February 22, 2022.

20. Rooney KP, Lahham S, Lahham S, et al. Pre-hospital assessment with ultrasound in emergencies: Implementation in the field. World J Emerg Med 2016;7(2):117. Available at: https://www-ncbi-nlm-nih-gov.ezproxy.neu.edu/pmc/articles/PMC4905867/. Accessed April 20, 2022.
21. Ketelaars R, Hoogerwerf N, Scheffer GJ. Prehospital chest ultrasound by a dutch helicopter emergency medical service. J Emerg Med 2013;44(4):811–7. Available at: https://www.sciencedirect.com/science/article/pii/S0736467912014175. Accessed April 2, 2022.
22. Huis in 't Veld, Maite A, Allison MG, et al. Ultrasound use during cardiopulmonary resuscitation is associated with delays in chest compressions. Resuscitation 2017;119:95–8. Available at: https://www.sciencedirect.com/science/article/pii/S0300957217303027. Accessed February 22, 2022.
23. Smith S. Chenkin. Checking the pulse in the 21st century: Interobserver reliability of carotid pulse detection by point-of-care ultrasound. Am J Emerg Med 2021;45:280–3.
24. Tibballs J, Russell P. Reliability of pulse palpation by healthcare personnel to diagnose paediatric cardiac arrest. Resuscitation 2009;80(1):61–4. Available at: https://pubmed.ncbi.nlm.nih.gov/18992985/. Accessed February 25, 2022.
25. Badra K, Coutin A, Simard R, et al. The POCUS pulse check: A randomized controlled crossover study comparing pulse detection by palpation versus by point-of-care ultrasound. Resuscitation 2019;139:17–23. Available at: https://www.sciencedirect.com/science/article/pii/S0300957219300759. Accessed February 22, 2022.
26. Cohen AL, Li T, Becker LB, et al. Femoral artery doppler ultrasound is more accurate than manual palpation for pulse detection in cardiac arrest. Resuscitation 2022. https://doi.org/10.1016/j.resuscitation.2022.01.030. Available at: https://www.resuscitationjournal.com/article/S0300-9572(22)00032-6/abstract. Accessed February 12, 2022.
27. Zengin S, Yavuz E, Al B, et al. Benefits of cardiac sonography performed by a non-expert sonographer in patients with non-traumatic cardiopulmonary arrest. Resuscitation 2016;102:105–9. Available at: https://www.clinicalkey.es/playcontent/1-s2.0-S0300957216001088.
28. Hu K, Gupta N, Teran F, et al. Variability in interpretation of cardiac standstill among physician sonographers. Ann Emerg Med 2018;71(2):193–8. Available at: https://www.sciencedirect.com/science/article/pii/S0196064417313768. Accessed February 22, 2022.
29. Qaseem A, Etxeandia-Ikobaltzeta I, Mustafa RA, et al. Appropriate use of point-of-care ultrasonography in patients with acute dyspnea in emergency department or inpatient settings: A clinical guideline from the american college of physicians. Ann Intern Med 2021;174(7):985–93. Available at: https://www.acpjournals.org/doi/full/10.7326/M20-7844. Accessed February 22, 2022.
30. Rg W, Mb S. Sensitivity of bedside ultrasound and supine anteroposterior chest radiographs for the identification of pneumothorax after blunt trauma. Acad Emerg Med 2010;17(1). https://doi.org/10.1111/j.1553-2712.2009.00628.x. Available at: https://pubmed-ncbi-nlm-nih-gov.ezproxy.neu.edu/20078434/. Accessed April 20, 2022.
31. D L. Lung ultrasound in the critically ill. Curr Opin Crit Care 2014;20(3). https://doi.org/10.1097/MCC.0000000000000096. Available at: https://pubmed-ncbi-nlm-nih-gov.ezproxy.neu.edu/24758984/. Accessed April 20, 2022.
32. Chou H, Tseng W, Wang C, et al. Tracheal rapid ultrasound exam (T.R.U.E.) for confirming endotracheal tube placement during emergency intubation.

Resuscitation 2011;82(10):1279–84. https://doi.org/10.1016/j.resuscitation.2011. 05.016. Available at: https://www.resuscitationjournal.com/article/S0300-9572(11)00331-5/abstract. Accessed February 13, 2022.

33. Hsieh K, Lee C, Lin C, et al. Secondary confirmation of endotracheal tube position by ultrasound image. Crit Care Med 2004;32(9 Suppl):374. https://doi.org/10. 1097/01.ccm.0000134354.20449.b2. Available at: https://pubmed.ncbi.nlm.nih. gov/15508663/. Accessed February 13, 2022.

Moving?

Make sure your subscription moves with you!

To notify us of your new address, find your **Clinics Account Number** (located on your mailing label above your name), and contact customer service at:

Email: journalscustomerservice-usa@elsevier.com

800-654-2452 (subscribers in the U.S. & Canada)
314-447-8871 (subscribers outside of the U.S. & Canada)

Fax number: 314-447-8029

Elsevier Health Sciences Division
Subscription Customer Service
3251 Riverport Lane
Maryland Heights, MO 63043

*To ensure uninterrupted delivery of your subscription, please notify us at least 4 weeks in advance of move.

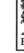

Printed and bound by CPI Group (UK) Ltd, Croydon, CR0 4YY

03/10/2024

01040475-0002